Essential Cases in Head and Neck Oncology

Essential Cases in Head and Neck Oncology

Edited by

MICHAEL G. MOORE, MD, FACS
Arilla Spence DeVault Professor
Vice Chair of Academic Affairs
Department of Otolaryngology-Head and Neck Surgery
Indiana University School of Medicine
Medical Director, IUH Joe & Shelly Schwarz Cancer Center
Indianapolis, IN, USA

ARNAUD F. BEWLEY, MD
Associate Professor
Department of Otolaryngology-Head and Neck Surgery
Chief of Head and Neck Surgery
University of California, Davis
Sacramento, CA, USA

BABAK GIVI, MD, FACS
Associate Professor, Section Chief
Patient Safety-Quality Improvement Officer
Department of Otolaryngology-Head and Neck Surgery
NYU Langone Health
New York, NY, USA

Endorsed by:
American Head and Neck Society
Los Angeles, CA, USA

WILEY Blackwell

Registered Office(s)
John Wiley & Sons, Inc., 111 River Street, Hoboken, NJ 07030, USA
John Wiley & Sons Ltd, The Atrium, Southern Gate, Chichester, West Sussex, PO19 8SQ, UK

Editorial Office
9600 Garsington Road, Oxford, OX4 2DQ, UK

For details of our global editorial offices, customer services, and more information about Wiley products visit us at www.wiley.com.

Wiley also publishes its books in a variety of electronic formats and by print-on-demand. Some content that appears in standard print versions of this book may not be available in other formats.

Library of Congress Cataloging-in-Publication Data

Names: Moore, Michael G. (Michael Geoffrey), 1976-editor.
  | Bewley, Arnaud F., editor. | Givi, Babak, editor. | American Head and Neck Society, issuing body.
Title: Essential Cases in Head and Neck Oncology / Edited by Michael
  G. Moore, Arnaud F. Bewley, Babak Givi
Description: First edition. | Hoboken, NJ : Wiley, 2022. | Includes
  bibliographical references and index.
Identifiers: LCCN 2021034618 (print) | LCCN 2021034619 (ebook) | ISBN 9781119775942 (paperback)
  | ISBN 9781119775959 (adobe pdf) | ISBN 9781119775966 (epub)
Subjects: MESH: Head and Neck Neoplasms–surgery | Otorhinolaryngologic
  Surgical Procedures–methods | Case Reports
Classification: LCC RF51 (print) | LCC RF51 (ebook) | NLM WE 707 | DDC
  617.5/1059–dc23
LC record available at https://lccn.loc.gov/2021034618
LC ebook record available at https://lccn.loc.gov/2021034619

Cover Design: Wiley
Cover Images: © (Top) courtesy of Babak Givi; (Bottom) courtesy of Dr. Charles Yates

Set in 10/12pt STIX Two Text by Straive, Pondicherry, India

Printed in Singapore
M114471_231221

Contents

List of Authors

Rizwan Aslam, DO, MScEd, MBA, FACS
Associate Professor
Department of Otolaryngology
Tulane University
New Orleans, LA, USA

Arnaud F. Bewley, MD
Associate Professor
Department of Otolaryngology-Head and Neck Surgery
Chief of Head and Neck Surgery
University of California
Davis, Sacramento, CA, USA

Kenneth Byrd, MD
Assistant Professor
Department of Otolaryngology-Head and Neck Surgery
Augusta University
Augusta, GA, USA

Brian Cervenka, MD
Assistant Professor
Department of Otolaryngology-Head and Neck Surgery
University of Cincinnati
Cincinnati, OH, USA

Raymond Chai, MD
Associate Professor
Department of Otolaryngology
Icahn School of Medicine
Mount Sinai, NY, USA

Charley Coffey, MD
Associate Professor
Department of Otolaryngology-Head and Neck Surgery
University of California San Diego
San Diego, CA, USA

Vasu Divi, MD
Associate Professor
Department of Otolaryngology-Head and Neck Surgery
Stanford University
Stanford, CA, USA

Antoine Eskander, MD
Assistant Professor
Department of Otolaryngology-Head & Neck Surgery
University of Toronto
Toronto, ON, Canada

Tanya Fancy, MD
Associate Professor
Department of Otolaryngology-Head & Neck Surgery
West Virginia University
Morgantown, WV, USA

Ian Ganly, MD
Attending Surgeon, Head and Neck Service
Memorial Sloan Kettering Cancer Center
Professor of Otolaryngology – Head and Neck Surgery
Weill Medical College
Cornell University
New York, NY, USA

Laureano A. Giraldez-Rodriguez, MD
Director, Voice and Swallowing Center of Puerto Rico
Adjunct Faculty Department of Otolaryngology –
   Head and
Neck Surgery, University of Puerto Rico School
   of Medicine
San Jaun, PR

Babak Givi, MD, FACS
Associate Professor of Otolaryngology-Head &
   Neck Surgery
Section Chief, Otolaryngology, Manhattan VA
   Medical Center
Department of Otolaryngology-Head & Neck Surgery
NYU Langone Health
New York, NY, USA

Glenn J. Hanna, MD
Assistant Professor
Harvard Medical School
Dana-Farber Cancer Institute
Boston, MA, USA

Catherine T. Haring, MD
Head & Neck Fellow
Department of Otolaryngology-Head and Neck Surgery
The Ohio State University Wexner Medical Center
Columbus, OH, USA

Chase Heaton, MD
Associate Professor
Department of Otolaryngology-Head & Neck Surgery
University of California
San Francisco, CA, USA

Basit Jawad, MD
Clinical Instructor
Department of Otolaryngology-Head & Neck Surgery
Tulane University
New Orleans, LA, USA

Lulia A. Kana
Medical Student
University of Michigan
Ann Arbor, MI, USA

Stephen Kang, MD
Associate Professor, Fellowship Director, Head and Neck
    Oncology and Microvascular Reconstruction
Department of Otolaryngology – Head and Neck Surgery
the Ohio State University Wexner Medical Center
the James Cancer Hospital and Solove Research Institute
Columbus, OH, USA

Jason I. Kass, MD, PhD
Reliant Medical Group
Head and Neck Surgeon
Worcester, MA, USA

Peter J. Kneuertz, MD
Assistant Professor
Division of Thoracic Surgery
the Ohio State University Wexner Medical Center
the James Cancer Hospital and Solove Research Institute
Columbus, OH, USA

Kevin J. Kovatch, MD
Head & Neck Fellow
Department of Otolaryngology/Head and Neck Surgery
Vanderbilt University Medical Center
Nashville, TN, USA

Luiz Paulo Kowalski, MD
Full Professor and Chairman, Director
Department of Head and Neck Surgery and
    Otorhinolaryngology
University of São Paulo Medical School
São Paulo, Brazil

Levi Ledgerwood, MD
Head & Neck Surgeon
South Sacramento Kaiser Permanente Medical Center
Sacramento, CA, USA

Avinash Mantravadi, MD
Associate Professor
Director, Head and Neck Surgical Oncology
Department of Otolaryngology - Head and Neck Surgery
Indiana University School of Medicine
Indianapolis, IN, USA

Michael G. Moore, MD, FACS
Arilla Spence DeVault Professor
Vice Chair of Academic Affairs
Department of Otolaryngology - Head and Neck Surgery
Indiana University School of Medicine
Medical Director, IUH Joe & Shelly Schwarz
    Cancer Center
Indianapolis, IN, USA

Fadi A. Nabhan, MD
Associate Professor
Endocrinology and Metabolism
Department of Medicine
Ohio State University College of Medicine
Columbus, OH, USA

David Neskey, MD
Director of Translational Research
Sarah Cannon Research Institute
Charleston, SC, USA

Paul O'Neill, MB, FRCSI, MMSc, MD, MBA, ORL-HNS
Professor
Otolaryngology-Head and Neck Surgery
Royal College of Surgeons – Ireland
Dublin, Ireland

Thomas J. Ow, MD, MS
Associate Professor
Department of Otolaryngology-Head and Neck
    Surgery/Pathology
Albert Einstein College of Medicine
Bronx, NY, USA

Aru Panwar, MD
Assistant Professor
Department of Otolaryngology-Head and Neck Surgery
University of Nebraska
Lincoln, NE, USA

Rusha Patel, MD
Associate Professor
Department of Otolaryngology-Head and Neck Surgery
The University of Oklahoma
Oklahoma City, OK, USA

Yash Patil, MD
Associate Professor
Program Director
Department of Otolaryngology-Head and Neck Surgery
University of Cincinnati
Cincinnati, OH, USA

Alok Pathak, MS, PhD
Professor, Director
Department of Surgery, Surgical Oncology Research
University of Manitoba
Winnipeg, MB, Canada

Daniel Pinheiro, MD, Phd
Department of Otolaryngology-Head and Neck Surgery
Cancer Center for the Ozarks, Mercy Hospital
Springfield, MO, USA

Liana Puscas, MD, MHS
Associate Professor
Department of Head and Neck Surgery & Communication
    Sciences
Duke University
Durham, NC, USA

Chris Rassekh, MD, FACS
Professor
Department of Otolaryngology-Head and Neck Surgery
University of Pennsylvania
Philadelphia, PA, USA

Camilo Reyes, MD
Assistant Professor
Department of Otolaryngology-Head and Neck Surgery
Medical college of Georgia
Augusta University
Augusta, GA, USA

Jesse Ryan, MD
Associate Professor
Department of Otolaryngology and Communication
    Sciences
SUNY Upstate Medical University
Syracuse, NY, USA

Zoukaa Sargi, MD, MPH
Professor of Otolaryngology and Neurosurgery
Residency Program Director
Department of Otolaryngology
University of Miami Miller School of Medicine
Miami, FL, USA

Daniel Sharbel, MD
Department of Otolaryngology
Augusta University
Augusta, GA, USA

Lucy Shi, MD
Department of Otolaryngology-Head and Neck Surgery
Ohio State University Wexner Medical Center
Columbus, OH, USA

Andrew G. Shuman, MD, FACS, HEC-C
Associate Professor, CBSSM
Department of Otolaryngology - Head and Neck Surgery
University of Michigan
Ann Arbor, MI, USA

Dustin A. Silverman, MD
Head & Neck Fellow
Department of Otolaryngology
University of California – Davis
Davis, CA, USA

Carl H. Snyderman, MD, MBA
Professor, Departments of Otolaryngology and
    Neurological Surgery
University of Pittsburgh School of Medicine
Co-Director, Center for Cranial Base Surgery
University of Pittsburgh Medical Center
Pittsburgh, PA, USA

Bharat Yarlagadda, MD
Division of Otolaryngology – Head and Neck Surgery
Lahey Hospital and Medical Center
Assistant Professor
Department of Otolaryngology – Head and Neck Surgery
Boston University School of Medicine
Boston, MA, USA

Charles Yates, MD
Associate Professor
Department of Otolaryngology – Head and Neck Surgery
University of Indiana
Bloomington, IN, USA

Jessica Yesensky, MD
Assistant Professor
Department of Otolaryngology – Head and Neck Surgery
University of Indiana
Bloomington, IN, USA

Chad Zender, MD, FACS
Associate Chief Medical Officer, UC Health
Center of Excellence Leader, Head and Neck, UC
    Cancer Institute
Professor Department of Otolaryngology – Head &
    Neck Surgery
University of Cincinnati College of Medicine
Cincinnati, OH, USA

SECTION 1

Oral Cavity

Chase Heaton

CASE 1

Babak Givi

History of Present Illness

A 53-year-old man presents with a 1-month history of tongue soreness and pain. He has not noticed any change in voice, difficulty swallowing, or a neck mass. However, the tongue pain is persistent and has not gone away with over-the-counter medications. His past medical history includes type II diabetes, controlled with oral agents, and hypertension. He does not smoke and has no history of tobacco or alcohol abuse. No other past medical history was identified.

Physical Examination

No palpable neck mass was identified. Oral cavity exam shows a slightly raised lesion on the right lateral tongue, which is soft and tender to palpation, measuring 1 cm in diameter (see Figure 1.1). There is no mass noted deep to the lesion. The rest of the exam, including fiberoptic laryngoscopy, is within normal limits.

Management

Question: What would you recommend next?

Answer: Tissue sampling with a punch or incisional biopsy of the lesion, preferably from the corner of the lesion.

Question: The biopsy shows squamous cell carcinoma (SCC), moderately differentiated, with a depth of invasion of at least 4 mm (punch biopsy specimen with tumor transected at the base). What would you recommend next in the workup?

Answer: Imaging of the neck is usually recommended to assess lymph node involvement. A computed tomography

(CT) scan with contrast or an ultrasound of the neck (which can be performed in the clinic) are both reasonable first options. The risk of distant metastases in early (T1 and T2) oral cavity SCC is extremely low. Therefore, extensive metastatic workup is not necessary. While positron emission tomography (PET)/CT has become more common, the evidence for its added benefit does not exist. Obtaining a chest CT to rule out lung metastases is considered adequate.

Question: A CT scan of the head and neck does not show any evidence of regional metastases. How would you clinically stage this disease?

Answer: Based on the AJCC staging manual, 8th Edition, the clinical stage is cT1N0Mx, stage I.

Question: What treatment would you recommend?

Answer: Early stage tongue cancer treatment is wide local excision of the primary tumor and addressing the regional lymph nodes. If the risk of regional lymph node metastases is presumed to be higher than 20%, an elective, selective neck dissection should be performed. Depth of invasion is a prognostic marker for the presence of occult nodal metastases in the cN0 neck. With a depth of invasion >3 mm, it is believed that the risk of occult nodal metastases is >20%, and therefore an elective neck dissection should be performed. In this scenario, the recommended treatment is wide local excision of the primary tumor with 1 cm margins and elective neck dissection (ipsilateral levels I–III, i.e., supra-omohyoid neck dissection). Alternatively, sentinel node biopsy could be offered if adequate expertise in the treating facility exists.

Question: Patient undergoes sentinel node mapping followed by wide local excision and sentinel node biopsy. The tongue defect is repaired with biologic dressing

(Continued)

Essential Cases in Head and Neck Oncology, First Edition. Edited by Michael G. Moore, Arnaud F. Bewley, and Babak Givi.
© 2022 American Head and Neck Society. Published 2022 by John Wiley & Sons Ltd.

CASE 1 (continued)

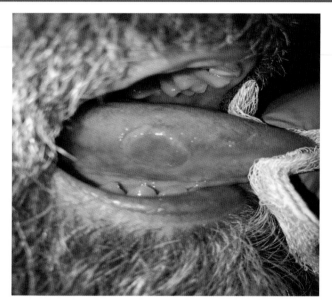

FIGURE 1.1 This photo demonstrates the patient's right lateral tongue ulceration.

and secondary intention closure. On lymphoscintigraphy, the sentinel node is located in an ipsilateral level II lymph node (Figure 1.2). Excisional biopsy and frozen section assessment shows metastatic SCC in the level II node. How would you proceed?

Answer: If the sentinel node is positive, completion lymphadenectomy (selective neck dissection, level I–IV) is recommended.

The patient recovers well from the operation. The final pathology report shows a 1.5 cm moderately differentiated SCC with a depth of invasion of 7 mm. All margins are free of tumor, with the closest margin being 8 mm from tumor. No lymphovascular or perineural invasion is identified. One out of 30 lymph nodes is positive for metastatic SCC without extranodal extension, measuring 1.9 cm (sentinel node).

Question: Based on these pathologic findings, what is the appropriate stage for this patient?

Answer: According to AJCC 8th Edition, tumors of the oral cavity with a depth of invasion of more than 5 mm are

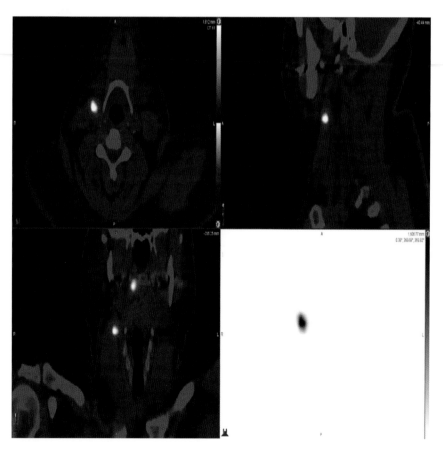

FIGURE 1.2 This image shows the patient's fused CT- lymphoscintigraphy image. Note the uptake at the injection site and a right level II lymph node.

CASE 1   (continued)

considered T2, even if the diameter is less than 2 cm. Therefore, the pathologic stage is pT2N1M0, stage III.

Question: What adjuvant treatment regimen, if any, would you recommend to this patient?

Answer: Since the disease is stage III, consideration of adjuvant treatment is warranted. Radiotherapy should be considered after discussion of the case at a multidisciplinary tumor board. The benefit of radiotherapy is not as clear in N1 disease; however, limited data exist that shows tumors with a depth of invasion of greater than 4 mm are at increased risk of regional failure without adjuvant therapy. Since there is no evidence of primary site positive margins or extranodal extension, there is no indication for adjuvant chemotherapy.

Question: The patient completes a course of adjuvant radiotherapy. What is your recommended regimen for follow-up and clinical surveillance?

Answer: Based on National Comprehensive Cancer Network (**NCCN**) guidelines, baseline imaging at 12 weeks after completion of adjuvant treatment should be obtained, followed by physical examination every 1–3 months in the first year post-treatment and then 4–6 months in the second year. In years 3–5, a physical exam every 4–8 months is recommended and annually after 5 years. Annual thyroid-stimulating hormone (**TSH**) testing is recommended since the neck has received radiotherapy. Dental, nutrition, and ongoing depression evaluation are also recommended.

Key Points

- Oral tongue SCC is the most common malignancy of the oral cavity. The most important risk factors are tobacco, alcohol, poor dentition, diets low in fruits and vegetables, and Fanconi anemia.
- The risk of occult metastases in early stage oral cavity cancers is usually upward of 20%. Level I clinical trial evidence exists in the survival benefit of elective neck dissection in early stage tongue cancer and clinically negative cervical nodes when the depth of invasion is >3 mm. Currently, imaging techniques are not sensitive enough to identify occult metastases, and a negative CT or PET scan does not rule out microscopic metastases.
- Sentinel node biopsy in oral cavity cancers has been studied and shown to be reliable enough to identify the majority of occult metastases. Sentinel node sensitivity is reported as 86% with a negative predictive value of 95% based on the European Organization for Research and Treatment of Cancer.
- Recommended primary treatment of oral cavity cancers is primarily surgical. Wide local excision with a 1 cm margin and lymph node dissection (selective node dissection in clinically negative neck) is the current recommendation.
- Depth of invasion is an important prognostic factor. A depth of invasion of more than 3 mm is associated with an increased risk of lymph node metastases.
- The current indications for adjuvant radiotherapy are (i) close or positive margins, (ii) nodal involvement, (iii) perineural invasion, and (iv) advanced stage tumor (T3–4).
- Concurrent chemotherapy with platinum-based agents is only recommended in positive margins or extranodal extension.

CASE 2

Babak Givi

History of Present Illness

A 64-year-old woman presents with a nonhealing ulcer of the right mandibular alveolus for the past month after extraction of the second molar. The lesion is not painful and does not bleed. She has a more than 40 pack-year history of smoking and drinking two alcoholic drinks a day for the past 30 years. She does not report any history of other medical problems or prior malignancy.

Physical Examination

No palpable neck mass is identified. Oral cavity exam shows an ulcerative lesion limited to the occlusal surface of the right mandibular alveolus measuring 2 × 1 cm. The lesion is not tender to touch, does not extend to the buccal mucosa or floor of the mouth (see Figure 2.1). The rest of the exam, including flexible laryngoscopy, is within normal limits.

(Continued)

CASE 2 (continued)

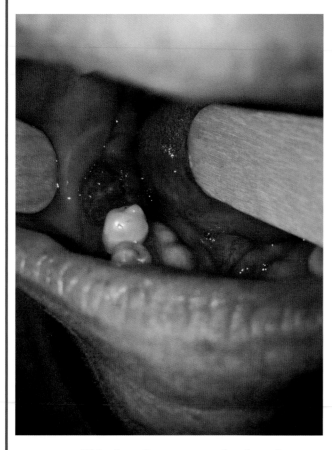

FIGURE 2.1 This photo demonstrates the ulcerative mucosal lesion of the right mandible gingiva.

Management

Question: What would you recommend next?

Answer: Since the lesion has been present for more than 2 weeks and a significant history of tobacco and alcohol abuse exists, tissue diagnosis via incisional or punch biopsy is warranted.

Question: The biopsy is performed and shows invasive, moderately differentiated keratinizing SCC. How would you stage this disease?

Answer: The clinical stage of the disease at this point is T2N0M0, stage II. However, the alveolar lesions can invade the mandible early in the process. Therefore, imaging of the mandible to better delineate osseous involvement is indicated.

Question: How would you determine the involvement of the mandible?

Answer: No imaging modality can offer 100% sensitivity and specificity. CT scanning, especially cone-beam CT, has been utilized as a modality with high sensitivity. Magnetic resonance imaging (MRI) could be useful in determining the involvement of the bone marrow. In the absence of any single definitive modality, attention to the overall clinical exam and imaging findings could guide the clinician to determine the extent of the disease. For oral cavity lesions with suspected mandibular involvement, most surgeons would start with a CT scan with contrast of the head and neck to evaluate the primary site lesion and regional lymphatics.

A PET/MRI and neck CT with IV contrast are obtained. The CT of the neck shows significant thinning of the lingual cortex of the mandible at the site of the lesion and the absence of the buccal cortex superiorly. The inferior alveolar canal appears intact (see Figure 2.2). The PET/MRI shows intense activity at the primary lesion without clear evidence of lymph node metastases. On MRI, there is an abnormal marrow signal at the location of the lesion, suspicious for marrow invasion. There is no evidence of involvement of the mandibular canal.

Question: Based on imaging findings, what is the clinical stage of the disease?

Answer: Since there is radiographic evidence of osseous invasion, the disease is upstaged to T4aN0M0, stage IVa.

Question: What is the recommended course of treatment?

Answer: Oral cavity SCC is primarily treated with surgery, followed by risk-adjusted adjuvant treatment. In this case, the recommended treatment is composite resection of the lesion with segmental mandibulectomy, selective neck dissection (levels I–III), and reconstruction with microvascular free tissue transfer, such as fibula free flap, to provide the best functional outcome.

The patient undergoes segmental mandibulectomy and selective neck dissection with fibula free flap reconstruction. The final pathology shows a 2×1 cm ulcerative SCC of the gingiva with invasion of the mandible. All margins are free of tumor (>5 mm). There is no perineural invasion. There is a microscopic focus of carcinoma present in 1 out of 32 lymph nodes (level Ib node, 2.3 cm) with no evidence of extracapsular extension.

Question: What is the pathologic stage?

Answer: Based on mandibular invasion and nodal involvement, the pathologic stage is pT4aN1M0, stage IVa.

Question: What adjuvant treatment regimen would you recommend to this patient?

Answer: In spite of negative margins and no perineural invasion, advanced T stage and involvement of regional nodes warrant adjuvant radiotherapy. There is no indication for chemotherapy (positive margins and extranodal extension). Therefore, adjuvant radiotherapy is adequate.

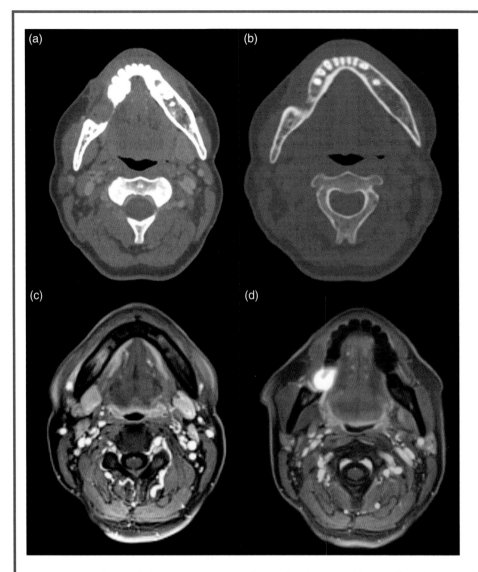

FIGURE 2.2 These axial images are from the patient's CT (a, b) as well as the T1-weighted MRI (c) and fused PET/MRI (d). Note the lesion of the right mandible with associated cortical erosion and hypermetabolism.

Key Points

- Alveolus SCC is less common than tongue or floor of mouth cancers.
- Achieving negative margin resection (>5 mm) is an extremely important objective in the treatment of alveolar cancers.
- To achieve negative margin resection, most alveolar tumors will require resection of the underlying bone. Determining the extent of the mandibulectomy required to achieve negative margins can be challenging.
- It is accepted that if there is no bone erosion on CT or MRI, and there is enough height of the bone, marginal mandibulectomy can achieve negative margin resection. The remaining mandible should have at least a height of 1 cm.

- If there is bone erosion on CT imaging or MRI shows changes in the bone marrow signal, segmental mandibulectomy is recommended.
- There is no level I data on the best method to determine bone involvement. Cone beam CT is considered a very sensitive method.
- In good risk candidates, osseous reconstruction with fibula, scapula, or iliac crest free flap is recommended.
- Osteocutaneous radial forearm or vascularized rib graft has been described and used in patients who are not good candidates for fibula or scapula. However, the harvested bone is not thick enough to host implants.

CASE 3

Michael G. Moore

History of Present Illness

A 68-year-old white male presents with a chief complaint of a painful sore around his right lateral maxillary teeth. He states he initially thought it was related to a dental infection, but after having a tooth pulled, the area has continued to enlarge.

Question: What are the other important points in history taking?

Answer:

- Presence of other adjacent loose teeth.
- Facial numbness.
- Difficulty in opening the mouth.
- Dysphagia, odynophagia.
- Voice changes.
- Presence of neck mass.

  For maxillary lesions, it is always important to determine the extent of the disease. Signs such as loose teeth, difficulty in opening the mouth (trismus), and facial numbness (perineural invasion) could provide critical clinical clues to the extent of disease and aggressive behavior.

Question: What additional aspects of the history and risk factors should be investigated?

Answer:

- Tobacco or alcohol use.
- Any history of head and neck cancers.
- Past medical history for significant diseases: peripheral vascular disease, diabetes, autoimmune diseases, chronic kidney disease, coagulation disorders, to name a few.

  This patient has a history of 10 pack-year smoking but quit 25 years ago. He drinks alcohol socially with no history of excessive drinking. There is no history of significant diseases or malignancy.

Physical Examination

Oral cavity examination shows a 3×2 cm ulcerative lesion on the buccal aspects of teeth #2 to #4 with slight extension onto the palatal aspect of these teeth. No obvious loose teeth, but there is fleshy tissue at the site of the previously extracted tooth #3. His upper teeth are otherwise intact.

Neck exam revealed a 1.5 cm, firm, mobile, slightly tender right level 1b neck mass. No other neck masses were noted. No trismus or paresthesias noted. The rest of the examination is within the normal limits. Cranial nerves II–XII are intact.

Management

Question: What would you recommend next?

Biopsy of the lesion is the first step and is recommended even before imaging.

An office biopsy is performed and shows a moderately differentiated invasive SCC.

Question: What is the clinical stage at this point?

Answer: T2N1M0, stage III, based on a larger than 2 cm lesion and one palpable node. However, in alveolar lesions, it is important to evaluate the involvement of the bone, and these lesions could be upstaged to T4. Therefore, it is better to obtain imaging before assigning a clinical stage.

Question: What imaging modality would be an appropriate next step in the evaluation and management of this patient?

Answer: A CT of the neck and chest with IV contrast is an excellent next step as this will allow for evaluation of the extent of the primary lesion and to look for bone erosion as well as for any pathologic lymphadenopathy. CT of the chest helps to complete the staging. Alternatively, a PET/CT would be reasonable, but it may not allow for as good of resolution of the primary lesion to evaluate for bone involvement. Given that there is no evidence of neural deficits or concern for orbital or infratemporal fossa extension on physical exam, an MRI is probably not necessary (see Figures 3.1 and 3.2).

Chest CT demonstrated no evidence of metastatic disease.

Oromaxillofacial prosthodontics is consulted to assist with a dental impression and the production of an obturator if maxillectomy is considered.

Question: Based on your current assessment, what would be this patient's clinical stage?

Answer: This patient has oral cavity cancer. The primary lesion is staged based on size and depth of invasion. Here, depth is not known. Size puts it in the T2 category. Of note, minor bone erosion or maxillary involvement through a tooth socket alone does not upstage it to T4a. The patient has multiple ipsilateral pathologic nodes, none of which are larger than 6 cm in size, making him cN2b. Therefore, the stage is T2N2bM0: stage IVa.

Question: Given the above information, what would be the most appropriate management approach for this patient?

Answer: This patient has stage IVa oral cavity cancer. The optimal treatment strategy in patients who are amenable to surgery is for upfront surgical resection of the primary lesion with a concomitant neck dissection. Given the N2b neck dissection, he would benefit from adjuvant radiation therapy (**RT**) or chemoradiation therapy, depending on the final margin status and the presence or absence of extracapsular spread.

Question: Figure 3.3 shows an intraoperative photo of the oral cavity defect after surgical resection of the primary tumor. What would you recommend for the reconstruction of the defects? What are the factors that should be considered in the reconstruction of the maxillary defect?

(a) (b)

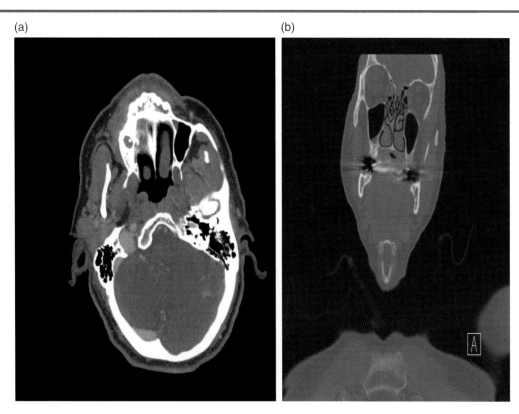

FIGURE 3.1   Axial (a) and coronal (b) cut of the primary lesion. Note there is minor bone erosion – no obvious extension into the pterygoid plates or muscles.

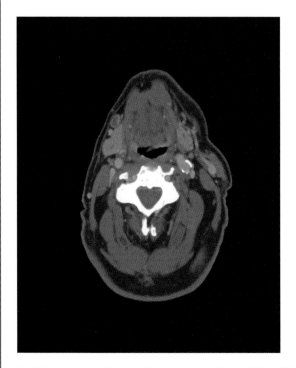

FIGURE 3.2   Axial cut of the neck portion of the CT demonstrating the pathologic node felt on physical examination. There was one additional node with evidence of central necrosis in right level 1b. Both lymph nodes were less than 3 cm in size.

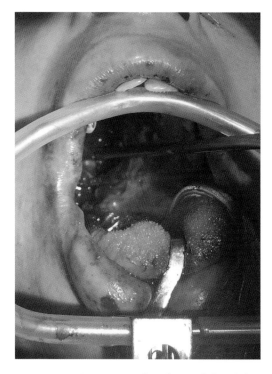

FIGURE 3.3   Intraoperative photo of the right oral cavity defect after surgical resection of the primary tumor.

(Continued)

CASE 3 (continued)

Answer: In a patient undergoing maxillectomy, it is critical to consider the best way to rehabilitate the defect. Limited defects, especially those with no communication to the sinonasal cavity, may require no reconstruction or simple adjacent tissue closure. For more extensive defects entering the sinonasal cavity, it is necessary to address this defect to allow for functional speech and swallowing. In this patient, an excellent option would be rehabilitation with a maxillofacial prosthesis. To do this, the patient must have adequate mouth opening and manual dexterity to allow for placement and removal. Moreover, retention is significantly improved when the ipsilateral canine tooth is maintained to allow for an adequate fulcrum for stability. Other contraindications to obturator use are resection of the orbital floor (unless a separate orbital floor repair is also performed) or resection of the anterior (premaxilla) or lateral (zygoma) projecting elements. Resection of the pterygoid plates does not significantly impact whether or not appropriate obturation can be achieved.

The patient's final pathology demonstrates a 3.2 cm primary tumor, resected closest margin is 4 mm, posteriorly.

There was only minor bone erosion seen. The neck dissection specimen showed 5 out of 58 lymph nodes positive. The largest lymph node was 2.7 cm, and there was evidence of extracapsular spread.

Question: What would be the recommended next step in this patient's management?

Answer: This patient has pT2N3bM0, stage IVb disease based on the 8th Edition of the AJCC staging system. The presence of a close margin at the primary site would indicate the need to consider adjuvant radiation therapy. However, the presence of extracapsular spread of cervical lymph nodes (or the presence of a positive margin at the primary that cannot be re-excised) is an indication for adjuvant chemoradiation therapy as this has been shown to improve overall survival and disease-free survival. Since the posterior margin was close but clear, re-excision would not be necessary. The patient will benefit from concurrent adjuvant chemoradiotherapy with platinum-based agents.

Key Points

- Evaluation of oral cavity cancer starts with a biopsy and typically a CT scan of the face and neck with IV contrast to assess the extent of the primary lesion and to evaluate for regional lymphadenopathy. An MRI may be indicated if there is concern for significant perineural invasion, deep tongue invasion, or extension near the orbit, skull base, or parapharyngeal space. The use of PET/CT should be in patients with stage III or IV disease.
- Management of tumors of the maxillary alveolus typically involves upfront surgery with removal of the primary tumor with clear surgical margins. A neck dissection should be performed for pathologic lymphadenopathy. For cN0 patients, elective neck dissection should be considered for advanced (T3 or T4) primary tumors as it may improve cancer control. more recent evidence suggests elective neck dissection in T2 tumors or consideration of sentinel node biopsy to determine the need for neck dissection.

- Adjuvant radiation therapy should be considered for advanced primary tumors, the presence of lymph node metastases, perineural invasion, lymphovascular invasion, or close surgical margins.
- Adjuvant chemoradiotherapy should be recommended in instances of positive surgical margins and/or the presence of extracapsular spread in cervical lymph nodes.
- In patients where a maxillectomy is considered, options for reconstruction include the use of a maxillofacial prosthesis or the use of a regional or free flap. If a maxillary obturator is planned, it is essential to have the patient see a maxillofacial prosthodontist soon after diagnosis to allow for a prosthesis to be made prior to the day of the resection.
- In instances when there is resection of the orbital floor or orbital exenteration, or when there will be inadequate remaining dentition to retain an obturator, reconstruction with free tissue transfer should be considered in suitable candidates.

CASE 4

Alok Pathak

History of Present Illness

A 75-year old man with a 35 pack-year smoking history presents for evaluation of a sore in the left side of his mouth. He quit tobacco 30 years ago but continues to drink two to three alcoholic drinks every day. He had extractions of tooth #17

and #18 3 months ago. However, the extraction site has not healed since then.

Physical Examination

Oral cavity examination demonstrates a 2.5 cm proliferative mass over the left retromolar trigone adherent to the underlying mandible with loss of sensation over the left chin (see

CASE 4 (continued)

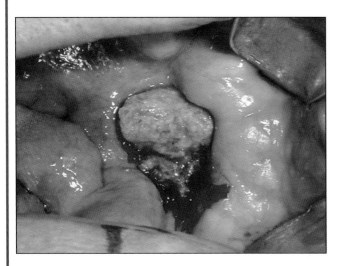

FIGURE 4.1 This intraoral photograph shows the lesion of the patient's left retromolar trigone extending on the left mandible body.

Figure 4.1). There is also a palpable 2 cm mobile left submandibular lymph node.

Question: What is the most likely clinical diagnosis?

Answer: In view of progressive proliferative growth, with loss of sensation over the distribution of mental nerve with the risk factors of past tobacco use and current alcohol, the most likely diagnosis is SCC. In the presence of a gingival growth, tooth extraction should be avoided as it provides easy access to the mandible through the tooth socket.

Management

Question: What is the best way to achieve preoperative tissue diagnosis?

Answer: Punch/incisional biopsy. Since the lesion is easily accessible in the oral cavity, transoral incisional biopsy in the clinic is the most appropriate and expeditious way to get a tissue diagnosis. Fine needle aspiration of the lymph node may also be performed. However, a negative cytology from the lymph node does not rule out malignancy. Any consideration of an open biopsy of the lymph node should be avoided as it can complicate further neck treatment.

Question: What would be the most appropriate next step in the evaluation of this patient?

Answer: Considering the extent of the symptoms, imaging is recommended. CT scan of the head and neck with contrast is the most appropriate first step. Mental paresthesia is an indicator of the involvement of the inferior alveolar nerve in the mandibular canal. CT scan with contrast is the most appropriate imaging modality to assess the extent of mandibular

invasion and cervical lymphadenopathy. If proximal extension of the tumor along the mandibular nerve is a concern on CT scan, an MRI could be obtained. For advanced oral cavity cancer, distant imaging is recommended, in the form of a CT chest with contrast or PET/CT.

Contrast-enhanced CT of the neck shows a 4.5 cm heterogeneous tumor centered in the left retromolar trigone with underlying osseous destruction through the inferior alveolar canal. The erosive component of the tumor crosses the midline at the mandibular symphysis (see Figure 4.2). There are multiple enlarged and round lymph nodes in the left neck, the largest measuring 3.1 cm in left level 1b.

Chest CT does not demonstrate any distant metastatic disease.

The incisional biopsy came back as moderately differentiated SCC.

Question: What is the clinical tumor stage?

Answer: cT4aN2bM0, stage IVa. Mandibular involvement upstages the T stage to T4a. With multiple ipsilateral nodes <6 cm, the N stage is N2b.

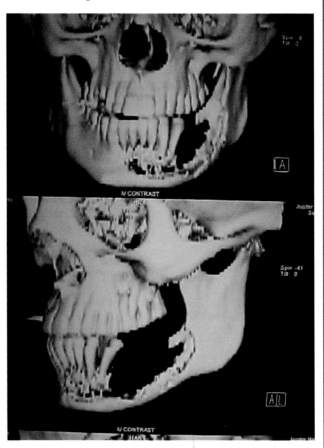

FIGURE 4.2 CT scan shows an extensive and destructive process of the left mandibular body.

(Continued)

CASE 4   (continued)

Question: What course of treatment would you recommend?

Answer: Treatment of advanced oral cavity SCC requires extirpation of the primary tumor with negative margins and addressing the lymphatics of the neck. Segmental mandibulectomy is required to obtain negative primary site surgical margins. The mandibular defect will require free tissue transfer reconstruction. The ipsilateral involved neck will require a neck dissection, level I–IV (skip metastases to level V in oral cavity carcinoma are uncommon). As the lesion crosses midline anteriorly, it is appropriate to consider or perform a contralateral selective (level I–III) neck dissection.

Question: What are the potential functional deficits after surgical treatment?

Answer: While rare, injuries to the spinal accessory nerve (CN XI) resulting in shoulder weakness, and marginal mandibular branch of the facial nerve (CN VII) resulting in lower lip depressor weakness, can occur but are not an expected outcome in experienced settings. Left chin numbness is to be expected after a segmental mandibulectomy as the inferior alveolar nerve is transected during the extirpation. Injury to the hypoglossal nerve (CN XII) is also rare and would be considered a complication. Treatment of alveolar cancer is not expected to result in significant dysphagia or aspiration postoperatively. However, when resection extends across the midline anteriorly, resulting in detachment of the genial muscular attachments, some loss of function can be observed.

Final pathology shows a 4.2 cm tumor centered in the left retromolar trigone with mandibular invasion, extensive perineural invasion, and a deep positive margin. In the right neck dissection specimen, 0/8 lymph nodes are involved with the tumor. In the left neck dissection specimen, 6/32 lymph nodes are involved with the tumor. There is a 3.1 cm level 1b lymph node that shows extranodal extension into the submandibular gland.

Question: Based on the final pathology, what is the pathologic stage and your recommended adjuvant treatment regimen?

Answer: pT4aN3bM0, stage IVb. Mandibular involvement results in pT4a staging. Any node with extranodal extension (ENE) results in an upstaging to N3b. There are many indications for radiation, including positive margins, perineural invasion (PNI), and multiple nodes involved. There are two indications for chemotherapy: positive surgical margins at the primary site and extranodal extension. In this case, considering that a large resection was performed and the defect is reconstructed with fibula flap, the expectation of re-resection is not realistic. Therefore, continuing with concurrent adjuvant chemoradiation with platinum-based agents is appropriate.

Key Points

- Evaluation of oral cavity cancer starts with a biopsy and typically a CT scan of the face and neck with IV contrast to assess the extent of the primary lesion and to evaluate for regional lymphadenopathy. An MRI may be indicated if there is concern for significant perineural invasion, deep tongue invasion, or extension near the orbit, skull base, or parapharyngeal space. The use of PET/CT should be in patients with stage III or IV disease.
- Management of tumors of the oral cavity typically involves upfront surgery with removal of the primary tumor with clear surgical margins. A neck dissection should be performed for pathologic lymphadenopathy. Contralateral selective neck dissections should be performed if the tumor crosses the midline.
- Adjuvant radiation therapy should be considered for advanced primary tumors, the presence of lymph node metastases, perineural invasion, lymphovascular invasion, or close surgical margins.
- Adjuvant chemoradiation therapy should be recommended in instances of positive surgical margins and/or the presence of extracapsular spread in cervical lymph nodes.

CASE 5

Arnaud Bewley

History of Present Illness

A 62-year-old white female is seen in the office with a 3-month history of a gradually enlarging lower lip mass. She has not had any previous biopsies, imaging, or treatment.

Her past medical history includes hypercholesterolemia, hypertension, appendectomy, and tonsillectomy. She takes Lisinopril and atorvastatin. She has a history of 30 pack-year smoking but quit 10 years ago. She drinks a glass of wine with dinner every night.

CASE 5   (continued)

Question: What are the other important points in history?

Answer:

- Pain and tenderness. This is an important question, as pain that is out of proportion with exam can be suggestive of perineural invasion.
- The presence of neck masses is an important finding, as advanced lower lip cancers have a high propensity for spread to the regional lymphatics.
- Voice change. It is important to screen for other head and neck cancer primaries in patients who are high risk.
- Weight loss, which is often associated with the duration and severity of symptoms.

The lesion is exquisitely painful, particularly along the right lower lip. She has not experienced any voice changes or weight loss and has not noticed any neck masses.

Physical Examination

An image of the patient's lower lip lesion is shown in Figure 5.1. The tumor is very tender to palpation and extends from the right commissure to about 3 mm from the left commissure. Intraorally, it is free from the fixed gingiva by about 1 cm. There is subcutaneous extension palpable at the right lateral aspect of the tumor. There is no palpable lymphadenopathy. The remainder of her head and neck examination is unremarkable.

Management

Question: What would you recommend next?

Answer: Punch biopsy of the lower lip lesion. Pathologic diagnosis is imperative and is the most appropriate next step

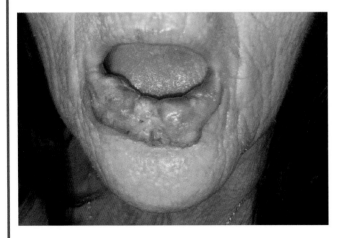

FIGURE 5.1   The patient's lower lip mass. The tumor extends from the right Commissure to about 3mm from the left Commissure.

in management. This would most easily be obtained with a punch biopsy at the time of her initial visit.

Question: What other tests or studies would you consider, if any?

Answer: A CT of the neck with IV contrast is an important next step in evaluating regional adenopathy. MRI of the neck could be considered, given the acute tenderness noted along the right lower lip. An MRI would be superior to a CT in evaluating for enhancement of the right mental nerve. An MRI would also allow for evaluation of the regional nodes, though less cost-effective than a CT scan. PET/CT scan could be considered. Also, a potential method of evaluating the regional nodal basin while also ruling out distant metastatic disease. For early stage disease (T1/T2) without clinical or radiographic evidence of regional disease, a PET/CT is usually unnecessary. If a PET/CT is considered, it is recommended that CT is performed with contrast and with adequate detail to delineate the neck anatomy.

A punch biopsy is performed and demonstrates SCC.

A contrast-enhanced CT scan is obtained with representative images shown below. No abnormal lymph nodes are reported. The tumor is measured around 5 cm on the CT scan (see Figure 5.2).

Question: Based on the patient's examination and radiographic findings, how would you stage this disease?

Answer: T3N0M0, stage III. Cancers of the lip mucosa continue to be staged as cancers of the oral cavity, while cancers of the external vermillion lip are now staged as cutaneous carcinomas, per AJCC 8th Edition. However, in advanced tumors, this can be a difficult distinction to make when tumors involve both the mucosal and external vermillion surface. In these cases, staging should be based on the tumor's historical origin when this can be deduced. In this case, the patient reports the tumor originated on the inner aspect of the lip, and this is corroborated by the greater degree of extension noted on the mucosal surface. The tumor is greater than 4 cm in diameter, therefore, it meets the criteria for a T3 primary. It would also likely meet the 1 cm depth of invasion criteria for T3 tumor. There is no clinical or radiographic evidence of regional metastatic spread; therefore, the patient should be staged as a T3N0M0, stage III.

Question: What is the appropriate treatment for this patient?

Answer: Primary surgical therapy is generally considered the standard of care for lip cancers as with oral cavity cancers. While the resection of lip cancer is relatively straightforward, the complex functional and aesthetic roles of the lip present major reconstructive challenges.

Due to the challenges of achieving acceptable functional and aesthetic outcomes with surgery for extensive lip

(Continued)

CASE 5 (continued)

(a)

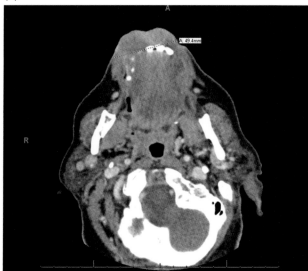

(b)

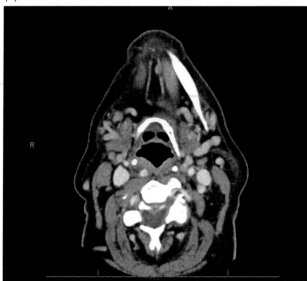

FIGURE 5.2 These representative axial cuts for the patient's neck CT with IV contrast demonstrate a large ill-defined soft tissue tumor of the lower lip (a) with rounded level Ia and (b) Ib lymph nodes without obvious necrosis.

cancer, radiotherapy is considered an acceptable alternative. In particular, extensive lower lip cancers that extend over a significant proportion of the surface of the lip are particularly amenable to this approach.

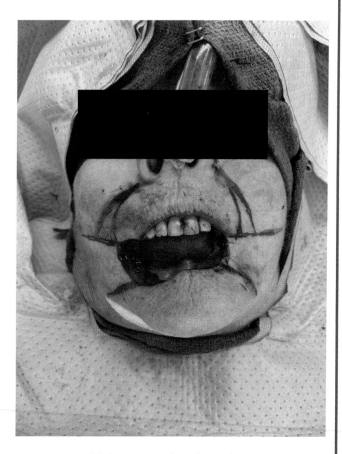

FIGURE 5.3 This intraoperative photo shows the patient's total lower lip defect.

In this patient's case, given the thickness of the tumor and soft tissue extension, she elected for definitive surgical resection, yielding the defect pictured below (see Figure 5.3).

Final pathology report showed SCC, 4.1 cm in greatest dimension, with a depth of invasion of 13 mm. Perineural invasion is present, but no lymphovascular invasion. The closest margin is 3 mm.

Question: How would you reconstruct the primary defect depicted in Figure 5.3?

Answer: While a Karapandzic flap is an excellent option for large lower lip defects, it relies entirely on the existing lip. As a result, some amount of preserved lower lip is needed to prevent severe microstomia. With a total lower lip defect, a Karapandzic flap would result in an unacceptable degree of microstomia.

Abbe/Estlander flaps are ideal for small lateral defects of the lip where sufficient lip can be recruited from the uninvolved

CASE 5   (continued)

lip to achieve a functional reconstruction. This defect is clearly too extensive to be amenable to these types of flaps.

Bernard/Webster flap could be used as an option. Total lower lip defects require the recruitment of additional tissue to recreate the lip, thereby minimizing the degree of microstomia. The Bernard and Webster flaps recruit tissue from the

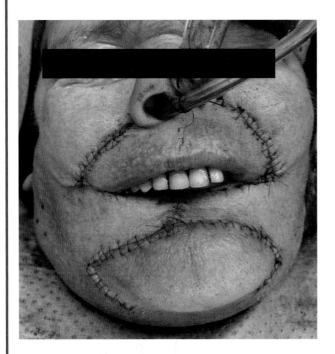

FIGURE 5.4   Bernard-Webster bilateral advancement flap reconstruction.

cheek and buccal mucosa to reconstruct the lower lip and are therefore ideal for total or subtotal lip defects. The reconstructed tissue is not contractile but maintains sensation with good skin match.

The radial forearm free flap is another method of creating a new lip and is best for mitigating microstomia. This is often performed with a palmaris longus tendon sling to aid with oral competence. Disadvantages are lack of contractility, lack of sensation, and poor skin match.

This patient was reconstructed with a Bernard-Webster bilateral advancement flap as pictured below (see Figure 5.4).

Question: How would you manage the patient's regional lymph node basin?

Answer: Bilateral supra-omohyoid neck dissection is an acceptable way to address the high risk for occult regional disease in locally advanced lower lip cancer. This is a particularly appealing approach in patients who may be able to avoid adjuvant RT. Given the tumor involvement of the bilateral lower lip, any elective nodal dissection should address both sides of the neck.

Sentinel lymph node biopsy (**SLNB**) has been shown to be feasible and effective in patients who may be at high risk of metastases based on tumor size and depth. However, given the extensive nature of this primary tumor, the specificity of a sentinel node identification may be lower as four-quadrant injection of the radiotracer would likely trace to a variety of nodes. This would, therefore, not be an ideal case for SLNB. In general, sentinel node biopsy is recommended in T1, T2 tumors.

Given the locally advanced nature of this patient's tumor (T3) and the presence of PNI, she would benefit from adjuvant radiation therapy to the tumor bed. The regional lymphatics could likewise be irradiated to an adjuvant dose without the need for elective neck dissection.

Key Points

- Cancers of the lip mucosa continue to be staged as cancers of the oral cavity, while cancers of the external vermillion lip are now staged as cutaneous carcinomas.
- Primary radiotherapy can offer equivalent oncologic outcomes to surgical resection for early stage tumors.
- Extensive, superficial lower lip cancers are good candidates for primary radiotherapy as they avoid the potential high morbidity of surgical resection.
- Total lower lip defects require the recruitment of additional tissue to recreate the lip, thereby minimizing the degree of microstomia.
- The Bernard and Webster flaps recruit tissue from the cheek and buccal mucosa to reconstruct the lower lip and are therefore ideal for total or subtotal lip defects.
- SLNB has been shown to be feasible and effective in patients with lip tumors who may be at high risk of metastases based on tumor size and depth.
- Due to extensive lymphatic drainage from the upper lip and commissure, tumors of these subsites have a higher incidence of lymph node metastases at the time of diagnosis.

CASE 6

Ian Ganly

Presentation

A 45-year-old man presents with a soft tissue swelling of the left hard palate and soft palate. He denies pain. The patient had previously been seen by his dentist, who initiated a course of antibiotics with no effect. The patient was referred for further investigation. Examination showed a diffuse swelling of the hard palate as shown in Figure 6.1.

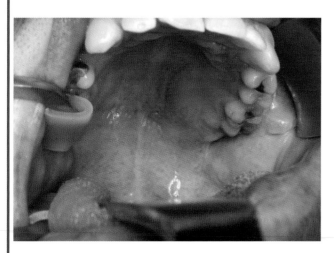

FIGURE 6.1 This transoral photograph shows mild submucosal fullness of the left aspect of the hard palate.

Question: What are the differential diagnoses for this mass?

Answer: Hard palate tumors are rare. The differential includes ameloblastoma, odontogenic keratocyst, and lymphoma, among others. However, the most common pathologies are minor salivary gland tumors.

Question: What is the most common minor salivary tumor in the oral cavity?

Answer: The most common minor salivary tumor of the oral cavity is mucoepidermoid carcinoma, followed by adenoid cystic carcinoma.

Question: What would you recommend next? What further investigations should be done for this patient?

Answer: Tissue diagnosis is the next step. Fine needle aspirate will most likely determine if this is a malignant versus benign tumor. However, core needle biopsy is often needed due to the heterogeneity in salivary gland pathology to establish the exact pathological diagnosis.

A contrast CT scan is a very reasonable first imaging study to determine the extent of bone invasion of the hard palate and upper alveolus and will determine if any neural foramens are widened in keeping with perineural invasion. An MRI scan might be necessary and is used more often to determine the extent of soft tissue invasion and to determine if any perineural invasion is present. MRI is also helpful in distinguishing between different salivary tumors.

A core biopsy was done and reported as adenoid cystic carcinoma. A CT scan and MRI scan were done. The results of the MRI scan are shown in Figure 6.2.

(a)

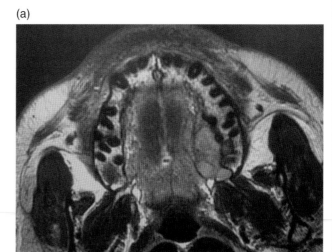

(b)

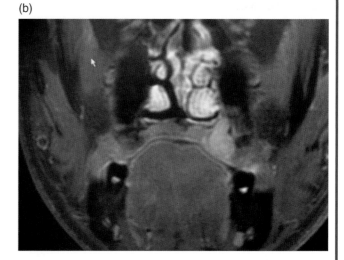

FIGURE 6.2 An axial T1-weighted MRI image without contrast (a) and a coronal T1-weighted MRI with contrast (b) show an enhancing submucosal lesion of the left hard palate.

CASE 6   (continued)

Question: What are the pertinent findings in MRI on your review?

Answer: The MRI shows widening of the palatine canal, which is most likely due to the perineural invasion of the greater palatine nerve.

Question: What is the recommended management for this patient?

Answer: Adenoid cystic carcinoma is best managed by wide surgical resection followed by adjuvant radiation unless the tumor is considered unresectable. In this particular case, the extent of perineural invasion was limited to the greater palatine nerve with no extension to the skull base or cavernous sinus. The tumor was, therefore, deemed to be resectable. Due to the presence of perineural invasion and high incidence of positive margins in adenoid cystic cancer, adjuvant radiotherapy is recommended in the majority of cases to improve local control.

Question: What is the extent of surgery? What approach would you recommend?

Answer: Based on the extent of the tumor on imaging and exam, peroral left infrastructure maxillectomy with resection of the hard palate, upper alveolus incorporating the palatine canal, and pterygoid plates appears to be a reasonable approach. The steps involved in the surgery are summarized in Figure 6.3.

An infrastructure maxillectomy is started by completing mucosal cuts to allow for at least a 1 cm soft tissue margin around the visible and palpable tumor. The next steps in the maxillectomy are accomplished by performing bone cuts. This is first done through the use of an oscillating saw. Due to the risk for bleeding, the posterior cut is often saved for last and is accomplished by the use of a curved osteotome followed by heavy curved scissors.

Question: What would you recommend for rehabilitation or reconstruction of this defect?

Answer: This patient could be rehabilitated with a dental obturator. The obturator allows for inspection of the resection site as well as for dental rehabilitation. The main disadvantage is the inability to eat without the prosthesis and nasal speech. An alternative method is with a free radial forearm flap, which allows for eating without a prosthesis and normal speech. However, a dental plate with teeth is still required for dental rehabilitation. In this particular case, a free radial forearm flap was used with donor vessels arising from the facial artery (see Figure 6.4).

Final pathology showed adenoid cystic carcinoma, predominantly tubular, 3.5 cm, no bone invasion, but with gross perineural invasion into the greater palatine nerve. All margins are free of tumor.

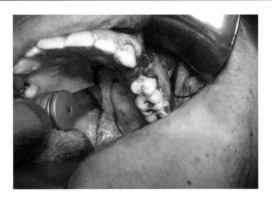

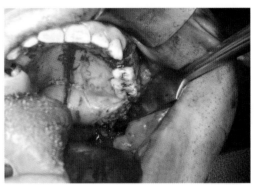

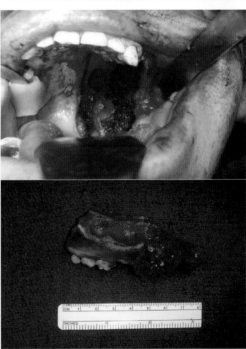

FIGURE 6.3   These intraoperative images show the surgical approach transorally and the resulting maxillectomy defect as well as the associated specimen.

(Continued)

CASE 6 (continued)

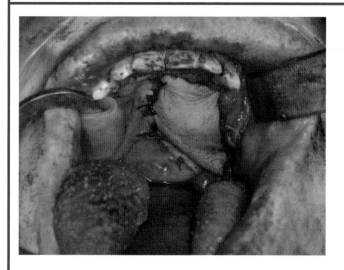

FIGURE 6.4 **This intraoperative photo shows the palate defect after reconstruction using a radial forearm free flap. An alternative approach would have been a maxillary obturator given the preservation of the ipsilateral canine tooth and adequate contralateral maxillary dentition.**

Question: What would you recommend next?

Answer: Although the tumor is completely excised, the risk of local failure is still significant in adenoid cystic carcinoma. Adjuvant radiotherapy is recommended. Since there are no adverse features (such as lymph node involvement, positive margins), adjuvant chemotherapy or consideration of clinical trials to add chemotherapy to radiotherapy are not appropriate in this case.

Question: What is the expected outcome for this patient?

Answer: Patients with minor salivary cancer tend to have a very good overall survival of 80% and disease-specific survival of 80–90%. The main predictors of outcome are stage III/IV disease and high-grade pathology. Female patients have a superior survival compared to male patients. Distant failure is more common and is the main cause of death.

This patient was treated with adjuvant radiation and remains disease-free at 3 years post-treatment.

Key Points

- The oral cavity is the most common location for the development of minor salivary gland tumors due to the high concentration of minor salivary gland tissue in this location.
- Adenoid cystic carcinoma is the most common minor salivary gland cancer.
- For minor salivary gland cancers of the palate, evaluation includes a detailed history, physical exam, a thorough cranial nerve exam, and a biopsy, often with a fine needle aspiration.
- For further assessment of palate salivary cancers, both CT and MRI are typically employed to assess for bone erosion and perineural invasion, respectively.
- Due to the close association of the mucosa of the hard palate and the underlying bone, infrastructure maxillectomy is often required.
- When considering a patient for an infrastructure maxillectomy, it is essential to consider the expected defect and discuss options for rehabilitation. If the use of a maxillary obturator is considered, a preoperative evaluation by a maxillofacial prosthodontist is crucial to get a surgical obturator created.
- To successfully retain an obturator, it is necessary to have adequate dentition to stabilize the prosthesis. Retention of the ipsilateral canine tooth typically allows for excellent obturator stability.
- In patients where a maxillary obturator is not appropriate or desired, more definitive reconstruction with a regional or free flap is needed.

Multiple Choice Questions

1. In managing a 52-year-old female patient with a cT1N0M0 SCC of the right lateral tongue, you offer a right partial glossectomy. Final pathology demonstrates invasive SCC with maximal dimension of 1.5 cm and 6 mm depth of invasion. What would be the most appropriate next step in management of this patient?

   a. Close observation of the neck with clinical exam and ultrasound every 3 months.

   b. A right-sided supraomohyoid neck dissection.

   c. A right-sided radical neck dissection.

   d. A bilateral supraomohyoid neck dissection.

   Answer: b. This patient has a pT2 lesion. With a depth of invasion greater than 3 mm, level I evidence shows improved disease control and overall survival when an ipsilateral supraomohyoid neck dissection is performed. Since they are cN0, a radical neck dissection would not be appropriate. Moreover, since it is a lateral tongue cancer, it would not be necessary to do a bilateral dissection.

2. In a patient who undergoes a left partial glossectomy and left neck dissection, final pathology shows a 3.2 cm primary lesion with 12 mm depth of invasion. There was 1 out of 37 lymph nodes positive in the neck dissection (2.2 cm maximal dimension and no ECS). What is the pathologic stage of this patient's cancer?

   a. pT2N1M0, stage III.

   b. pT3N1M0, stage III.

   c. pT3N1M0, stage IVa.

   d. pT4aN1M0, stage IVa.

   Answer: b. Due to the depth of invasion being greater than 10 mm but the overall lesion size being less than 4 cm, this would be a T3 tumor. T3N1M0 carries a group stage of III.

3. A 67-year-old male presents for evaluation of persistent pain in the left jaw following a tooth extraction. On exam he is found to have granular tissue emanating from the extraction site of his second left mandibular molar. He expresses progressive left lip, chin, and tongue numbness. Biopsy is consistent with SCC. Which of the following would **not** be an appropriate next step in the evaluation of this patient?

   a. A neck MRI with and without gadolinium.

   b. A neck CT with IV contrast.

   c. A neck ultrasound.

   d. A PET/CT from the skull base to midthighs.

   Answer: c. In this patient, there seems to be significant tumor extension beyond what is identifiable clinically. A CT of the neck will provide good detail of the bone involvement, but an MRI will also be needed as the tongue numbness suggests there may be perineural invasion tracking proximally on V3. A PET/CT is also helpful in completing the staging for this patient. A neck ultrasound, while it may be helpful in looking for cervical lymphadenopathy, would not be able to assess the mandible and would be redundant if other studies were ordered.

4. The lingual nerve runs in what relationship with the pterygoid muscles?

   a. It runs medial to both muscles.

   b. It runs between the medial and lateral pterygoid muscles.

   c. It runs lateral to both the medial and lateral pterygoid muscles.

   d. It has a variable relationship with the two muscles.

   Answer: b. This is an important landmark on tumor resections with extension into the infratemporal fossa. The lingual nerve can also be traced proximally to identify foramen ovale.

5. Retention of which tooth on a right posterior maxillectomy will have the biggest impact on whether or not they can be rehabilitated with an obturator?

   a. Tooth #4.

   b. Tooth #5.

   c. Tooth #6.

   d. Tooth #7.

   Answer: c. Retention of the ipsilateral canine tooth for posterior infrastructure maxillectomies has been shown to significantly reduce the fulcrum effect and improve obturator retention.

6. A 76-year-old male patient presents with a T4aN1M0 SCC of the left ventral tongue and floor of mouth with involvement of the left mandible body. On history, the patient has a history of lower extremity claudication with walking of 1.5 blocks. It is anticipated that resection will require a left hemiglossectomy and a segmental mandible resection of 9 cm. What would be the most appropriate donor site for reconstruction in this patient?

   a. Left scapula osseocutaneous flap.

   b. Right fibula osseocutaneous flap.

   c. Left radial forearm osseocutaneous flap.

   d. Anterolateral thigh musculocutaneous free flap.

   Answer: a. This patient has a segmental mandibulectomy defect and a considerable soft tissue defect as well. Due to the soft tissue requirements as well as the lower extremity claudication, a fibula free flap would not be ideal. The radial forearm free flap with bone is a reasonable option, but the concern here is an inadequate amount of soft tissue. Scapular or parascapular free flap can be harvested with a large amount of soft tissue with adequate bone to reconstruct up to 14 cm of bone. The subscapular system tends to be less impacted by atherosclerosis than flaps from the extremity.

7. Which of the following is true:

   a. Tumors in the upper lip and commissure have a higher incidence of lymph node metastases at the time of diagnosis.

   b. Tumors of the lower lip have a higher rate of lymph node metastasis than those of the upper lip and commissure.

   c. Tumors of the local commissure have the highest rate of lymph node metastasis of all lip cancers.

   d. All locations of lip cancer result in the same rate of lymph node metastasis.

Answer: a. Due to extensive lymphatic drainage from the upper lip and commissure, tumors of these subsites have a higher incidence of lymph node metastases at the time of diagnosis.

8. You evaluate a patient with a 1.5 cm, thin-appearing SCC of the left lower lip. His clinical exam and recent CT imaging do not demonstrate any enlarged adenopathy. How would you counsel the patient regarding the efficacy of surgery versus primary radiotherapy as definitive treatment for his tumor?

   a. Primary surgical resection offers a higher chance of local control and overall survival.

   b. Primary surgical resection offers a higher chance of local control but equivalent overall survival.

   c. Primary surgical resection offers equivalent local control and overall survival.

   d. Primary surgical resection offers inferior local control and overall survival.

   Answer: c (see de Visscher et al. 1999). A retrospective study of 99 patients treated with definitive radiotherapy versus surgery for stage I lower lip cancers found that rates of survival and disease control were equivalent between treatment groups. Tumor size was independently associated with poorer outcomes.

9. The above patient elects for primary surgical resection, and the final pathology demonstrates a 1.7 cm SCC with a 6 mm depth of invasion and positive perineural invasion. How would you stage the patient, and what additional treatment would you offer, if any?

   a. T1N0: elective neck dissection, no adjuvant RT if cN0.

   b. T1N0: adjuvant RT only.

   c. T2N0: observation only.

   d. T2N0: adjuvant RT only.

   Answer: d. This patient's tumor should be staged according to the AJCC oral cavity staging criteria. With a depth of invasion >5 mm, this tumor therefore meets the criteria for a T2N0. Perineural invasion has been described as a strong predictor of locoregional failure for lip cancers and is considered an indication for adjuvant RT. Management of this patient with adjuvant RT only would therefore be appropriate. Elective ND followed by potential avoidance of RT if cN0 could be considered. However, the patient would be at increased risk of local failure.

10. Which of the following is true regarding minor salivary gland cancer tumors?

    a. More common in advanced age.

    b. Are more common in women.

    c. Cervical lymph node metastases are common.

    d. The most common site is the oropharynx.

    Answer: b. The most common site for minor salivary gland cancer is the oral cavity, accounting for 68% of cancers, followed by the oropharynx in 21%, sinonasal tract in 8%, and larynx/trachea in 3%. A particularly common location is the junction between the hard and the soft palate due to the high concentration of minor salivary tissue in this location. These tumors are more common in women and younger groups. The most common pathology of minor salivary gland cancers in the oral cavity is mucoepidermoid carcinoma. Cervical lymph node metastases are rare.

11. In minor salivary glands tumors:

    a. The most common salivary gland cancer of the trachea is mucoepidermoid carcinoma.

    b. The most common salivary gland cancer on the hard palate is adenoid cystic carcinoma.

    c. Perineural invasion is a feature of acinic cell carcinoma.

    d. The most common pathology that develops distant metastases is adenoid cystic carcinoma.

    Answer: d. The most common pathology that develops distant metastases is adenoid cystic cancer (lungs). The most common tracheal tumor is adenoid cystic carcinoma. The most common minor salivary gland tumor of the hard palate is polymorphous low-grade adenocarcinoma. Perineural invasion is a feature of adenoid cystic carcinoma.

12. Which of the following statements regarding the outcome of minor salivary gland cancers is true?

    a. The overall survival of minor salivary gland cancer is poor with 5-year disease-specific survival of 50–60%.

    b. Distant failure is more common than local or regional failure.

    c. Patients with high-grade pathology have similar outcomes to those with low-grade pathology.

    d. The main predictor of outcome is the presence of perineural invasion.

    e. Female patients have a poorer survival to male patients.

    Answer: b. Patients with minor salivary cancer tend to have a very good overall survival of 80% and disease-specific survival of 80–90%. The main predictors of outcome are stage III/IV disease and high-grade pathology. Female patients have a superior survival compared to male patients. Distant failure is more common and is the leading cause of death.

13. Which of the following statements is correct with regards to the primary site of a minor salivary gland cancer?

    a. Tumors of the sinonasal tract have a poorer outcome.

    b. The most common site in the oral cavity is the floor of the mouth.

    c. Tumors of the oropharynx tend to be mucoepidermoid cancer.

    d. Tumors arising from the oropharynx have superior outcome to those of the oral cavity.

    Answer: a. Of all of the subsites, tumors arising from the sinonasal tract tend to have poorer outcomes. This is because they present with a more advanced local stage (T3, T4) and are more likely to have positive margin resection. Within the oral cavity, the most common subsite is the hard palate. In the trachea, the most common pathology is adenoid cystic cancer. Patients with tumors in the oropharynx have similar outcomes to those with oral cavity cancers.

Reference

de Visscher, J.G., Botke, G., Schakenraad, J.A., and van der Waal, I. (1999). A comparison of results after radiotherapy and surgery for stage I squamous cell carcinoma of the lower lip. *Head Neck* 21: 526–530. Available at: http://www.ncbi.nlm.nih.gov/pubmed/10449668.

Suggested Readings

Amin, M.B., Edge, S., Greene, F. et al. (2017). *AJCC Cancer Staging Mannual*, vol. 8. Chicago IL: American Joint Committee on Cancer, Springer.

Barttelbort, S.W. and Ariyan, S. (1993). Mandible preservation with oral cavity carcinoma: rim mandibulectomy versus sagittal mandibulectomy. *Am. J. Surg.* 166 (4): 411–415. https://doi.org/10.1016/s0002-9610(05)80344-7. PMID: 8214304.

Bernier, J., Ozsahin, M., Lefebvre, J.L. et al. (2004). Postoperative ioncomitant chemotherapy for locally advanced head and neck cancer. *New Engl. J. Med.* 350 (19): 1945–1952.

Bernier, J., Cooper, J.S., Pajak, T.F. et al. (2005). Defining risk levels in locally advanced head and neck cancers: a comparative analysis of concurrent postoperative radiation plus chemotherapy trials of the EORTC (#22931) and RTOG (# 9501). *Head Neck* 27 (10): 843–850. https://doi.org/10.1002/hed.20279.

Brown, J.S., Lowe, D., Kalavrezos, N. et al. (2002). Patterns of invasion and routes of tumor entry into the mandible by oral squamous cell carcinoma. *Head Neck* 24 (4): 370–383.

Cooper, J.S., Pajak, T.F., Forastiere, A.A. et al. (2004). Postoperative concurrent radiotherapy and chemotherapy for high risk squamous cell carcinoma of the head and neck. *New Engl. J. Med.* 350 (19): 1937.

D'Cruz, A.K., Vaish, R., Kapre, N. et al. (2015). Elective versus therapeutic neck dissection in node-negative oral cancer. *N. Engl. J. Med.* 373: 521–529. https://doi.org/10.1056/NEJMoa1506007.

Ferris, R.L., Blumenschein, G. Jr., Fayette, J. et al. (2016). Nivolumab for recurrent squamous-cell carcinoma of the head and neck. *N. Engl. J. Med.* 375 (19): 1856–1867. https://doi.org/10.1056/NEJMoa1602252.

Futran, N.D. and Mendez, E. (2006). Developments in reconstruction of midface and maxilla. *Lancet Oncol.* 7: 249–258.

Givi, B., Eskander, A., Awad, M.I. et al. (2015). Impact of elective neck dissection on the outcome of oral squamous cell carcinomas arising in the maxillary alveolus and hard palate. *Head Neck* 38 (Suppl 1): E1688–E1694. https://doi.org/10.1002/hed.24302.

Hanasono, M.M. (2014). Reconstructive surgery for head and neck cancer patients. *Adv. Med.* 2014: 795483.

Huang, S.H., Hwang, D., Lockwood, G. et al. (2009). Predictive value of tumor thickness for cervical lymph-node involvement in squamous cell carcinoma of the oral cavity: a meta-analysis of reported studies. *Cancer* 115 (7): 1489–1497. https://doi.org/10.1002/cncr.24161.

Linz, C., Müller-Richter, U.D.A., Buck, A.K. et al. (2015). Performance of cone beam computed tomography in comparison to conventional imaging techniques for the detection of bone invasion in oral cancer. *Int. J. Oral Maxillofac. Surg.* 44 (1): 8–15.

McCombe, D., MacGill, K., Ainslie, J. et al. (2000). Squamous cell carcinoma of the lip: a retrospective review of the Peter MacCallum Cancer Institute experience 1979-88. *Aust. N. Z. J. Surg.* 70: 358–361. Available at: http://www.ncbi.nlm.nih.gov/pubmed/10830600.

Pfister DG, Spencer S, Adelstein D, et al (2018). NCCN Clinical Practice Guidelines in Oncology, Head and Neck Cancers, (version 2, 2018). Available at: https://www.kankertht-kepalaleher.info/wp-content/uploads/2019/02/NCCN-Clinical-Practice-Guidelines-in-Oncology-2018.pdf.

Okay, D.J., Genden, E., Buchbinder, D., and Urken, M. (2001). Prosthodontic guidelines for surgical reconstruction of the maxilla: a classification system of defects. *J. Prosthet. Dent.* 86 (4): 352–363.

Poeschl, P.W., Seemann, R., Czembirek, C. et al. (2012). Impact of elective neck dissection on regional recurrence and survival in cN0 staged oral maxillary squamous cell carcinoma. *Oral Oncol.* 48: 173–178.

Schilling, C., Stoeckli, S.J., Haerle, S.K. et al. (2015). Sentinel European node trial (SENT): 3-year results of sentinel node biopsy in oral cancer. *Eur. J. Cancer* 51 (18): 2777–2784. https://doi.org/10.1016/j.ejca.2015.08.023.

Sollamo, E.M., Ilmonen, S.K., Virolainen, M.S., and Suominen, S.H. (2016). Sentinel lymph node biopsy in cN0 squamous cell carcinoma of the lip: a retrospective study. *Head Neck* 38 (Suppl. 1): E1375–E1380. Available at: https://www.ncbi.nlm.nih.gov/pubmed/26514547.

de Visscher, J.G., Grond, A.J., Botke, G., and van der Waal, I. (1996). Results of radiotherapy for squamous cell carcinoma of the vermilion border of the lower lip: a retrospective analysis of 108 patients. *Radiother. Oncol.* 39: 9–14. Available at: http://www.ncbi.nlm.nih.gov/pubmed/8735488.

de Visscher, J.G., van den Elsaker, K., Grond, A.J. et al. (1998). Surgical treatment of squamous cell carcinoma of the lower lip: evaluation of long-term results and prognostic factors – a retrospective analysis of 184 patients. *J. Oral Maxillofac. Surg.* 56: 814–820. Available at: http://www.ncbi.nlm.nih.gov/pubmed/9663570.

SECTION 2

Oropharynx

Liana Puscas

CASE 7

Raymond Chai

History of Present Illness

A 62-year-old Caucasian male is seen in the office with a 2-month history of a palpable left neck mass.

Question: What additional questions would you want to ask?

- Is it painful? Patient denies.
- Is it tender to the touch? Patient denies.
- Is it growing? Patient denies.
- Any trouble swallowing? Patient denies.
- Any voice changes? Patient denies.
- Any throat pain? Patient denies.
- Any ear pain? Patient denies. Base of tongue/tonsil tumors may produce referred ear pain.
- Any skin changes over the mass? No. Erythema or induration could indicate extranodal extension of a malignancy or an infectious etiology (e.g., scrofula).
- Has he received any treatment for this? Yes. He has undergone two rounds of antibiotic therapy and steroids without decrease in the size of the mass.

Past Medical History

Hypercholesterolemia, hypertension.

Past Surgical History

Appendectomy and tonsillectomy as a child.

Medications

Atorvastatin, lisinopril.
No known drug allergies.

Social History

- Tobacco use? Patient denies.
- Alcohol use? The patient has a glass of wine with dinner on a regular basis.

Physical Examination

Well-developed male in no distress. Voice strong.
Skin: no suspicious lesions.
Oral cavity examination shows teeth in good condition. No lesions seen or palpated.
Oropharynx: tonsils surgically absent; no lesions palpated in the base of tongue but exam limited due to gag reflex.
Neck exam: salivary gland exam normal. He has a 3 cm left level IIA neck mass that is mobile on palpation.
Cranial nerves II–XII intact.
Flexible laryngoscopy is performed without obvious lesions seen of the upper aerodigestive tract. The true vocal folds move well.

Management

Question: Which of the following would be appropriate next steps in the evaluation and management of this patient?

- Fine needle aspiration biopsy: **yes**/no. This is probably the best next step as it will likely yield a diagnosis. The use of ultrasound guidance is often helpful as these lesions may have a significant cystic component.
- Excisional biopsy of the neck mass: yes/**no**. Open surgical biopsies should be avoided, when possible, due to the concern for tumor seeding and disruption of surgical tissue planes. In instances where the clinical presentation

(Continued)

CASE 7   (continued)

suggests lymphoma and a fine needle aspiration shows lymphoid tissue, without evidence of carcinoma, an excisional biopsy can be considered. In these instances, the surgeon should discuss the option of sending the mass for a frozen section and if cancer is found intra-operatively, a completion neck dissection and endoscopy should be performed.

- Computed tomography (CT) of the neck with IV contrast: **yes**/no. This is a potential next step as this will allow for evaluation of the neck and the upper aerodigestive tract.
- Neck ultrasound: **yes**/no. This is a potential next step as this will allow for evaluation of the neck mass and may be used to confirm correct needle placement during the FNA. Newer techniques have also allowed for transcervical evaluation of the oro-pharynx for potential primary lesions.
- Magnetic resonance imaging (MRI) of the neck: **yes**/no. This is a potential next step as this will allow for evaluation of the neck and the upper aerodigestive tract.
- Positron emission tomography (PET)/CT neck: **yes**/no. This is a potential next step as this will allow for eval-uation of the neck and the upper aerodigestive tract as well as provide assessment of metastatic disease. It is important to note that typically a biopsy should dem-onstrate malignancy before obtaining a PET/CT.

Question: What additional testing may be performed of an FNA specimen to aid in diagnosis of an unknown primary?

Answer: Assessment for p16 and EBER. Molecular diagnostic testing should be performed to assist in identifying potential occult primary sites. Per the AJCC 8th Edition guidelines, p16 should be performed as a surrogate for human papillomavirus (HPV)-associated oropharyngeal carcinoma. Likewise, Ep-stein–Barr virus-encoded RNA (EBER) should be performed to evaluate for an occult nasopharyngeal primary carcinoma.

Question: What threshold for p16 immunohistochemis-try (IHC) is typically used to define p16 positive disease?

Answer: 70%. Per the College of American Pathologists guide-lines for HPV testing in head and neck carcinoma, patholo-gists should report p16 IHC positivity as a surrogate for HPV when there is at least 70% nuclear and cytoplasmic expression with at least moderate to strong intensity.

Fine needle aspiration is performed in the office under ultrasound guidance. The final pathology reveals nonkera-tinizing squamous cell carcinoma (SCC) that is p16+.

Question: What imaging modality has the highest sen-sitivity for detecting the primary site in carcinoma of unknown primary?

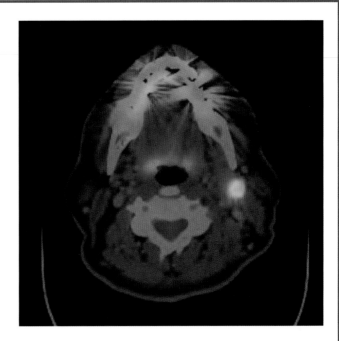

FIGURE 7.1   This is a fused axial image of a PET/CT scan at the level of the oropharynx. Note the hypermeta-bolic left level II neck mass. There is fairly symmetric low-intensity uptake in the patient's lingual tonsil tissue.

Answer: PET/CT. Multiple studies have demonstrated that PET/CT compared with contrast-enhanced CT alone has a significantly improved rate of detecting the primary site of carcinoma. A prior systematic review of 7 studies demonstrates a sensitivity of 44% and a specificity of 97% with PET/CT.

PET/CT neck is performed showing a solid left level IIA lymph node without extranodal extension measuring $22 \times 27 \times 29$ mm that demonstrates high-grade hypermetabolism with max SUV of 16.4 (see Figure 7.1). No other lymph nodes meet the radiographic criteria for significance or demonstrate hypermetabolism. Symmetric FDG uptake is seen when com-paring the left tongue base to the right (max SUV 4.2). There are no imaging findings to suggest systemic metastatic disease.

Question: Which of the following would be appropriate treatment options in the management of this patient?

- Panendoscopy: **yes**/no. This is an essential compo-nent of the patient's treatment since a primary site must be investigated.
- Tonsillectomy: **yes**/no. The palatine and lingual tonsils often harbor occult primary tumors. This particular patient has already undergone palatine tonsillectomy as a child but lingual tonsillectomy should be performed.
- Treatment with surgical resection: **yes**/no. As the patient has only one lymph node that is PET avid,

CASE 7   (continued)

surgical resection of the primary tumor (if identified) and left neck dissection may be curative.

- Treatment with radiation: **yes**/no. This disease may be cured with XRT to the neck and primary site (if identified).
- Treatment with chemotherapy: yes/**no**. Treatment with chemotherapy alone would have no role here. If upfront surgery is performed, the addition of chemotherapy to XRT is not indicated unless significant extracapsular spread or positive margins of the primary tumor are observed on final pathology. Clinical trials are currently underway to evaluate the safety and efficacy of de-escalation of therapy.

After discussion in the multidisciplinary tumor board, an upfront surgical approach is advocated. The patient is taken to the operating room for panendoscopy, left selective II–IV neck dissection, and bilateral lingual tonsillectomy. Palatine tonsillectomy is not performed given the patient's prior tonsillectomy as a child and lack of residual tonsil tissue. No obvious primary site is identified on panendoscopy.

The final pathology report shows one out of 54 positive nodes. The pathologic node is 2.7 cm in maximum diameter without evidence of extranodal extension. A 0.7 mm primary tumor is identified within the left lingual tonsillectomy specimen with negative margins. There is no evidence of perineural invasion or lymphovascular invasion.

Question: Per the AJCC 8th Edition guidelines, what is the TNM stage for this carcinoma?

Answer: T1N1M0, Stage I. For HPV-positive oropharyngeal SCC, there are separate staging systems for clinical versus pathologically confirmed disease following surgery. A 0.7 mm primary is staged as T1 disease. Following neck dissection, the presence of only one positive 2.7 cm node is staged as N1 disease. This disease is staged as T1N1M0 (given negative PET/CT for distant metastases) and is an overall stage I given the HPV positive nature of the cancer.

The patient is rediscussed in the multidisciplinary tumor board. Given the staging and clear margins, consensus decision is made for observation following surgery without the need for adjuvant therapy.

Key Points

- Presentation of a neck mass in an adult should be considered cancer until proven otherwise. All patients should have a thorough assessment of the upper aerodigestive tract at the time of the initial office evaluation.
- PET/CT is the best imaging modality for thorough assessment of the neck and upper aerodigestive tract when assessing a patient with an unknown primary carcinoma.
- Viruses are an etiologic factor in head and neck carcinoma, and testing for HPV and EBV can be performed on the FNA specimen to yield valuable additional information.

- Patients with a single lymph node and without evidence of extranodal extension of disease may be successfully treated with a surgical approach involving complete resection of the primary and neck dissection if there is no perineural or lymphovascular invasion and if the primary site is small and has negative margins.
- Lingual tonsillectomy and palatine tonsillectomy should be performed in cases of an unknown primary as the tonsils are often the site of unknown primary tumors.

CASE 8

Jason I. Kass and Glenn J. Hanna

History of Present Illness

A 55-year-old man presents with a 6-month history of a persistent sore throat, which did not improve with antibiotics. He presented to his local otolaryngologist, who identified a right anterior tonsil mass. Biopsy of this mass showed nonkeratinizing, invasive, poorly differentiated SCC, which was p16 positive by immunostaining.

Question: What additional questions would you want to ask?

- Any trouble opening his mouth? Yes. He reports right-sided jaw pain that limits his mouth opening.
- Any trouble swallowing? Patient denies., but he does have a globus sensation in his throat.
- Any voice changes? Patient denies.
- Any other lumps that have been noticed? Patient denies.
- Any ear pain? Yes. He has pain in his right ear that radiates to his shoulder.
- Has he received any treatment for this? Yes. He is taking acetaminophen-oxycodone every 3 hours for relief.

(Continued)

CASE 8 (continued)

Past Medical History

Type II diabetes mellitus and hypertension.

Past Surgical History

Cholecystectomy 10 years ago.

Social History

50 pack-year history of tobacco use.
A glass of wine with dinner on a regular basis.

Physical Examination

Well-developed middle-aged male in no distress. Voice strong.
Skin: no suspicious lesions.
Oral cavity: limited mouth opening to 2.5 cm. Teeth in good condition. No lesions seen or palpated.
Oropharynx exam: 2.5 cm mass in the right anterior tonsillar pillar extending to the retromolar trigone. The mass is firm and fixed.
Neck exam: salivary gland exam is normal and there is no adenopathy.
Cranial nerves II–XII intact.
Flexible laryngoscopy: right oropharynx mass producing some displacement of the right palate superiorly, but no other lesions noted in any level of the pharynx or larynx. The true vocal folds move well.

Management

Question: Which of the following imaging studies would be appropriate next steps in the evaluation and management of this patient?

- A CT of the neck and chest with IV contrast: **yes**/no. This is a potential next step as this will allow for evaluation of the neck and the upper aerodigestive tract. CT chest will complete the metastatic workup. CT images are rapidly obtained and provide both soft tissue and bone detail. For patients being considered for transoral robotic resection, it is important to evaluate for a retropharyngeal carotid artery.
- Neck ultrasound: **yes**/no. Neck ultrasound may be helpful here to assess for pathologic cervical lymphadenopathy and to assist with FNA, if needed. Newer techniques have also been described using transcervical ultrasound to assess for primary tumors of the palatine and lingual tonsil tissue. If a CT of the neck is performed, neck ultrasound would likely provide little additional benefit.
- MRI of the neck: **yes**/no. This is a potential next step as this will allow for evaluation of the neck and the upper aerodigestive tract. MRI is particularly helpful in assessing for soft tissue extension to the base of tongue and/or the parapharyngeal space.
- PET/CT neck: **yes**/no. This is a potential next step as this will allow for evaluation of the neck and the upper aerodigestive tract as well as provide assessment for metastatic disease. This study should typically be performed after confirming the presence of a malignancy.

A neck CT with IV contrast and PET/CT are both performed that show a 2.5 × 1.5 cm PET avid mass in the right tonsil with involvement of the right medial pterygoid muscle (see Figure 8.1). There is no suspicious cervical lymphadenopathy or evidence of distant disease.

Question: What is the clinical stage of this patient?

Answer: cT4N0M0. The involvement of the pterygoid musculature seen on the CT and his evolving trismus make this clinically a T4 tumor using the AJCC 8th Edition staging for HPV+ oropharyngeal tumors.

Question: What would be the most appropriate treatment option for this patient?

Answer: This is not a primary tumor best approached using transoral robotic surgery (TORS) for two reasons: (i) With the advanced nature of this tumor, and extension to the pterygoid musculature, obtaining a clean resection with negative margins is very challenging unless an open approach is used: (ii) this disease likely extends beyond the superior constrictor muscle, as evidenced by the effacement of the parapharyngeal fat plane. Negative surgical margins are important to consider in this setting because postoperative adjuvant therapy for positive resection margins warrants consideration of concurrent chemoradiotherapy – which commits the patient to a trimodality approach for therapy. While a traditional mandibular split approach will allow complete access to the tumor, this approach has its own morbidity, and due to the extent of the disease, postoperative radiation therapy is still required.

Question: What is the first line treatment plan for non-operative disease in this scenario?

Answer: Radiotherapy with concurrent bolus cisplatin (dose: 100 mg/m² IV every 21 days for three cycles). For locoregionally advanced cancers of the oropharynx treated nonoperatively, concurrent chemoradiotherapy remains the standard of care. Cisplatin is a potent radiosensitizer. The MACH-NC meta-analysis clarified the survival benefit of a combined chemoradiation approach with greater benefit for platinum-containing chemotherapies.

The bolus schedule (every 3 weeks at higher dosing), however, more than doubles the risk of severe toxicities including mucositis, fibrosis, nausea and vomiting. It has been shown that increased toxicity occurs when cumulative dosing reaches 200–300 mg/m². To limit the toxicities of cisplatin, a weekly

CASE 8 (continued)

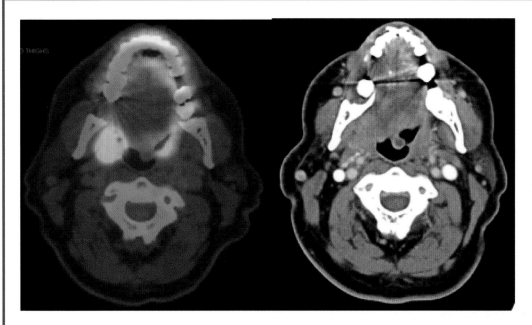

FIGURE 8.1 These axial images of the fused PET/CT (left) and CT of the neck with IV contrast (right) demonstrate a right-sided tonsillar mass with involvement of the right medial pterygoid muscle.

schedule has been adopted by many. Prospective data by Noronha et al. (2018) comparing weekly and bolus schedules demonstrated that a weekly schedule (30 mg/m², as opposed to 40 mg/m²) was inferior in terms of locoregional control. Many institutions in the United States and Europe use 40 mg/m² weekly, and retrospective data support similar response rates to bolus dosing with fewer toxicities. This is still an active area of study as there are no prospective studies comparing a bolus schedule to 40 mg/m² weekly dosing.

While radiotherapy with concurrent cetuximab was previously considered an appropriate alternative to cisplatin among platinum-ineligible patients, RTOG 1016 and the European De-ESCALaTE HPV studies both demonstrated the superiority of cisplatin in low-risk, locoregionally advanced HPV+ oropharyngeal cancer patients, with improved overall

survival and locoregional control rates with platinum compared to EGFR inhibitor therapy.

The use of pembrolizumab is indicated in unresectable locoregionally recurrent head and neck cancer and/or distant metastatic disease. Its mechanism is to bind to the PD-1 receptors on lymphocytes to disrupt the local immune-suppression generated by the cancer. The use of immunotherapy in the primary treatment of cancer is an area of active investigation.

Following definitive chemoradiation therapy, a post-treatment PET/CT was performed 12 weeks after completion of treatment showing no evidence of local, regional or distant disease. The patient was started on regular surveillance follow-up with visits every 3 months.

Key Points

- The presence of trismus in a patient with an oropharyngeal carcinoma reflects either perineural invasion or direct extension to the pterygoid muscles. The presence of either would predict aggressive behavior.
- It is important to completely and accurately assess a patient for surgical resectability prior to undertaking a surgical approach. A large tumor at risk of excision with positive margins obligates the patient to receive trimodality therapy if surgery is pursued.

- If there is concern regarding resectability, the patient is best treated nonoperatively to decrease morbidity.
- PET/CT after chemoradiation therapy must be obtained at least 12 weeks after completion of treatment to allow for accurate assessment of treatment response.
- A negative PET/CT at the completion of therapy is a reliable predictor of a complete response.
- Platinum-based chemotherapy is the mainstay of head and neck SCC treatment, but there are other effective options for those patients who cannot receive platinum-based agents.

CASE 9

Aru Panwar

History of Present Illness

A 52-year-old man who works on a farm presents with an asymptomatic right upper neck mass for 6 weeks.

Question: What additional questions would you want to ask?

- Is it painful? Patient denies.
- Is it tender to the touch? Patient denies.
- Is it growing? Patient denies.
- Any trouble swallowing? Patient denies.
- Any voice changes? Patient denies.
- Any throat pain? Patient denies.
- Any ear pain? Patient denies.
- Any skin changes over the mass? Patient denies. Erythema or induration could indicate extranodal extension of a malignancy or an infectious etiology (e.g., scrofula).
- Has he received any treatment for this? Patient denies.

Past Medical History

None.

Past Surgical History

None.

Social History

Nonsmoker.

Physical Examination

Well-developed male in no distress. Voice strong.
Skin: no suspicious lesions.
Oral cavity examination shows teeth in good condition. No lesions seen or palpated.
Oropharynx: slight fullness of the right tonsil. Difficult to palpate due to gag reflex.
Cervical exam: firm, 3 cm right level IIA neck mass that is mobile on palpation. Salivary gland exam is normal. No other neck masses. Cranial nerves II–XII intact.
Flexible laryngoscopy is performed and is pictured below (see Figure 9.1).

Management

Question: Which of the following would be appropriate options in the management of this patient?

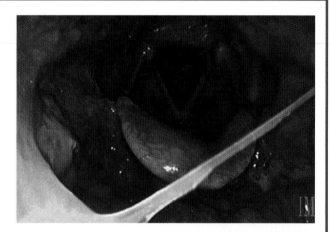

FIGURE 9.1 This image from a transnasal fiberoptic laryngoscopy shows no obvious primary lesion. The true vocal folds are fully mobile, bilaterally.

- CT with contrast or MRI: **yes**/no. A contrast-enhanced CT or MRI of the neck should also be ordered to characterize the suspected primary neoplastic site, identify regional anatomy and extent of regional nodal disease. CT allows for rapid image acquisition with less motion artifact and also evaluates for bone erosion (see Figure 9.2). MRI provides improved soft tissue detail for tumors with deep tongue and/or parapharyngeal space extension and also may be helpful in identifying perineural invasion.
- Fine needle aspiration of neck mass: **yes**/no. Determination of etiology may hinge on cytologic identification of malignancy through fine needle aspiration of an enlarged lymph node. Fine needle aspiration is safe, cost-effective, and highly accurate (sensitivity 89.6%, specificity 96.5%, positive predictive value 96.2%, and negative predictive value 90.3%).
- PET/CT imaging: **yes**/no. A PET/CT may be requested in appropriately selected patients after a diagnosis of malignancy has been established as it may help guide the workup for the primary lesion. It is primarily indicated in patients with significant cervical nodal disease and/or in those patients with no identifiable primary lesion (see Figure 9.3).
- Antibiotic treatment for 2 weeks, followed by repeat examination: yes/**no**. A persistent neck mass in older adults that persists for greater than 2 weeks or is of uncertain duration should raise significant concern for underlying malignancy. Other concerning

CASE 9   (continued)

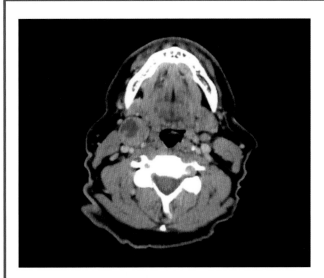

FIGURE 9.2   A contrast-enhanced CT of the neck demonstrates a solitary, enlarged, partially cystic right level II cervical lymph node. CT exam of the oropharynx is obscured by dental artifact.

features associated with the presentation include absence of infectious etiology, firm consistency, neck mass >1.5 cm, and tonsil asymmetry. Patients who present with neck masses and high suspicion for underlying malignancy should not be routinely offered antibiotics unless there are signs and symptoms of bacterial infection.

- Open incisional biopsy of right neck mass: yes/**no**. Incisional biopsy of neck masses should be avoided in favor of fine needle aspiration. In some circumstances, an excisional biopsy of a neck mass may be considered when diagnosis remains elusive despite appropriate clinical examination, imaging, fine needle aspiration cytology, comprehensive examination under anesthesia, and biopsy of alternative sites including sites suspected to harbor a primary neoplasm do not provide a definitive diagnosis. If an open biopsy is needed, the patient should also be consented for a neck dissection if the frozen section shows carcinoma.

A fine needle aspiration of the neck mass reveals the diagnosis of SCC with basaloid appearing cells in a background of necrosis.

Question: What is the next appropriate ancillary test for this patient?

Answer: p16 expression tested by IHC is widely available, cost-sensitive and a reliable surrogate for HPV status (sensitivity 94–97%, specificity 83–84%). The AJCC 8th Edition uses p16 status as the agreed upon biomarker to determine TNM class and prognostic stage grouping specific to HPV-associated oropharyngeal SCCs (OPSCC). Distinction between p16 posi-

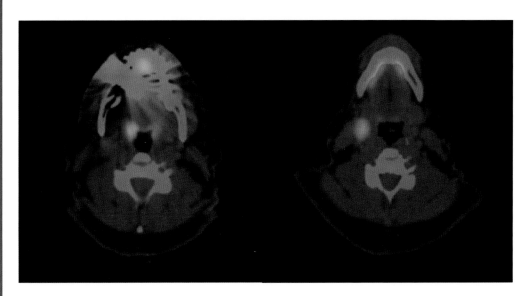

FIGURE 9.3   A PET/CT demonstrates no distant metastatic sites but shows focal uptake in the right palatine tonsil and in the solitary right level II cervical lymph node.

(Continued)

CASE 9 (continued)

tive (defined as >70% nuclear and cytoplasmic staining on IHC) and p16 negative OPSCC is critical to choosing the appropriate staging schema and determination of prognosis. The p16 IHC and polymerase chain reaction (PCR)-based assays have high sensitivity, although ISH boasts the highest specificity. Epstein–Barr virus testing should be considered for patients presenting with suspected nasopharyngeal carcinoma and patients with unknown primary site where nasopharyngeal malignancy is part of the differential diagnosis.

This Patient undergoes panendoscopy and biopsy from tonsil reveals invasive SCC.

IHC test for p16 suggests >70% positive nuclear and cytoplasmic staining (Figure 9.4). On palpation in the OR, the tumor lesion is limited to the tonsil and the base of tongue is soft and without evidence of tumor. A biopsy of the base of tongue adjacent to the tonsil primary is negative for carcinoma.

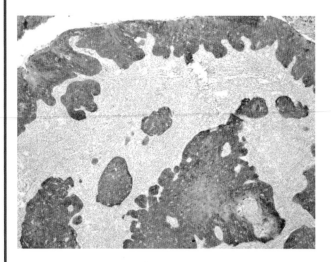

FIGURE 9.4 **Histologic images of a poorly differentiated squamous cell carcinoma with >70% nuclear and cytoplasmic staining for p16.**

Question: What is the most appropriate stage assignment?

Answer: cT1N1M0, prognostic stage I. The demographics of patients affected by p16+ OPSCC are distinct from those affected by p16 negative OPSCC. Patients affected by p16+ OPSCC are often younger, have limited or no exposure to tobacco and alcohol, and have fewer comorbidities compared to patients affected by p16 negative disease. These tumors also are significantly more responsive to radiotherapy. As a result, the prognosis of patients with p16+ OPSCC is markedly better. A study by Ang et al. (2010) highlighted that tumor HPV status is a strong, independent prognostic factor for survival in OPSCC (3-year overall survival for patients with HPV-positive tumors was 82.4% vs. 57.1% for patients with HPV-negative tumors, $P < 0.001$, and HPV-positive tumors were associated with a 58% reduction in the risk of death [hazard ratio, 0.42; 95% CI, 0.27 to 0.66]). This distinct, favorable prognostic behavior has been recognized in the creation of a separate staging system specific to p16+ OPSCC, which reorganizes the TNM classification and prognostic stage grouping. As a result, a patient with a p16+ T1 or T2 primary neoplasm, and ipsilateral lymph node involvement <6 cm in greatest dimension (irrespective of number of nodes), and no distant metastases, is classified as cT1N1M0, and assigned prognostic stage I.

Question: What is/are the appropriate treatment recommendations for this patient?

Answer: Patients with p16+ OPSCC with small primary neoplasms (T1–2) and single ipsilateral lymph node ≤3 cm, without adverse features on pathology may be treated using single modality treatment (surgery or radiotherapy). It is important to recognize that while there is significant interest in de-escalation of therapy to minimize treatment-related morbidity, especially in the context of expected favorable prognosis in patients affected by p16+ OPSCC, any efforts toward de-escalation should be pursued strictly in the context of clinical trials. The treatment algorithms are best determined by extent and burden of disease, and not on the basis of revised prognostic groups that have been newly assigned to this unique disease.

Key Points

- Surgical treatment of oropharyngeal carcinoma is appropriate in patients with transorally accessible early-stage cancers without pathologically concerning features and no more than one ipsilateral lymph node.
- Surgical treatment of oropharyngeal carcinoma can be done through transoral traditional, laser and robotic techniques. Patient factors such as trismus or having a narrow mandible or torus mandibularis may limit exposure. Moreover, a retropharyngeal internal carotid artery is a contraindication for transoral surgery for tumors involving the palatine tonsils.
- Patients with obvious indications for postoperative chemoradiation should be given strong consideration for treatment with nonsurgical means to avoid trimodality therapy and reduce treatment burden.
- Ipsilateral versus bilateral neck dissection depends on the location of the oropharyngeal tumor. Tumors limited to the palatine tonsil can be managed with ipsilateral dissection, whereas base of tongue cancers or those with significant soft palate extension should be considered for bilateral treatment.

CASE 10

Daniel Sharbel and Kenneth Byrd

History of Present Illness

A 67-year-old Caucasian male with a history of cT2N1M0 SCC of the right tongue base treated with chemoradiation 3 years ago presented to his primary care physician complaining of several weeks of severe pain in his right upper neck, right cheek, and ear.

Past Medical History

Coronary artery disease with history of stenting 2 years prior, and peripheral vascular disease.
Nonsmall-cell lung cancer treated with chemoradiation therapy fifteen years ago.

Past Surgical History

History of prior cervical spine surgery.

Social History

Former smoker with 40 pack-year history, quit more than 20 years ago. Former drinker, quit more than 20 years ago.

Question: What additional questions would you want to ask?

- Any trouble swallowing? Yes.
- Any recent infection? Patient Denies.
- Any hemoptysis or hematemesis? Patient Denies.
- Any difficulty opening and closing the mouth? Patient denies.
- Any other masses in the neck that have been noticed? Patient denies.
- Any sexually transmitted diseases? None known. The presence of these may increase likelihood of HPV exposure.
- History of tracheostomy or gastrostomy? Patient denies. The presence of these may suggest dependence postoperatively.
- Performance status? ECOG 1.

Physical Examination

Thin, adult male in mild distress from pain but breathing comfortably.
Skin: no suspicious lesions.
Oral cavity and oropharynx: 3 cm right-sided nodular tumor arising from the tonsillar bed.

Neck: cervical exam reveals no palpable lymphadenopathy or salivary lesions.
Cranial nerves II–XII intact.
Flexible fiberoptic laryngoscopy: large right tonsillar mass. The epiglottis is displaced inferiorly and posteriorly on exam. The view of the glottis is limited but without any apparent involvement, and the true vocal folds are bilaterally mobile.
Contrasted CT of the neck was performed (see Figure 10.1).

Question: What is the next appropriate step in management?

Answer: Histopathologic diagnostic confirmation is recommended prior to proceeding with next steps in treatment. In this instance, this can likely be performed via a transoral office biopsy. If exposure is a challenge and/or there are concerns for significant bleeding due to the tumor appearance or a patient being on anticoagulation, a panendoscopy under general anesthesia could be performed.

Biopsy confirms diagnosis of SCC, p16 negative.

Question: Are any further imaging studies appropriate?

- PET/CT: **yes**/no. This is an ideal imaging study as it will reveal the extent of the recurrence, evaluate for regional and distant disease, and assess for a second primary lesion.

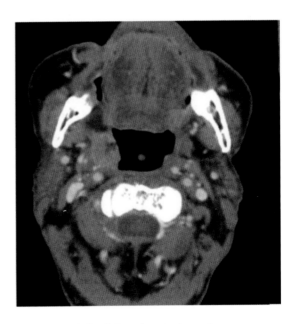

FIGURE 10.1   AxialAxial CT image.

(Continued)

CASE 10 (continued)

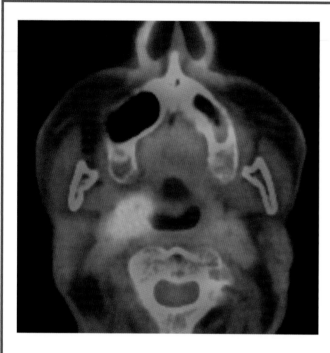

FIGURE 10.2 ¹⁸FDG-PET/CT axial view demonstrating an intense right tonsil tumor with an SUV of 16.6. No regional or distant lesions were noted.

- MRI neck: **yes**/no. MRI can provide increased soft tissue detail when evaluating cancers of the oropharynx. This may be particularly beneficial in this case when assessing for parapharyngeal space extension. Evaluation for retropharyngeal lymphadenopathy is also important. An MRI is unlikely to yield more information in this patient that will alter management compared with the information available from the CT neck with contrast. Although not strictly contraindicated its value is limited in this patient.
- Ultrasound: yes/**no**. This study is not indicated because given the location of the primary tumor adjacent to the mandible, the bone would preclude complete evaluation of the primary cancer.
- Chest CT: **yes**/no. If a PET scan is not obtained, a chest CT would be helpful to assess for distant disease or a recurrence of his lung cancer.

An ¹⁸FDG-PET/CT was performed from skull base to midthigh (see Figure 10.2) due to the recurrent oropharyngeal cancer, as well as the history of lung cancer. The patient was then presented at a multidisciplinary tumor board.

Question: What is the most appropriate therapeutic management for this patient?

Answer: Open radical tonsillectomy with clear margins, ipsilateral neck dissection and free flap reconstruction. Due to the proximity of the lesion to the internal carotid artery, the risk of life-threatening hemorrhage, and the patient's prior definitive treatment with chemoradiation, open approach is favored over TORS. While TORS has been shown to be a safe and effective alternative to open resection of oropharyngeal malignancies in the salvage setting, this patient's anatomy is better suited for an open approach, which will allow dissection directly on the vessel, as well as proximal and distal control. Reirradiation, palliative chemotherapy, or hospice may be considered in poor operative candidates, in those with more advanced disease, or in patients who refuse surgery.

The patient's case was presented at the institutional Multidisciplinary Head and Neck Tumor Board, and open resection with right neck dissection and reconstruction via lip split and mandibulotomy approach, tracheostomy, and percutaneous endoscopic gastrostomy were undertaken. Sacrifice of the lingual nerve was necessary due to the location of the tumor, but the hypoglossal nerve was preserved. The specimen was removed en bloc, and the defect exposed the parapharyngeal carotid and radiated fat of the parapharyngeal space and the prevertebral fascia. Right neck dissection required resection of some branches of the external carotid artery, but all tumor was removed from the neck, and the internal jugular vein and the internal carotid artery were preserved.

Question: What is the best reconstructive option for this patient?

Answer: Due to the history of prior radiation therapy, the proximity to the carotid artery as well as the wide communication of the primary site resection and the neck, a vascularized flap reconstruction is required. Free tissue transfers have largely supplanted regional flaps for large oropharyngeal and oral cavity reconstruction in appropriate candidates, but because of this patient's comorbidities and poor recipient vessels, a regional flap reconstruction with the pectoralis major myocutaneous flap was performed (see Figure 10.3). A segment of skin with the flap is required for approximation with pharyngeal mucosa to ensure a water-tight closure. Despite the favorability of free tissue transfer in oropharyngeal reconstruction, the pectoralis major myocutaneous flap remains a viable reconstructive alternative in patients who are not candidates for free flaps. A nonvascularized repair such as a skin graft or acellular dermal autograft would be inappropriate here given the large communication with the neck wound, poor tissue quality, the prior radiation, and the proximity to the internal carotid artery.

CASE 10   (continued)

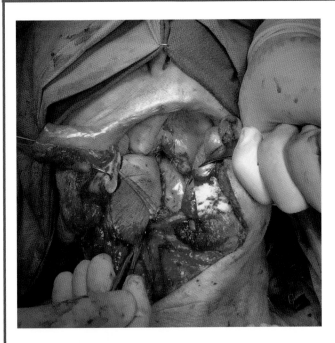

The patient failed a follow-up modified barium swallow study and remained PEG-dependent after surgery.

Final pathologic evaluation of the surgical specimens revealed a pT2N0M0 moderately differentiated SCC that was completely excised with >5 mm margins. Perineural invasion was present, but there was no lymphovascular invasion. Tumor immunohistochemical staining for p16 was negative. Reirradiation was discussed at tumor board, but observation was favored due to clear margins.

FIGURE 10.3   This intraoperative photo demonstrates an open approach to the oropharynx via lip split and paramedian mandibulotomy. The tumor has been excised and the defect reconstructed using a pectoralis major myocutaneous flap.

Key Points

- Surgical salvage of oropharyngeal cancers in patients who have already received radiation therapy increases the risk of significant problems with swallowing and secretion management. Patients may end up being tracheostomy tube or gastrostomy tube dependent according to the exact location of the cancer and the nature of the prior treatment.

- In the setting of operating on irradiated tissue in the pharynx, vascularized tissue in the form of a pedicled or free flap provides healthy tissue for closure.
- Reirradiation of oropharyngeal cancer can predispose to soft tissue necrosis of the pharynx, carotid rupture and/or injury to the spinal cord. The additional benefit of improving the chance for cure through reirradiation must be balanced against the significant morbidity of another full course of radiation.

CASE 11

Daniel Pinheiro

History of Present Illness

A 73-year-old woman presents with a 2-month history of right-sided sore throat. She has mild dysphagia but eats a mostly unrestricted diet. She attributes her dysphagia to dry mouth because of prior radiation.

Past Medical History

Hypertension, hypercholesterolemia.

Past Surgical History

History of prior cervical spine surgery.

Social History

30 pack-year smoking history.
She drinks alcohol on occasion with approximately one beer/week.

Question: What additional questions should you want to ask?

(Continued)

CASE 11 (continued)

- Any trismus? Patient denies.
- Any otalgia? Patient denies.
- Any neck masses? Patient denies.
- Any prior head and neck cancer? She has a remote history of nasopharyngeal carcinoma for which she was treated with external beam radiotherapy to the nasopharynx and bilateral neck 24 years prior to presentation.

Physical Examination

Well-developed female in no distress. Voice strong.
Skin: no suspicious lesions.
Well-aerated middle ears without effusions.
Oral cavity: limited mouth opening to 2.5 cm. Teeth in good repair. No lesions seen or palpated.
Oropharynx exam: small asymmetry in right tonsil with an ulcerative area that measures approximately 1.5 cm; both tonsils are small. Right tonsillar lesion is firm, but the tonsil is mobile. There is no trismus and the soft palate moves symmetrically. No lesions are palpable in the base of tongue. Vallecula is clear on mirror indirect laryngoscopy. The nasopharynx was incompletely visualized.
Neck exam: normal salivary glands with no adenopathy. The patient does have radiation changes in the neck but no woody induration.
Cranial nerves II–XII intact.

Management

Question: Which of the following steps would be appropriate?

- Flexible fiberoptic nasopharyngoscopy: **yes**/no. This is appropriate for full evaluation of nasopharynx (given prior history) and to examine the inferior extent of lesion in the right tonsil and rule out other lesions in larynx or hypopharynx.

    In this patient, exam showed no lesions in nasopharynx with a patent fossa of Rosenmuller bilaterally and radiation changes of the pharynx.
- Tonsil biopsy in office: **yes**/no. This is appropriate since a visible lesion is apparent and is accessible for office biopsy.

    Pathology demonstrated invasive well-differentiated SCC. Stains for p16 on immunohistochemistry were negative.
- CT neck with contrast or MRI neck with contrast: **yes**/no. Kidney function may not permit administration of contrast, and, in general, MRI can be performed in patients with lower GFR who may not tolerate the contrast required for a CT.

    This patient was found to have normal kidney function with estimated GFR = 90 and so a CT of the neck with contrast is obtained (see Figure 11.1).

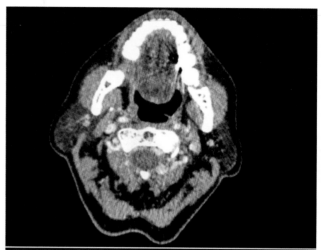

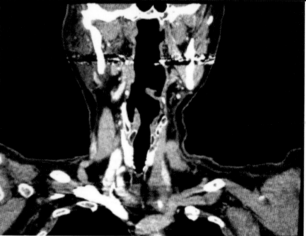

FIGURE 11.1   A CT of the neck was performed with intravenous contrast. There is a 1.5 cm right tonsil primary tumor with normal fat plane observed in the right parapharyngeal space. Left submandibular gland is not visualized. Right submandibular gland is small. There is no pathologic lymphadenopathy.

- PET scan: **yes**/no. PET scan is appropriate in staging head and neck cancer and to identify distant disease and possibly second primaries (see Figure 11.2). This is particularly important in patients with a history of smoking >40 pack-years who have significant risk of lung primaries. CT chest with contrast may also be obtained. Consideration should be given to renal function when additional contrast is given for a CT chest shortly after administration of contrast for a CT neck.

Question: Based on your assessment, what would be this patient's clinical staging?

Answer: HPV- oropharynx T1N0M0. It is an oropharynx primary since the lesion is in the tonsil. The nasopharynx is clear

CASE 11   (continued)

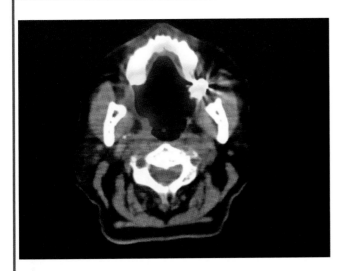

FIGURE 11.2   This is an axial cut of the patient's PET/CT. There is slight soft tissue thickening of the right tonsillar pillar with a maximal SUV of 2.6. The SUV of the left tonsil bed is 2.3. No lymphadenopathy is noted.

and the history is so remote that recurrence is not likely. Given her history of tobacco use, prior mucosal primary and lack of concurrent adenopathy, her tumor is most likely not HPV-associated. A p16 immunohistochemical stain was performed as a surrogate marker for HPV, and the tumor cells did not stain. The oropharynx subsite has a sized-based staging system for the primary tumor. Since it is less than 2 cm, it is a T1 lesion.

Question: What is the next appropriate step in her management?

Answer: Multidisciplinary consultation and/or tumor board. It is always a good idea to obtain multidisciplinary input especially when there are several treatment options. This patient's case of a cT1N0M0 right tonsil cancer was reviewed at the institution's Multidisciplinary tumor board. Due to her prior radiation treatment for nasopharyngeal cancer, consensus opinion was that therapeutic dose of reirradiation could not be given because of concern over overlapping fields and increased toxicity. Surgery was therefore recommended.

Question. The decision is made to manage the patient with definitive surgical resection. What is the best surgical therapy to address the primary tumor?

Answer: Radical tonsillectomy with removal of the constrictor muscle lateral to the tumor. A simple tonsillectomy is not an oncologic operation and should not be performed in the presence of a known malignancy. The goal is to obtain margins of normal tissue around the tumor. The deep margin is the most challeng-

ing in the oropharynx because the constrictor muscle itself can be <5 mm. A radical tonsillectomy includes resection of the underlying superior constrictor muscle. In this radiated patient, if the lesion is superficial, it may be advisable to maintain the deep aspect of the muscle or fascia to optimize healing and minimize the risk to the adjacent neck vessels. If the patient is at high risk for carotid exposure from the resection, reconstruction with a regional tissue or a free flap should be considered.

Question: How should the neck be treated in this patient?

Answer: An ipsilateral selective neck dissection should be performed. The risk of neck metastasis is still significant for a small primary such as this. As mentioned before, reirradiation is not advisable due to the risk to the carotid artery and spinal cord. Contralateral neck dissection is not necessary because risk of contralateral metastases in tonsil cancer is very low when there are no metastases seen in the ipsilateral neck.

The patient undergoes surgery: transoral partial pharyngectomy and right selective neck dissection – levels I–IV (see Figure 11.3).

Question: Based on the pathological findings, what additional treatment would you recommend?

Answer: Close observation. In general, margins greater than 5 mm are considered ideal. However, in the tonsillar fossa it may be hard to achieve greater than 5 mm. This patient now has a history of two head and neck cancers and mucosal dysplasia associated with a second primary. She should have close clinical follow-up.

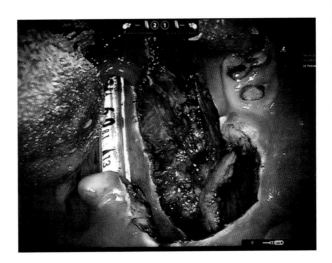

FIGURE 11.3   This intraoperative photo shows the resection bed following a robotic right-sided radical tonsillectomy. Pathology reveals no tumor identified in 25 lymph nodes (0/25). The primary tumor is a 1.2 cm well- to moderately differentiated SCC. All margins free of cancer by at least 5 mm. Reconstruction of intraoral soft palate defect is performed with a pedicled buccal fat flap.

(Continued)

Key Points

- SCC of the oropharynx is still often associated with tobacco and alcohol use.
- Treatment for HPV negative cancer follows the same general principles as treatment for HPV positive cancer. The goal is to achieve cure with the fewest modalities of treatment possible.
- Extent of neck dissection is dictated by the size of the tumor and the exact location within the pharynx. For cN0 patients, ipsilateral selective neck dissection is considered adequate.
- Surgical treatment alone of HPV negative cancer is limited to those patients with early-stage primary tumor and no more than one involved lymph node at the time of evaluation and no pathologic features such as lymphovascular invasion and perineural invasion.

Multiple Choice Questions

1. You are evaluating a 52-year-old male patient with a 3 cm left neck lymph node where an ultrasound guided fine needle aspiration confirms p16+ SCC. Your office exam, including fiberoptic laryngoscopy, as well as a PET/CT fails to yield an identifiable primary tumor. What would be the most appropriate step in the management of this patient?

   a. A left-sided selective neck dissection followed by close observation.

   b. A left-sided selective neck dissection followed by radiation therapy to the neck and oropharynx.

   c. A left-sided selective neck dissection with direct laryngoscopy. If no primary tumor is seen, palatine and lingual tonsillectomies should be performed.

   d. Definitive chemoradiation therapy.

   Answer: c. In this patient with left neck cancer, unknown primary, the fact that the neck node is p16+ suggests a likely oropharyngeal primary site. While both nonsurgical and surgical treatment options should be discussed with the patient in all instances, additional evaluation for potential primary sites is indicated. With the increased visualization offered by transoral robotic surgical systems, both lingual and palatine tonsillectomies should be performed as these sites are the most common locations to find occult primary tumors. Choice b is a reasonable option, but ideally, attempts would be made to find the primary tumor to focus any radiotherapy.

2. Which of these patients is NOT suitable for transoral resection of the primary neoplasm?

   a. A patient with T1 primary neoplasm located in the palatine tonsil and inter-incisor opening of 2 cm.

   b. Edentulous patient, excellent neck extension, T4 primary neoplasm located in the palatine tonsil.

   c. Patient with T1 primary neoplasm located in the palatine tonsil with medially located (retropharyngeal) internal carotid artery.

   d. a and c.

   e. All of the above.

   Answer: e. Patients being considered for transoral resection of primary oropharyngeal neoplasm require careful selection. Factors that should be considered include availability of physician and institutional experience in transoral surgery, extent of disease and anatomical factors among other considerations. Anatomical factors that may be considered as absolute contraindications include trismus, large primary tumor (including most T3 and all T4 tumors), inability to obtain adequate exposure due to limitations of neck extension, trismus, presence of mandibular tori, or sequelae of prior therapy. Other factors that may suggest relative contraindications for transoral resection include direct extension of primary neoplasm across the midline of the base of tongue, extension beyond the midline of the soft palate or the posterior pharyngeal wall, or extension out to involved level II nodes and/or major vessel encasement. Patients with medialized retropharyngeal carotid arteries may experience vascular exposure with resection of the primary site and may present a relative contraindication especially when expertise for advanced reconstruction including free tissue transfer is unavailable. The ideal candidate for transoral resection is an edentulous patient with well-lateralized, small (T1 or T2) primary, with no trismus and good neck extension. When the candidacy for transoral resection is ambiguous, clinicians may consider performing an exam under anesthesia before determining care plans.

3. Which of the following is a potential side effect of the chemotherapy agent cisplatin?

   a. Sensorineural hearing loss.

   b. Polyneuronal distal neuropathy.

   c. Renal insufficiency.

   d. All of the above.

   Answer: d. These are well-known complications of this agent.

4. When should one consider taxane-based chemotherapy as an alternative to platinum-based regimens?

   a. Always, as taxane-based regimens have superior efficacy, albeit with greater toxicity.

   b. Never, as taxane-based regimens have inferior oncologic efficacy when compared to radiation alone.

   c. Only considered when there is a contraindication to platinum.

   d. As a first-line therapy for patients with unresectable locoregionally recurrent and/or distant metastatic disease.

   Answer: c. Carboplatin plus paclitaxel is generally inferior to platinum-based chemotherapy. However, studies have demonstrated favorable locoregional control and short-term survival rates; therefore, this could be considered in platinum-ineligible patients such as those with compromised baseline renal function. Immunotherapy (not taxane-based chemotherapy) is considered first-line therapy for unresectable locoregionally recurrent and/or distant metastatic disease.

5. What is the current standard of care for post treatment restaging following nonoperative management of oropharyngeal cancer?

   a. 8-week post-treatment PET/CT.

   b. 12-week post-treatment PET/CT.

c. 16-week post-treatment PET/CT.

d. Planned salvage neck dissection.

Answer: b. Mehanna et al. (2016) performed a prospective study of 564 patients and evaluated a 12-week PET/CT scan as compared with a planned neck dissection to understand the role of image-guided surveillance post-treatment. While there was no significant survival difference in the two groups, the group managed by PET/CT surveillance had noticeably fewer operations, and the strategy was more cost-effective. Obtaining a PET/CT prior to 12 weeks runs the risk of false positive results, while delaying imaging may allow for disease progression.

6. When might one consider induction chemotherapy?

   a. Desire for rapid initiation of therapy.

   b. Rapid disease progression in a healthy patient who can tolerate the potential toxicity.

   c. Potential oligometastatic disease that is not amenable to biopsy.

   d. All of the above.

Answer: d. While there is no survival benefit to adding induction chemotherapy prior to definitive concurrent chemoradiation, it represents a noninferior approach compared with concurrent chemoradiation alone. Often it is an option to start therapy immediately, particularly when a patient cannot wait 2 weeks for radiation planning. It has been useful in the setting of low (level III/IV) cervical nodal involvement where the risk of distant metastatic spread is high, and in oligometastatic disease that is not amenable to biopsy where one wants to use chemotherapy to select patients that may respond to treatment. Chemoselection has been best studied in SCC of the larynx, where it has been shown to be an effective strategy.

7. What role does immunotherapy or immune checkpoint blockade currently have in nonoperative HPV-associated oropharyngeal cancer?

   a. There is currently no role in the definitive setting.

   b. In platinum-refractory patients regardless of tumor HPV status.

   c. As an adjunct for taxane-based therapy.

   d. a and b.

Answer: d. The role of immunotherapy in the management of head and neck cancer is an area of active investigation. There is currently no role in the curative setting, although trials are underway. Current indications for immunotherapy are for unresectable locoregionally recurrent disease and/or distant metastases with both HPV-positive and HPV-negative squamous cell cancers of the head and neck.

8. In patients with a history of prior head and neck radiation therapy, which additional tests should be performed prior to surgery?

   a. Creatinine.

   b. Total cholesterol.

   c. EKG.

   d. Thyroid-stimulating hormone (TSH).

Answer: d. In patients with a history of prior external beam radiation to the neck, there is a significant risk of hypothyroidism. A TSH should be obtained unless recently performed. If a patient is hypothyroid, this should be corrected prior to surgical intervention because the risk of wound complications is significantly higher in patients who are hypothyroid.

References

Ang, K.K., Harris, J., Wheeler, R. et al. (2010). Human papillomavirus and survival of patients with oropharyngeal cancer. *N. Engl. J. Med.* 363: 24–35.

Mehanna, H., Wong, W.L., McConkey, C.C. et al. (2016). PET-CT surveillance versus neck dissection in advanced head and neck cancer. *N. Engl. J. Med.* 374: 1444–1454.

Noronha, V., Joshi, A., Patil, V.M. et al. (2018). Once-a-week versus once-every-3-weeks cisplatin chemoradiation for locally advanced head and neck cancer: a phase III randomized noninferiority trial. *J. Clin. Oncol.* 36: 1064–1072.

Suggested Reading

Amsbaugh, M.J., Yusuf, M., Cash, E. et al. (2016). Distribution of cervical lymph node metastases from squamous cell carcinoma of the oropharynx in the era of risk stratification using human papillomavirus and smoking status. *Int. J. Radiat. Oncol. Biol. Phys.* 96 (2): 349–353. https://doi.org/10.1016/j.ijrobp.2016.06.2450.

Bernier, J., Domenge, C., Ozsahin, M. et al. (2004). Postoperative irradiation with or without concomitant chemotherapy for locally advanced head and neck cancer. *N. Engl. J. Med.* 350: 1945–1952.

Bots, W.T., Bosch, S., Zwijnenburg, E.M. et al. (2017). Reirradiation of head and neck cancer: long-term disease control and toxicity. *Head Neck* 39: 1122–1130. https://doi.org/10.1002/hed.24733.

Cooper, J.S., Pajak, T.F., Forastiere, A.A. et al. (2004). Postoperative concurrent radiotherapy and chemotherapy for high-risk squamous-cell carcinoma of the head and neck. *N. Engl. J. Med.* 350: 1937–1944.

Gillison, M.L., Trotti, A.M., Harris, J. et al. (2019). Radiotherapy plus cetuximab or cisplatin in human papillomavirus-positive oropharyngeal cancer (NRG oncology RTOG 1016): a randomised, multicentre, non-inferiority trial. *Lancet* 393 (10166): 40–50.

Hay, A., Migliacci, J., Karassawa Zanoni, D. et al. (2018). Haemorrhage following transoral robotic surgery. *Clin. Otolaryngol.* 43 (2): 638–644.

Hinni, M.L., Zarka, M.A., and Hoxworth, J.M. (2013). Margin mapping in transoral surgery for head and neck cancer. *Laryngoscope* 123 (5): 1190–1198. https://doi.org/10.1002/lary.23900.

Kubik, M., Mandal, R., Albergotti, W. et al. (2017). Effect of transcervical arterial ligation on the severity of postoperative hemorrhage after transoral robotic surgery. *Head Neck* 39 (8): 1510–1515.

Lee, J.R., Kim, J.S., Roh, J.L. et al. (2015). Detection of occult primary tumors in patients with cervical metastases of unknown primary tumors: comparison of 18(F) FDG PET/CT with contrast-enhanced CT or CT/MR imaging-prospective study. *Radiology* 274: 764–771.

Lewis, J.S., Beadle, B., Bishop, J.A. et al. (2018). Human papillomavirus testing in head and neck carcinomas: guideline from the College of American Pathologists. *Arch. Pathol. Lab. Med.* 142 (5): 559–597.

Lim, Y.C., Koo, B.S., Lee, J.S. et al. (2006). Distributions of cervical lymph node metastases in oropharyngeal carcinoma: therapeutic implications for the N0 neck. *Laryngoscope* 116: 1148–1152. https://doi.org/10.1097/01.mlg.0000217543.40027.1d.

Lydiatt, W.M., Patel, S.G., O'Sullivan, B. et al. (2017). Head and neck cancers – major changes in the American Joint Committee on Cancer Eighth Edition Cancer Staging Manual. *CA Cancer J. Clin.* 67: 122–137.

Mehanna, H., Robinson, M., Hartley, A. et al. (2019). Radiotherapy plus cisplatin or cetuximab in low-risk human papillomavirus-positive oropharyngeal cancer (De-ESCALaTE HPV): an open-label randomized controlled phase 3 trial. *Lancet* 393 (10166): 51–60.

Mehta, V., Johnson, P., Tassler, A. et al. (2013). A new paradigm for the diagnosis and management of unknown primary tumors of the head and neck: a role for transoral robotic surgery. *Laryngoscope* 123: 146–151.

Nichols, A.C., Kneuertz, P.J., Deschler, D.G. et al. (2011). Surgical salvage of the oropharynx after failure of organ-sparing therapy. *Head Neck* 33 (4): 516–524.

Pignon, J.P., le Maître, A., Maillard, E., and Bourhis, J. (2009). MACH-NC collaborative group. *Radiother. Oncol.* 92 (1): 4–14.

Pilouze, P., Peron, J., Poupart, M. et al. (2017). Salvage surgery for oropharyngeal squamous cell carcinoma: a retrospective study from 2005 to 2013. *Head Neck* 39: 1744–1750.

Pollei, T.R., Hinni, M.L., Moore, E.J. et al. (2013). Analysis of post-operative bleeding and risk factors in transoral surgery of the oropharynx. *JAMA Otolaryngol. Head Neck Surg.* 139 (11): 1212–1218.

Pynnonen, M.A., Gillespie, M.B., Roman, B. et al. (2017). Clinical practice guideline: evaluation of the neck mass in adults. *Otolaryngol. Head Neck Surg.* 157 (2S): S1–S30.

Sinha, P., Karadaghy, O.A., Doering, M.M. et al. (2018). Survival for HPV-positive oropharyngeal squamous cell carcinoma with surgical versus non-surgical treatment approach: a systematic review and meta-analysis. *Oral Oncol.* 86: 121–131.

Szturz, P., Wouters, K., Kiyota, N. et al. (2017). Weekly low-dose versus three-weekly high-dose cisplatin for concurrent chemoradiation in locoregionally advanced non-nasopharyngeal head and neck cancer: a systematic review and meta-analysis of aggregate data. *Oncologist* 22 (9): 1056–1066.

White, H., Ford, S., Bush, B. et al. (2013). Salvage surgery for recurrent cancers of the oropharynx comparing TORS with standard open surgical approaches. *JAMA Otolaryngol. Head Neck Surg.* 139 (8): 773–778.

Zafereo, M.E., Hanasono, M.M., Rosenthal, D.I. et al. (2009). The role of salvage surgery in patients with recurrent squamous cell carcinoma of the oropharynx. *Cancer* 115 (24): 5723–5733.

SECTION 3

Nasopharynx

Chad Zender

CASE 12

Levi Ledgerwood

History of Present Illness

A 49-year-old South Chinese man presents to an otolaryngologist for evaluation of left-sided hearing loss. He had seen his primary care physician, and an audiogram was ordered. Audiogram showed asymmetric, mild–moderate conductive hearing loss on the left side and normal hearing on the right side. On further questioning, the patient endorses intermittent bloody drainage from his left nostril. He also has started to notice some increased nasal congestion, particularly pronounced on the left side. He was recently on antibiotics for a dental infection and concomitant left neck enlarged lymph node for about 2 months, though now he feels that this has gotten a bit smaller.

Question: What additional questions would you want to ask?

- Any voice changes or hoarseness? Important to ask because a vocal cord paralysis could mean that there is vagal nerve/jugular foramen involvement. He denies any hoarseness.
- Any difficulty breathing? Patient denies.
- Any facial numbness? Patient denies. Important to ask because in instances where deficits are noted, there would be concern for significant perineural invasion (trigeminal nerve).
- Any difficulty with opening the mouth? Patient denies. Important to ask because either perineural invasion or direct extension to the pterygoid muscles can contribute to trismus.
- Any trouble swallowing? Patient denies, but again could indicate cranial nerve involvement at the skull base and aggressive/advanced disease.

- Any other lumps or bumps in the head or neck? Patient states he has noticed a left neck mass.

Past Medical History

Significant for chronic hepatitis B and asthma. No previous surgeries.

No family history of cancer or other medical issues.

Social History

Positive for smoking a half-pack per day for 25 years. No history of alcohol abuse.

Physical Examination

General: pleasant and well-appearing male in no acute distress.
Eyes: extraocular motions intact, vision grossly normal.
Ears: bilateral external auditory canals are clear, tympanic membranes are intact, no evidence of fluid on right side, left with serous effusion and TM not mobile on pneumatic otoscopy.
Nose: external nose normal. Anterior rhinoscopy shows straight septum, no lesions.
Oral cavity: no lesions or masses. Poor dentition.
Oropharynx: no lesions or masses visible, soft to palpation throughout, tonsils are 2+ and symmetric.
Face: symmetric, no lesions or masses.
Neck/lymph: left neck mass in level II, firm, nontender, mobile, trachea midline, parotid and thyroid beds are soft to palpation with no masses.
Neuro: cranial nerves are grossly intact including facial sensation, facial motion, tongue motion, and shoulder shrug.
Respiratory: no abnormal effort of breathing, voice strong and clear, no stridor.

(*Continued*)

Essential Cases in Head and Neck Oncology, First Edition. Edited by Michael G. Moore, Arnaud F. Bewley, and Babak Givi.
© 2022 American Head and Neck Society. Published 2022 by John Wiley & Sons Ltd.

CASE 12 (continued)

(a)

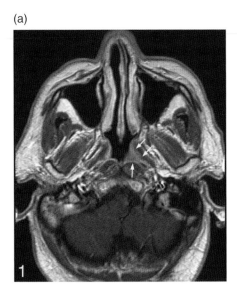

(b)

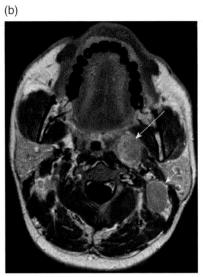

FIGURE 12.1 This axial cut of a T1-weighted MRI of the skull base demonstrates (a) an enhanced 2 cm mass in the left fossa of Rosenmuller (arrows) and (b) an enlarged retropharyngeal node on the left side (long arrow) and an enlarged 2.5 cm left level II lymph node (short arrow).

Fiberoptic nasopharyngolaryngoscopy was performed; there is a 2 cm growth in the left fossa of Rosenmuller, no other lesions.

Management

Question: What first steps would you take in the evaluation and management of this patient?

- Magnetic resonance imaging (MRI) of the neck with and without gadolinium: **yes**/no (see Figure 12.1).
- Ultrasound guided fine needle aspiration (FNA) of the neck lymph node: **yes**/no. This was done before a biopsy of the nasopharynx. It revealed a poorly differentiated carcinoma.
- Positron emission tomography (PET)/computed tomography (CT) scan: **yes**/no. This was performed once a histological diagnosis was confirmed and demonstrated hypermetabolism in the nasopharyngeal mass and enlarged lymph nodes in the left neck with no evidence of any other hypermetabolic focus. PET/CT scans are typically ordered *after* there has been histologic confirmation of malignancy.
- Biopsy of the nasopharynx: **yes**/no. A directed biopsy of the nasopharyngeal mass demonstrated nonkeratinizing squamous cell carcinoma (SCC), consistent with an Epstein–Barr virus (EBV)-positive nasopharyngeal carcinoma (NPC). Additional tissue can allow for immunostains and molecular testing, which can help with the diagnosis and prognosis.

- Thyroid function tests: yes/**no**. This testing would not be appropriate in the absence of symptoms or a large mass involving the hypophysis.

Qustion: Based on this description, what is the patient's clinical TNM stage?

Answer: cT1N1M0, stage II.

The tumor is confined to the nasopharynx, making it a T1 tumor. Ipsilateral lymph nodes less than 6 cm in size above the level of the cricoid make this N1 disease. No distant metastases confer the M0 staging. Overall staging makes this a stage II tumor.

Question: Given this diagnosis and staging, what would be the most appropriate treatment strategy?

Answer: Given his nodal disease, treatment with definitive chemoradiation therapy is the most appropriate choice. Generally, this is a platinum-based regimen along with definitive radiation dosing of 66–70 Gy.

The patient underwent chemoradiation therapy and had an uneventful course. The patient did well for 2 years until he noted a swelling of his anterior frontal scalp. He reported mild pain and headache. No skin changes. No other complaints.

On focused examination, he had a firm, fixed mass immediately deep to the skin and fixed to the underlying bone. Minimally tender to palpation. No other masses or lesions present. Repeat MRI imaging was performed.

CASE 12   (continued)

MRI brain showed a 3 cm infiltrative mass within the left frontal sinus extending through the bone to the skin. This mass abuts the superior orbit and penetrates the bone of the superior lamina papyracea. There was no connection to the nasopharyngeal mucosa and no recurrent tumor in that location.

Transcutaneous biopsy of this mass was performed and consistent with metastatic, nonkeratinizing SCC. Follow-up PET scan demonstrated this single focus of intense FDG-avidity in the frontal sinus. The patient wished to be as aggressive as possible regarding additional treatment.

Question: Given the described recurrence, how would you proceed with treating this patient?

Answer: The patient wishes to pursue surgical treatment and his original tumor had a complete locoregional response to chemoradiation previously. Given the infiltrative nature of this lesion and involvement of the orbital contents along with the fact that the lesion is technically a distant metastasis given the lack of communication with the primary site, surgical resection was not offered initially. The patient was given the option for a palliative care consult, which he refused. Immunotherapy has not yet been validated as a treatment strategy for NPC, except on clinical trials.

The patient underwent chemoradiation therapy directed at the frontal sinus mass, which he tolerated without undo consequences. He had a good response with his post-treatment PET showing complete response of the tumor. Three months after this, the patient developed swelling in the left parotid gland and imaging demonstrated a new mass. No facial nerve weakness or pain. Biopsy of this mass demonstrated recurrent nonkeratinizing SCC, consistent with regional recurrence of his NPC. Repeat PET/CT scan shows a focus of FDG-avidity within the left parotid gland and an additional small questionable focus within the left level II. The patient still desires further treatment that could prevent further decline in function and/or increase quantity of life.

Question: At this stage, what is the best next treatment option for this patient?

Answer: The patient developed a regional recurrence in a field that was already covered by his radiation therapy previously and no new tissue has been placed within this field. Therefore, repeat radiation therapy is not feasible. If the patient was no longer inclined to be aggressive with treatment, palliative care/Hospice referral is reasonable. The recommendation for a neck dissection along with the parotidectomy is based on the fact that his original tumor was metastatic to the left neck and he has new questionable uptake in the neck, most likely representing new metastatic disease.

The patient underwent parotidectomy and neck dissection with one node positive within the parotid and three cervical lymph nodes involved with microscopic metastatic disease. Patient is now over 2 years out from parotidectomy and neck dissection and currently no evidence of disease.

Key Points

- Patients presenting with a unilateral ear effusion should be assessed for a nasopharyngeal mass.
- History and physical exam are extremely important and can help the clinician gauge the extent/aggressiveness of the disease.
- The clinical staging of NPC includes appropriate imaging, typically in the form of MRI and CT scanning, in addition to imaging of the chest (PET/CT or CT chest).
- The primary treatment for NPC is radiation therapy for early stage disease and chemoradiation for advanced-stage disease.
- When considering radiation therapy for recurrent disease, the primary dose to the affected tissue must be considered.
- Surgery can play a role in the setting of recurrent NPC.

CASE 13

Jesse Ryan and Alice Tang

History of Present Illness

A 62-year-old male presents for evaluation of nasal congestion that has been present for several years. He reports that he had a septoplasty, inferior turbinate reduction, and adenoid reduction by another physician about 4 years ago. He had relief of congestion for several months, but then symptoms recurred. His insurance coverage changed, so he was subsequently seen by a second otolaryngologist. He was diagnosed at that time with chronic sinusitis and a sinus procedure was performed about 2 years ago. Again, symptoms of nasal congestion improved for a period of time.

For the past 6 months, patient reports change in tone of his voice, sensation of tightness with swallowing, plugged sensation in left ear, and nasal congestion worse on the left side.

(Continued)

CASE 13 (continued)

Question: What additional questions would you want to ask?

- Any facial numbness? Patient denies. Important to ask because in instances where deficits are noted, there would be concern for significant perineural invasion (trigeminal nerve).
- Any difficulty with opening the mouth? Patient denies. Important to ask because either perineural invasion or direct extension to the pterygoid muscles can contribute to trismus.
- Any other lumps or bumps in the head or neck? Patient denies. Important to ask as this would suggest pathologic lymphadenopathy.

Past Medical/Surgical History

Significant for diabetes, obstructive sleep apnea, gastroesophageal reflux disease, and hypertension.

Tonsillectomy as a child, septoplasty/turbinoplasty/adenoid reduction 4 years ago, and the sinus procedure 2 years ago.

Social History

Patient is a never smoker and nondrinker.

Physical Examination

General: healthy male in no apparent distress, though overweight with large neck.
Voice: muffled tone to voice but no difficulty breathing.
Ears: right TM normal. Left side shows a serous effusion with no mobility of TM.
Nasal cavity: septum straight, clear anteriorly, no masses visualized.
Oral cavity/oropharynx: no masses seen, absent tonsils, normal palate, large tongue, Friedman class III.
Neck: no palpable lymph nodes but patient has a large neck.
Cranial nerve exam: no deficits identified.
You proceed with a flexible nasopharyngolaryngoscopy exam. This shows enlarged adenoid tissue obstructing nasal cavity posteriorly on the left side. Lingual tonsils are significantly enlarged bilaterally. The larynx is visualized and noted to be normal appearance with intact bilateral vocal fold motion.
Photos of the nasopharynx and base of tongue are shown in Figure 13.1.

Management

Question: Which of the following are appropriate steps in the evaluation and management of this patient? (Choose all that apply.)

- MRI of the head and neck with contrast: **yes**/no. This is reasonable as certain head and neck tumor sites, including the nasopharynx, benefit from MRI imaging, to assess for skull base or cranial nerve involvement for instance.

(a)

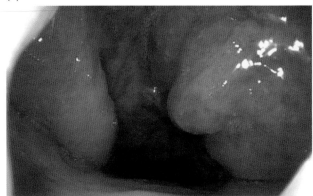

(b)

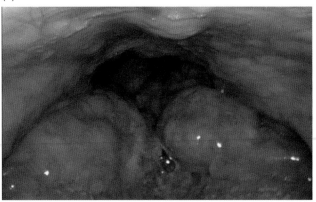

FIGURE 13.1   (a) and (b) These photos from the patient's fiberoptic nasopharyngolaryngoscopy demonstrate diffuse enlargement of the Waldeyer's ring tissue.

- CT scan of the neck with IV contrast: **yes**/no. A CT should be performed whenever the is concern for clival, skull base involvement as CT scans is optimal for delineating bony involvement.

In this case, a CT scan of the neck with contrast is ordered. Representative axial and sagittal images from the CT neck are shown in Figure 13.2.

Question: Based on the history, physical examination, and imaging characteristics, what is the most likely diagnosis for this patient?

Answer: Lymphoma.

The recurrence of lymphoid hypertrophy in an adult after prior adenoid surgery 4 years ago, involvement of multiple anatomic locations, and bilateral nature support a more diffuse process like lymphoma.

CASE 13   (continued)

(a)

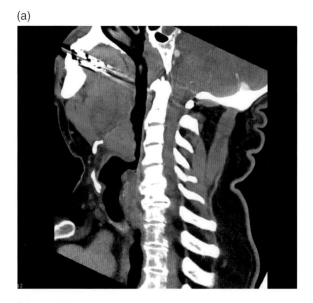

(b)

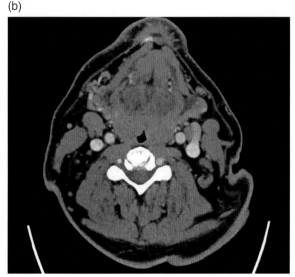

FIGURE 13.2   This figure shows enlargement of the adenoid tissue and lingual tonsils, consistent with your exam (a). Multiple enlarged bilateral lymph nodes are noted up to 2 cm in size (b). There are no pharyngeal or laryngeal masses.

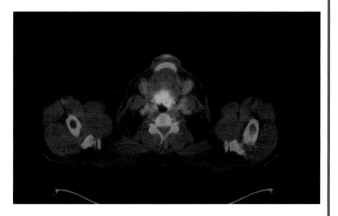

FIGURE 13.3   This is a representative fused axial image from the patient's PET/CT, demonstrating increased FDG uptake in the lingual tonsil tissue (bright yellow area) as well as in the nasopharynx and in bilateral level II cervical lymph nodes (not shown).

Question: What would be an appropriate next step in the evaluation/management of this patient?

Answer: Given high suspicion for lymphoma, tissue from base of tongue and nasopharynx should be sent fresh for lymphoma protocol. This means biopsy would likely need to be done in the operating room for availability of pathology services.

The patient undergoes a direct laryngoscopy/nasopharyngoscopy with biopsies. Pathology from the bilateral base of tongue and left nasopharynx shows Mantle cell lymphoma. After return of the pathology result, a PET/CT scan is performed (see Figure 13.3).

Question: What would be the most appropriate next step in the management of this patient?

Answer: Management of Mantle cell lymphoma, a type of non-Hodgkin's lymphoma (NHL), is with chemotherapy under the direction of medical oncology. Surgery does not have a role in treatment unless it is to aid in obtaining a diagnosis or to assist with airway management.

Key Points

- Lymphoma of Waldeyer's ring can mimic a mucosal malignancy of nasopharynx or oropharynx and must be considered in the differential diagnosis of any oropharyngeal or nasopharyngeal mass.
- Laryngoscopy and nasal endoscopy with biopsy should be considered early in the management of adult patients with persistent lymphoid hypertrophy after conservative management.
- B-cell lymphomas (NHL) are the most common type of lymphoma to develop in Waldeyer's ring, with large B-cell lymphoma being the most common subtype, followed by Mantle cell lymphoma.

CASE 14

Bharat Yarlagadda

History of Present Illness

A 62-year-old male presents for evaluation of a right-sided neck mass. This has been present for the past 3 months and has been slowly growing since then. He feels that additional masses may have developed on the same side recently as well.

Question: What additional questions would you want to ask?

- Any pain related to the mass? Patient denies. Appropriate question to ask.
- Any throat pain or problems swallowing? Patient denies. Appropriate question to ask.
- Any changes in your voice? Patient denies. Appropriate question to ask as this may signify a primary tumor in the larynx or pharynx, or involvement of the vagus or recurrent laryngeal nerve by a malignant process.
- Any previous cancer diagnoses? Yes. He has a history of multiple nonmelanoma skin cancers that have been treated in the past with topical therapies and Mohs surgery. This includes lesions of the face and scalp.
- Any prior head and neck surgery? Important to ask. Patient denies other history of head and neck surgery (other than skin cancer excisions) or radiation exposure.

Question: What additional aspects of the history are important?

- Tobacco or alcohol use? He is a lifelong nonsmoker. He has a history of alcohol abuse and is currently sober.
- Any unusual travel or exposures? Patient denies. He was born in the United States and is of Scotch-Irish descent.
- Any occupational exposures? Patient denies. Certain environmental exposure have been shown to predispose to head and neck malignancies. Nickel exposure and woodworking, for example, have been shown to lead to an increased incidence of certain sinonasal cancers.

Past Medical History

Past medical history is significant for hepatitis C, diverticulitis, panic disorder, and hypertension.

Physical Examination

General: pleasant and well-appearing male in no distress. Eyes: extraocular motions intact, vision grossly normal.

Ears: canals are clear, tympanic membranes are intact, no evidence of fluid.

Nose: external nose normal. Anterior rhinoscopy shows straight septum, no lesions.

Oral cavity: no lesions or masses. Healthy dentition.

Oropharynx: no lesions or masses visible, soft to palpation throughout, tonsils are 2+ and symmetric.

Face: symmetric, no lesions or masses.

Neck/lymph: there are multiple firm, hypomobile right neck masses in levels II–IV, trachea midline, parotid and thyroid beds are soft to palpation with no masses.

Neuro: cranial nerves are grossly intact including facial sensation, facial motion, tongue motion, and shoulder shrug.

Respiratory: no abnormal effort of breathing, voice strong and clear, no stridor.

Fiberoptic nasopharyngolaryngoscopy performed in the office did not show any apparent mucosal abnormalities. Vocal fold function was intact.

Management

Question: Which of the following would be appropriate steps in the evaluation and management of this patient? (Choose all that apply.)

- CT scan of the neck with IV contrast: **yes**/no. A CT scan of the neck with contrast was obtained (see Figure 14.1). This indicates the presence of multiple enlarged right-sided lymph nodes, the largest of which measures 3.3 cm. There is supraclavicular fossa involvement with abnormal lymph nodes below the caudal border of the cricoid cartilage. There are no abnormal lymph nodes on the left. There are no pharyngeal or laryngeal masses, and the nasopharynx appears grossly normal.
- FNA: **yes**/no. FNA is obtained of the largest right-sided lymph node is obtained. This indicates the presence of SCC.
- MRI of the head and neck with contrast: **yes**/no. This is reasonable as certain head and neck tumor sites, including the nasopharynx, benefit from MRI imaging, to assess for skull base or cranial nerve involvement for instance. This patient requires identification of the primary source of his nodal disease as the next step – the MRI can assist if that primary happens to be in the nasopharynx.
- PET/CT scan: **yes**/no. PET/CT imaging can be quite helpful in the identification of an occult primary tumor in the head and neck and to evaluate distant sites for metastatic disease. This is typically done after a diagnosis of malignancy is obtained (see Figure 14.2).

Question: The PET/CT scan suggests a primary tumor of the right nasopharynx. What additional workup would be helpful to complete your evaluation?

- In situ hybridization studies for EBV-encoded RNA (EBER): EBV RNA levels are strongly positive in the cytology specimen previously obtained with FNA. In this case, this strongly suggests a nasopharyngeal source, but is not considered confirmatory. Elevation of serum biomarkers, including EBV DNA and anti-EBV capsid antigen IgA are highly sensitive for the presence of NPC. This panel is used as a screening mechanism in endemic locales, and also can be used as a means of post-treatment surveillance.

CASE 14 (continued)

(a)   (b)

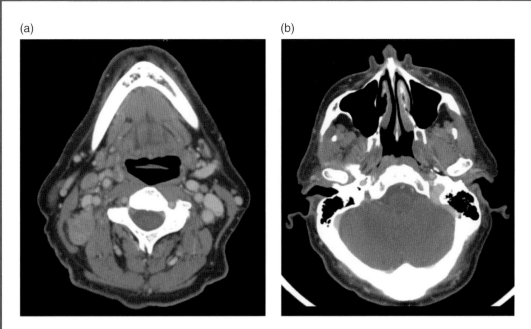

FIGURE 14.1 (a) and (b) On these representative contrast-enhanced axial cuts from the patient's CT of the neck, multiple right-sided abnormal lymph nodes are noted (a). There were no other lesions referable to the upper aerodigestive mucosa (b).

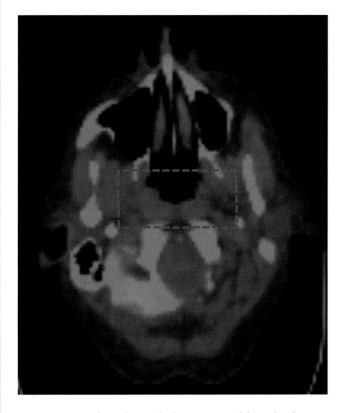

FIGURE 14.2 There is no obvious mucosal-based primary tumor, but there is a faint asymmetry in FDG avidity of the right nasopharynx.

(Continued)

CASE 14 (continued)

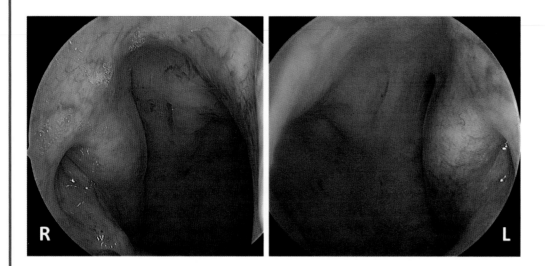

FIGURE 14.3 Operative nasopharyngolaryngoscopy indicates a slight fullness and irregularity of the right Fossa of Rosenmuller, ipsilateral to the cervical lymphadenopathy.

- Nasopharyngolaryngoscopy: Nasopharyngolaryngoscopy is needed to identify and confirm the primary tumor with biopsy (see Figure 14.3). This can be done in the office with adequate topical anesthesia, or in the operating room. In this case, biopsies of the right nasopharynx indicate nonkeratinizing undifferentiated carcinoma with lymphoid stroma, consistent with lymphoepithelial-type NPC.
- MRI of the neck and skull base with and without gadolinium contrast: An MRI of the skull base was ultimately obtained and there are no abnormalities of the cranial nerves or skull base foramina, and the parapharyngeal fat appears preserved.

Question: What is the TNM and group staging of this patient's nasopharyngeal cancer?

Answer: cT1N3M0, stage IVA.

This patient presents with a small primary tumor with no extension into the oropharynx, cranial nerve involvement, or parapharyngeal involvement. The T stage is thus T1 (see Table 14.1). A unique feature of the T staging of nasopharyngeal cancer is the use of T0 designation. The patient does have a significant nodal burden. There are multiple ipsilateral nodes, none are greater than 6 cm, but there is extension of the nodal disease below the caudal border of the cricoid cartilage. The N stage is thus N3 (see Table 14.2). It is important to recall that the nodal staging is different than what is used for other mucosal head and neck neoplasms (ex: larynx, hypopharynx, etc.). The group staging for this patient is stage IVA (see Table 14.3).

TABLE 14.1	T staging of nasopharyngeal cancer per AJCC 8.
TX	Primary tumor cannot be assessed
T0	No tumor identified, but EBV-positive cervical lymph node involvement
Tis	Carcinoma in situ
T1	Tumor confined to the nasopharynx, or extension into the oropharynx or nasal cavity, with no parapharyngeal space involvement
T2	Tumor with extension to the parapharyngeal space, and/or adjacent soft-tissue involvement of the medial or lateral pterygoid or prevertebral muscles
T3	Tumor with infiltration of skull base bone, cervical vertebrae, pterygoid plates, or sinuses
T4	Tumor with intracranial extension, involvement of the cranial nerves, hypopharynx, orbit, or soft-tissue infiltration beyond the lateral pterygoid muscle

CASE 14   (continued)

TABLE 14.2   N staging of nasopharyngeal cancer per AJCC 8.

NX	Nodal staging cannot be assessed
N0	No regional lymph node metastasis
N1	Unilateral metastasis in cervical lymph nodes and/or unilateral or bilateral metastasis in retropharyngeal lymph nodes, all nodes 6 cm or less, all nodes above the caudal border of the cricoid
N2	Bilateral cervical metastasis, all nodes 6 cm or less, all nodes above the caudal border of the cricoid
N3	Unilateral or bilateral cervical nodal metastasis, larger than 6 cm in greatest dimension, or any node below the caudal border of the cricoid cartilage

TABLE 14.3   Group staging of nasopharyngeal cancer per AJCC 8.

Stage 0	Tis	N0	M0
Stage I	T1	N0	M0
Stage II	T0, T1	N1	M0
	T2	N0, N1	M0
Stage III	T0, T1, T2	N2	M0
	T3	N0, N1, N2	M0
Stage IVA	T4	N0, N1, N2	M0
	Any T	N3	M0
Stage IVB	Any T	Any N	M1

Question: Which epidemiologic factor is the most relevant risk factor for development of non-keratinizing nasopharyngeal cancer?

Answer: EBV infection.

The most relevant epidemiologic risk factor is the presence of EBV. A large body of evidence supports EBV as a primary etiologic factor in the development of NPC. EBV is a ubiquitous virus, infecting over 90% of the worldwide population, most commonly producing an asymptomatic self-limited infection early in life, and the syndrome of infectious mononucleosis if infection occurs later. A small proportion of patients with a chronic infection go on to develop malignancy associated with EBV, and this transformation is considered to be multifactorial and epigenetic.

The World Health Organization (WHO) has classified NPC into three types:

Keratinizing:

- WHO type I – considered a sporadic form. Histologically, this subtype is akin to a classic pharyngeal SCC. This subtype has the weakest association with EBV and the strongest with tobacco use and has the worst prognosis.

Nonkeratinizing:

- WHO type II – differentiated subtype. Strong association with EBV.
- WHO type III – undifferentiated nonkeratinizing subtype, also known as a lymphoepithelioma. Strong association with EBV. The endemic forms of NPC are of this variety. Considered to have the most favorable prognosis.

EBV serum titers are used as a marker of treatment response, and can also be used as a marker of recurrence. The use of serum markers for screening is not yet defined.

Tobacco and alcohol abuse are considered etiologic factors for WHO type I variety of NPC. These exposures may promote carcinogenesis in patients with EBV who are otherwise at risk of type II and III, but this relationship is equivocal.

Globally, areas to which NPC is endemic include Southern China including Hong Kong, North Africa and the Middle East, the Arctic including Alaska and Greenland, and Southeast Asia. Geographic predilection is due to genetic factors, including HLA-associated risk for mainland Chinese individuals, and dietary including the consumption of smoked fish and nitrite-rich foods.

Question: In this patient with cT1N3M0, WHO type III, nasopharyngeal cancer, what is the recommended initial therapy?

Answer: Concurrent chemoradiation followed by chemotherapy.

This patient is counseled to proceed with concurrent chemoradiation followed by adjuvant chemotherapy. When available, enrollment into clinical trials is recommended. Early stage NPC (cT1N0) is addressed with radiation alone. For any more advanced T stages, or with any nodal involvement, the most common approach is concurrent chemoradiation followed by adjuvant chemotherapy. The traditionally described regimen is a platinum-based radio-sensitizing agent provided with radiation, followed by three cycles of cisplatin/5-FU. Surgery, neck dissection and/or nasopharyngeal resection, is generally reserved for salvage if there is persistent or recurrent disease.

46 SECTION 3 Nasopharynx

- Cervical lymphadenopathy with what appears to be an unknown primary can be related to clinically occult nasopharyngeal cancer. Diagnosis can be aided by EBER in situ hybridization of nodal aspiration samples, serum EBV biomarker measurements, PET imaging, and nasopharyngeal biopsies.
- EBV infection is an etiologic factor in many cases. EBER polymerase chain reaction (PCR) is considered a component of initial workup. Serum EBV titers can be used to assess response to therapy and may be used to monitor for recurrence, especially given the propensity of distant metastatic failure in NPC patients.
- Nodal staging of NPC is unique. Upstaging factors include bilateral nodal disease or nodal involvement below the level of the cricoid, namely the supraclavicular fossa, and lymph nodes larger than 6 cm in size.
- Early stage NPC (cT1N0M0) is treated with radiation alone. Locally or regionally advanced disease is treated upfront concurrent chemoradiation with adjuvant chemotherapy (cisplatin +5-FU). Surgery is used in the salvage setting.

CASE 15

Brian Cervenka

History of Present Illness

A 65-year-old Japanese male with a history of T2N1M0 NPC presents 2 years following concurrent cisplatin/intensity-modulated radiation therapy (IMRT). He presents with recent small-volume epistaxis and pain.

Question: What additional questions would you want to ask?

- Nasal obstruction? Patient denies. This is an appropriate question.
- Quantify the amount and frequency of bleeding? One to two times daily, low volume, stops spontaneously, has been occurring for the past month.
- Describe the pain: deep-seated pain, frontal, constant.
- Any new neck masses: Patient denies. This is an important question.
- When was the most recent post-treatment scan? 3 months following completion, negative, was lost to follow-up after.
- Dysphagia, aspiration? Patient denies. This is an appropriate question.
- Ear pain or fullness? Yes, right side, this is recent within last 2 months.

Question: What additional aspects of the history are important?

- Tobacco or alcohol use? Patient denies.
- Any history of head and neck cancers? Yes as mentioned above.
- Where was the previous treatment given? This is an important question. You will want to get outside records for the patient's prior treatment.

Past Medical History

Coronary artery disease, well controlled.
Type II diabetes mellitus, controlled on oral medications.

Physical Examination

Well-developed in no distress. Voice strong.
Skin: no suspicious lesions.
Salivary: no fullness or masses within parotid or submandibular glands.
Oral cavity: good dentition, no mucosal lesions, tonsils present.
Cervical exam reveals no lymphadenopathy.
Cranial nerves II–XII intact.
Nasal endoscopy reveals an endophytic ulcerative lesion on the right lateral aspect of the nasopharynx, obstructing the eustachian tube, mass appears to extend lateral toward the parapharyngeal space (see Figure 15.1)

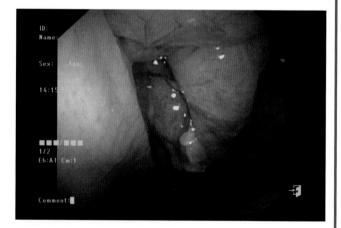

FIGURE 15.1 Endophytic ulcerative lesion on the right lateral aspect of the nasopharynx.

CASE 15 (continued)

Management

Office biopsy is taken demonstrating a recurrent poorly differentiated NPC. It is important to recognize that there may be imaging findings suggestive of recurrence but these may be located submucosally. Operative deep biopsies with frozen section are the next step if an awake biopsy fails. This can also be a first step if there is a concern for a submucosal tumor. For all biopsies of the lateral nasopharynx, it is important to obtain imaging with contrast to discern the location of the internal carotid artery. Vessels with a medial course may be at risk from biopsies. If there is concern, the biopsy should be performed under general anesthesia to optimize safety.

Question: Which of the following would be appropriate next steps in the evaluation and management of this patient? (Choose all that apply.)

- MRI with and without contrast: **yes**/no. This is an excellent next step as this will allow for evaluation of the soft-tissue extension, parapharyngeal involvement, cranial nerve involvement, brain involvement. In the post-treatment setting, differentiating fibrotic tissue and recurrent cancer can be challenging, as both enhance with contrast. Diffusion weighted imaging can be used to distinguish between the two.

MRI demonstrates an enhancing mass involving the soft tissue of the nasopharynx, centered on the right with extension into the parapharyngeal space but not abutting/involving the carotid artery. It does not extend to the paranasal sinuses or posteriorly into the musculature or clivus. No brain involvement. DWI window consistent with recurrent tumor.

- CT neck with contrast: **yes**/no. If there is a concern for clival, skull base involvement, a CT scan is optimal for delineating bony involvement. If there is just soft-tissue extension, a CT may add little additional detail to the MRI.

A contrast-enhanced CT is performed and does not demonstrate any bone erosion (see Figure 15.2). Tumor extension is as described in the MRI.

- A PET/CT: **yes**/no. In the setting of recurrent NPC, a PET/CT is a critical adjunct. Up to 20% of patients will have distant metastasis at recurrence diagnosis. In addition, MRI and CT may not delineate post-treatment fibrosis from recurrence. PET/CT can greatly improve the diagnostic sensitivity of the imaging.

A PET/CT is performed and demonstrates no evidence of regional or distant metastases.

- Plasma EBV level: **yes**/no. In the setting of recurrent disease, it is not a sensitive test as levels can be low even with recurrent disease. That said, it can be helpful as

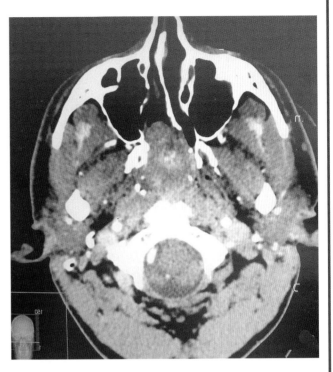

FIGURE 15.2   Right nasopharyngeal mass on CT scan without bony invasion.

those with higher levels are at increased risk for aggressive distant disease. In addition, can be used as a reference following treatment.

This patient's plasma EBV titers are elevated.

- Consultation with medical oncology and radiation oncology and discussion at multidisciplinary tumor board: **yes**/no. This is a critical step for all malignancies but it is particularly important for patients with complex recurrent disease.
- Modified barium swallow: **yes**/no. Speech and swallowing assessment is critical here given the patient's disease and prior treatment history. This patient may have baseline deficits from prior therapy. Nutrition and dental follow-up can be considered as well.

Question: Imaging demonstrated a nasopharyngeal mass with involvement of the parapharyngeal space on the right without involvement of the clivus, skull base, carotid, paranasal sinuses, vertebrae. No nodal disease. Based on your current assessment, what would be this patient's clinical stage?

Answer: rT2N0M0.

T2 is defined as a tumor with extension to the parapharyngeal space and/or adjacent soft-tissue involvement

(Continued)

CASE 15   (continued)

of the medial or lateral pterygoid or prevertebral muscles. A T3 tumor would demonstrate infiltration of skull base bone, cervical vertebrae, pterygoid plates, or sinuses.

Question: Given the recurrent nature of the patient tumor and his stage, what is the best management option for this patient?

- Definitive surgical resection.
  This would be the most appropriate management option for this patient if the tumor is amenable to surgical resection.
- Reirradiation.
  Given that most recurrent nasopharyngeal tumors are considered unresectable, reirradiation is often the treatment of choice. What is clear is from published series describing these patients is that reirradiation is associated with significant short and long-term morbidity. Leong et al. (2018) looked at 1768 patients in a meta-analysis who underwent reirradiation and found that the 5-year overall survival (OS) was 41% but the grade 5 toxicity occurred in 33% of patients with a high rate of treatment related mortality. Mucosal necrosis and massive hemorrhage accounted for 40% of the deaths and failure to thrive and encephalopathy accounting for the rest. Therefore, surgical resections to negative margins should be considered first. The diagram below is a flow sheet that helps delineate treatment options.

Question: If the tumor is deemed resectable, what are the possible surgical approaches to the nasopharynx?

- Maxillary swing: **yes**/no.
- Transpalatal: **yes**/no.
- Transcervical: **yes**/no.
- Endoscopic: **yes**/no.
- Transoral robotic: **yes**/no.
- Infratemporal fossa: **yes**/no.

All of the listed approaches are viable surgical options. Each approach has certain benefits and based on tumor location the approach that gives the safest access for complete tumor removal should be selected. The maxillary swing approach yields fantastic access to the nasopharynx and ipsilateral parapharyngeal space. Removing the posterior nasal septum can provide access to the contralateral nasopharynx. There is limited exposure to the contralateral parapharyngeal space. Transpalatal can be used alone or with robotic/endoscopic assist. This is good for lesions without parapharyngeal involvement. Endoscopic approaches alone are emerging as a major treatment modality for T1–2 limited recurrent NPCs. In retrospective case matched series, similar local salvage rates have been described with less treatment morbidity, improved QOL, and less complications than IMRT. For limited recurrences not approaching internal carotid, this has become a preferred approach. Transcervical is often used in concert with endoscopic assist or other approaches. It is especially helpful (i) for any nodal disease, including retropharyngeal and (ii) for control of the internal carotid prior to resecting the tumor endoscopically. In these large resections with exposure of the great vessels, clivus, skull base, a vascularized free flap is typically needed so neck exposure is required. Transoral robotic in concert with a longitudinal soft palate split has been described. Infratemporal fossa with carotid transposition is described, though not often used.

Key Points

- Local, recurrent NPCs are rare due to the overall superb treatment response to IMRT alone or IMRT + cisplatin for advanced disease. In addition, recurrence often occurs with metastatic disease.
- Available treatment modalities include surgery, reirradiation with or without chemotherapy, or palliative chemotherapy, and treatment decisions should be made in the context of a multidisciplinary tumor board discussion.
- A thorough evaluation of the previous IMRT plan by the radiation oncologist should be performed to identify patients that can tolerate additional radiation to surrounding structures without significant morbidity.
- Surgery, when feasible and able to obtain negative margins, achieves good local control rates and limits morbidity, when compared to reradiation.
- Surgical approaches should limit morbidity while giving necessary visualization for safe resection with negative margins. Special consideration should be given to protection of the internal carotid artery with lateral tumors in the parapharyngeal space.
- Proton and carbon ion therapy are promising new options that can significantly limit the radiation dose to surrounding structures for reirradiation candidates.

Multiple Choice Questions

1. Which of the following World Health Organization type of NPC is **not** linked with infection with the Ebstein-Barr Virus?

   a. WHO type I.

   b. WHO type II.

   c. WHO type III.

   d. All of the above are linked with EBV infection.

   Answer: a. NPCs that are keratinizing are classified as WHO type I. For these tumors, tobacco use is the more common risk factor and they are not typically related to EBV infection. WHO type II and III tumors are both EBV-related cancers.

2. On evaluating a patient with a right ear effusion, the patient has a complaint of double vision on looking to the right. What is the most likely structure to be involved?

   a. The right oculomotor nerve.

   b. The right lateral rectus muscle.

   c. The right trochlear nerve.

   d. The right abducens nerve.

   Answer: d. Tumor extension from nasopharyngeal cancer can directly involve the cavernous sinus. Loss of abducens nerve function is common in this setting, which results in paralysis of the lateral rectus muscle (rather than direct muscle involvement by tumor). While the third (oculomotor) and fourth (trochlear) cranial nerves can be involved, this typically would occur after the abducens nerve and would not be expected to result in diplopia with right lateral gaze.

3. A 55-year-old female presents with hyponasal voice and sterdor on physical exam and inability to lie flat due to difficulty breathing. Scope exam shows enlarged but nonobstructive adenoid tissue and prominent lingual tonsil tissue. You are planning for a general anesthesia. What would be the most appropriate way to induce general anesthesia?

   a. Awake transoral intubation in the supine position using a fiberoptic scope.

   b. Asleep intubation in the supine position using a video laryngoscope (example being a glide scope).

   c. Awake transnasal fiberoptic intubation in the sitting position.

   d. None of the above.

   Answer: c. In this patient, due to her prominent lingual tonsil tissue, she is at risk for airway obstruction when lying supine. As a result, an awake transoral intubation would be contraindicated as would an asleep intubation in the supine position. For most video laryngoscopes, the blade is placed in the vallecula and in this patient and others with base of tongue masses, it is likely to either initiate bleeding and/or have the view obscured by the mass. A controlled transnasal intubation with topical anesthesia is often the safest route to establish an airway.

4. In evaluating a patient for lymphoma of the palatine tonsil, which of the following would **not** be an appropriate part of the workup?

   a. Oral and serum human papillomavirus (HPV)-DNA levels.

   b. Bone marrow biopsy.

   c. Peripheral blood smear.

   d. Tonsillectomy to achieve a tissue diagnosis.

   Answer: a. Lymphoma of Waldeyer's ring typically requires a tissue biopsy to achieve a diagnosis. It is recommended to get at least a 1 cm³ sample to be able to also run flow cytometry. Since NHLs are the most common types to affect this area, systemic workup with a bone marrow biopsy and a peripheral blood smear are also important. Oral and serum HPV-DNA levels, while they may be abnormal in patients with HPV-related oropharyngeal cancer, have not been shown to have diagnostic benefit in and of themselves.

5. A 44-year-old male patient presents with a rT2N0M0 keratinizing SCC of the nasopharynx with minimal extension into the parapharyngeal space. After discussion at multidisciplinary tumor board, it is recommended for the patient to undergo definitive surgical resection. What would be your approach in this patient?

   a. Endoscopic with ipsilateral R transcervical for parapharyngeal space assist and control of the internal carotid artery (ICA).

   b. Maxillary swing osteocutaneous.

   c. Transpalatal robotic.

   d. Endoscopic alone.

   Answer: a. Given the parapharyngeal space involvement and limited extent within the nasopharynx this tumor is resectable via an endoscopic approach. That said, for control of the ICA and exposure and resection of parapharyngeal involvement, an ipsilateral transcervical approach would be ideal. Certainly, a maxillary swing could be considered, but there is additional patient morbidity in this approach.

6. In patients with recurrent NPC after prior definitive radiation of chemoradiation therapy, when would reirradiation therapy with chemotherapy be considered? (Choose all that apply.)

   a. For patients with limited local recurrence of their primary tumor.

   b. For patients with unresectable tumors.

   c. For patients found to have microscopically positive margins following resection.

   d. None of the above.

   Answer: b and c. Radiation is considered the primary treatment with or without chemotherapy depending on stage for most primary NPC. That said, the patients that fail primary radiation therapy are likely somewhat radioresistant. In addition, the significant morbidity of treatment must be discussed with the patient and strongly considered. As discussed before, reirradiation is an appropriate option for unresectable recurrent NPC patients, and patients who are unable or unwilling to undergo surgical resection. There are emerging modalities other than IMRT that have been shown to reduce the acute and long-term toxicity of treatment. Proton or carbon ion therapy is unique in that the Bragg peak has such a precipitous drop off that the radiation exposure to surrounding structures can be significantly decreased. Access to this therapy is limited and there is still minimal data, but this should certainly be considered in this patient group when available.

Chemotherapy is often used in the neoadjuvant or adjuvant setting with reirradiation to decrease tumor size (when bulky) to limit surrounding structure dose exposure and as a radiosensitizer. In addition, patients with metastatic disease are candidates for chemotherapy alone as palliative therapy. Cisplatin is typically used in combination with gemcitabine but there are multiple other drug combinations that have been studied. There are small series looking at targeted therapy to epidermal growth factor receptor (EGFR) and vascular endothelial growth factor (VEGF) as well as immunotherapy and vaccine therapy.

Suggested Reading

Al-Sarraf, M., LeBlanc, M., Giri, P.G. et al. (1998). Chemoradiotherapy versus radiotherapy in patients with advanced nasopharyngeal cancer: phase III randomized intergroup study 0099. *J. Clin. Oncol.* 16 (4): 1310–1317.

Chan, J.Y. (2014). Surgical management of recurrent nasopharyngeal carcinoma. *Oral Oncol.* 50 (10): 913–917.

Galloway, T.J. and Ridge, J.A. (2015). Management of squamous cancer metastatic to cervical nodes with an unknown primary site. *J. Clin. Oncol.* 33 (29): 3328–3337.

Hao, S.P., Tsang, N.M., and Chang, C.N. (2002). Salvage surgery for recurrent nasopharyngeal carcinoma. *Arch. Otolaryngol. Head Neck Surg.* 128: 63–67.

Koletsa, T., Markou, K., Ouzounidou, S. et al. (2013). In situ mantle cell lymphoma in the nasopharynx. *Head Neck* 35 (11): E333–E337. https://doi.org/10.1002/hed.23206. Epub 2012 Dec 22. Review. PubMed PMID: 23280758.

Laskar, S., Mohindra, P., Gupta, S. et al. (2008). Non-Hodgkin lymphoma of the Waldeyer's ring: clinicopathologic and therapeutic issues. *Leuk. Lymphoma* 49 (12): 2263–2271. https://doi.org/10.1080/10428190802493686. Review. PubMed PMID: 19052973.

Lee, A.W.M., Ng, W.T., Chan, J.Y.W. et al. (2019). Management of locally recurrent nasopharyngeal carcinoma. *Cancer Treat. Rev.* 79: 101890.

Leong, Y.H., Soon, Y.Y., Lee, K.M. et al. (2018). Long-term outcomes after reirradiation in nasopharyngeal carcinoma with intensity-modulated radiotherapy: a meta-analysis. *Head Neck* 40 (3): 622–631.

Niedobitek, G. (2000). Epstein–Barr virus infection in the pathogenesis of nasopharyngeal carcinoma. *Mol. Pathol.* 53: 248–254.

Perri, F., Della Vittoria Scarpati, G., Caponigro, F. et al. (2019). Management of recurrent nasopharyngeal carcinoma: current perspectives. *Onco. Targets. Ther.* 12: 1583–1591.

Picard, A., Cardinne, C., Denoux, Y. et al. (2015). Extranodal lymphoma of the head and neck: a 67-case series. *Eur. Ann. Otorhinolaryngol. Head Neck Dis.* 132 (2): 71–75. https://doi.org/10.1016/j.anorl.2014.07.005. Epub 2014 Dec 29. PubMed PMID: 25553969.

Wei, I.W. and Mok, V.W.K. (2007). The management of neck metastases in nasopharyngeal carcinoma. *Curr. Opin. Otolaryngol. Head Neck Surg.* 15: 99–102.

You, R., Zou, X., Hua, Y.J. et al. (2015). Salvage endoscopic nasopharyngectomy is superior to intensity-modulated radiation therapy for local recurrence of selected T1–T3 nasopharyngeal carcinoma – a case-matched comparison. *Radiother. Oncol.* 115 (3): 399–406.

Yu, M.C. and Yuan, J.M. (2002). Epidemiology of nasopharyngeal carcinoma. *Semin. Cancer Biol.* 12: 421.

SECTION 4

Laryngeal Cancer

Bharat Yarlagadda

CASE 16

Bharat Yarlagadda

History of Present Illness

A 72-year-old man is referred to your clinic by a primary care physician for progressive dysphagia over 6 months that has not responded to antibiotics and reflux medication. No further workup has been performed.

Question: What additional questions would you want to ask in the initial evaluation?

- Any pain? Location? Yes, the patient has right-sided throat pain radiating to the ear.
- Any masses in the neck? No, he does not notice this.
- Voice change and/or breathing difficulty? He thinks his voice is more raspy
- Dysphagia to solids? Liquids? Both? Solid foods get "stuck", no issues with liquids.
- Any problems breathing? He has difficulty with exertion, but no new changes.
- Coughing with swallow? Recent pneumonia? No coughing or recent pneumonia.
- Weight loss? His weight is stable.
- Tobacco or alcohol use? He is a current pack-per-day smoker, and has been for 45 years. He has a history of social alcohol use.

Question: What additional aspects of the history are important?

- Any history of head and neck cancer? He denies this for himself and any of his family members.
- Any prior radiation exposure? No.

Past Medical History

- Moderate COPD, uses a steroid inhaler.

- Formerly active outdoorsman, retired city worker.

Physical Examination

Appears older than his stated age, slightly cachectic. Vital signs are normal. He is breathing comfortably without stridor. Upon speaking, you notice a slightly garbled, "hot potato" voice, with some breathiness. He is handling his secretions without issue.

Skin/scalp: no lesions.

Ears: within normal limits.

Nose: normal anterior rhinoscopy.

Cranial nerves: intact bilaterally.

Oral cavity: poor dentition, smells of smoke, no mucosal lesions.

Neck: Enlarged right level II lymph node, nontender, firm, mobile. No masses on the left.

Fiberoptic nasolaryngoscopy reveals an exophytic mass that appears to emanate off of the side of the epiglottis and onto the aryepiglottic (AE) fold. The right vocal cord is obscured, but on a brief glimpse of it you see that it appears to be mobile.

Management

Question: Which of the following would be appropriate next steps in the evaluation and management of this patient? (Choose all that apply.)

- Computed tomography (CT) scan of the neck with IV contrast: **yes**/no.

This is an appropriate initial step for evaluation of this patient's laryngeal and neck masses. One can presume a diagnosis of neoplasm based on this patient's medical history and presentation. The CT scan will provide information regarding extent of the laryngeal mass, and nodal disease beyond what is palpable.

(Continued)

Essential Cases in Head and Neck Oncology, First Edition. Edited by Michael G. Moore, Arnaud F. Bewley, and Babak Givi.
© 2022 American Head and Neck Society. Published 2022 by John Wiley & Sons Ltd.

CASE 16   (continued)

A CT scan of the neck and chest is performed and the patient returns for follow-up (see Figure 16.1). There is a 2.5 cm exophytic mass centered on the right AE fold extending onto the laryngeal surface of the epiglottis. There is no cartilage erosion, and no invasion of the pre-epiglottic, or paraglottic spaces. There are multiple ipsilateral (right) -sided enlarged lymph nodes, largest 2.1 cm in level III.

- CT scan of the chest with IV contrast: **yes**/no. Chest shows no evidence of metastatic nodules or primary tumors.

This is reasonable to perform in addition to the CT scan of the neck. Again, presuming a neoplastic diagnosis, the chest imaging will provide information regarding the possibility of pulmonary metastasis, as well as assess for primary lung tumors given the patient's smoking history.

- Fine needle aspiration (FNA) of the neck mass: **yes**/no.

This can be performed in the office setting or ambulatory procedure suite, with or without ultrasound guidance if the mass is readily palpable. FNA can provide a cytologic diagnosis of the mass and expedite workup with minimal risk. For this patient, an FNA of a neck node reveals squamous cell carcinoma (SCC), p16 negative.

- Examination under anesthesia (EUA) via direct laryngoscopy: **yes**/no.

In general, EUA is recommended for mucosal head and neck malignancies when the entirety of the mass cannot be fully delineated in the office. Generally, laryngeal and pharyngeal tumor characteristics are better assessed under anesthesia with the exception of vocal fold mobility. One purpose is to assess for surgical candidacy. Biopsy of the mass can confirm the index site of cancer, but is not necessary for diagnosis given the FNA results.

EUA via direct laryngoscopy indicates an exophytic mass arising from the right AE fold and extending onto the larynx (see Figure 16.2). The false vocal fold is involved but the glottis itself appears spared. The pyriform sinus mucosa and vallecula are spared.

- 18F-FDG positron emission tomography (PET)/CT scan: **yes**/no.

PET/CT scan is helpful for complete staging and is generally indicated for stage III and IV disease. PET/CT is not mandatory if a distant metastatic workup is otherwise completed, for example with a chest CT scan. Many multidisciplinary groups will obtain PET/CT scans routinely, however, for reasons including design of postoperative adjuvant therapies. In this current patient, the PET/CT scan corroborates the findings of the initial CT scans.

- Modified barium swallow (MBS): **yes**/no.

This patient did complain of solid food dysphagia. This study is helpful to evaluate for laryngeal dysfunction with regards to the patient's smoking history ongoing pretreatment aspiration. This patient's study does not indicate the presence of aspiration or penetration into the airway.

- Magnetic resonance imaging (MRI) of the neck with contrast: **yes**/no.

Given the workup done to this point, MRI of the neck would not offer additional information or change management. In some circumstances, MRI can assist

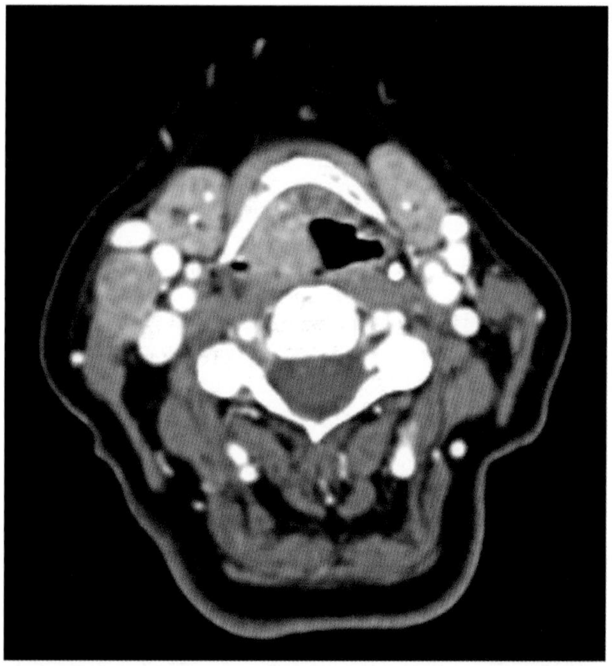

FIGURE 16.1   CT scan with contrast demonstrated exophytic mass of the right AE fold.

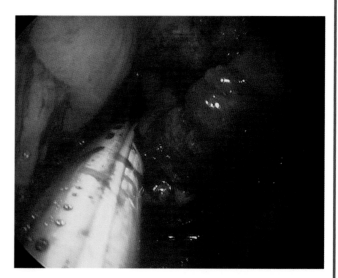

FIGURE 16.2   Direct laryngoscopy demonstrating an exophytic mass arising from the right AE fold and extending onto the larynx.

CASE 16   (continued)

with better definition of local invasion by laryngeal cancers including involvement of the base of tongue, paraglottic and pre-epiglottic spaces, or cartilaginous involvement, when not fully assessed with CT scan.

Question: Based on your examination and imaging, what is the cancer stage?

Answer: cT2N2b, stage IVa.

This patient has a supraglottic mass involving more than one subsite. There is no pre-epiglottic/paraglottic involvement or cartilage involvement, and the vocal folds are noted to be mobile. The T stage is T2. Multiple ipsilateral pathologic nodes not larger than 6 cm result in N stage N2b. There is no clinically overt extranodal extension, which would otherwise upstage to N3b.

The patient undergoes multidisciplinary evaluation including radiation oncology and medical oncology consultations. He is interested in an "organ preservation" approach.

Question: What type of "organ preservation" treatment would you recommend for this patient?

Answer: If a nonsurgical approach is chosen, upfront concurrent chemoradiation would be appropriate for advanced-stage laryngeal cancer. Generally, either radiosensitizing platinum regimen or concurrent epidermal growth factor receptor inhibitors are recommended. Initial radiation alone would not be recommended in the setting of multiple involved lymph nodes unless there was a contraindication to concurrent systemic therapies. If systemic therapy is not an option for a patient, upfront surgery and adjuvant radiation therapy should be seriously considered as this would offer the best chance for disease control. In general, this patient would be eligible for either upfront surgery with adjuvant radiation +/− chemotherapy, or for upfront concurrent chemoradiation with surgery for salvage if needed.

The VA larynx trial initially described that a laryngeal preservation approach, via induction chemotherapy followed by radiation, demonstrated a similar 2-year overall survival of 68% compared to upfront total laryngectomy with adjuvant radiation. There was a 64% rate of "laryngeal preservation" in patient with nonsurgical upfront treatment. Subsequent trials, such as RTOG 91-11 intergroup, demonstrated similar 2-year overall survival rates between induction chemo followed by radiation, radiation alone, and concurrent chemoradiation therapy. There was no benefit to the administration of induction chemotherapy. There was a higher rate of local failure requiring salvage laryngectomy with radiation alone compared to concurrent chemoradiation. In addition, there was a higher rate of distant metastatic disease when chemotherapy was not administered in any form. Currently, induction chemotherapy as a means to assess tumor responsiveness is not routinely practiced. Neoadjuvant chemotherapy prior to concurrent chemoradiation is controversial due to a lack of

reproducible benefit amongst studies but with significant increase in toxicities. Thus, for advanced laryngeal cancer without gross extralaryngeal spread, destruction of the laryngeal framework, or loss of laryngeal function, most institutions recommend an upfront nonsurgical approach as a means of "laryngeal preservation."

The patient has decided to proceed with upfront concurrent chemoradiation. Full dose radiation with weekly platinum based radiosensitizing chemotherapy is completed without interruption. He develops severe dysphagia and aspiration during treatment requiring gastrostomy placement.

Question: At 8 weeks post-treatment, the patient reports persistent throat pain. Endoscopy with biopsies of the larynx reveal persistent carcinoma of the supraglottis. The nodal disease appears resolved per CT imaging. What is the appropriate next step in therapy in this patient who desires a curative approach?

- Partial laryngectomy via transoral approach: yes/**no**.

Partial laryngectomy can be performed in the salvage setting for selected patients. Favorable features for this approach include small volume disease with relatively intact swallowing function. Our patient has developed worsening aspiration issues and is now NPO. This development along with the history of COPD would make this a challenging approach from an aspiration and pneumonia standpoint.

- Total laryngectomy, bilateral neck dissection, pectoralis flap reconstruction: **yes**/no.

The curative option for this patient is to proceed with total laryngectomy, primarily for oncologic control, and secondarily for aero-digestive separation. In the salvage setting, a comprehensive nodal dissection is recommended when there is detectable residual disease in the neck. Elective neck dissection remains controversial in the salvage setting. Studies have demonstrated 17% overall rate of occult nodal metastasis when neck dissections are performed for locally recurrent laryngeal cancer. The highest rates of occult nodal disease are associated with advanced T stage and the supraglottic subsites. In this patient, bilateral neck dissection is a reasonable component of the salvage procedure.

- Reirradiation: yes/**no**
  Reirradiation at a short interval, as in this patient, is not advised.
- Immunotherapy via the use of checkpoint inhibitors: yes/**no**

PD-1 or PD-L1 inhibitors are currently approved for the use of refractory recurrent or metastatic head and neck SCC. The rate of response is relatively low, but these agents can produce increases in overall survival. Currently this approach is considered palliative rather than curative.

(Continued)

Key Points

- Early stage supraglottic laryngeal SCC is generally treated with single modality therapy, either radiation alone or partial laryngeal surgery.
- Partial laryngeal surgery can be offered ideally for early stage disease in patients with intact swallowing function, pulmonary reserve, and who are anticipated to proceed with single modality therapy, such as those with limited nodal involvement.
- Advanced-stage laryngeal SCC requires multimodality therapy. In the absence of extralaryngeal spread, bulky T3 or T4 disease, or laryngeal destruction or dysfunction, a laryngeal preservation approach with concurrent chemoradiation is often appropriate.
- Salvage laryngectomy has a considerable risk profile with regards to postoperative complications including the development of a pharyngocutaneous fistula. The use of vascularized tissue reconstruction has been shown to decrease the rate of fistula formation and also decrease the duration of a fistula when it occurs.

CASE 17

Bharat Yarlagadda

History of Present Illness

A 57-year-old female presents to clinic with a diagnosis of a laryngeal tumor and was previously seen by an otolaryngologist. She has been having increasing throat pain and difficulty swallowing.

Question: What additional questions would you want to ask in the initial evaluation?

- What are the characteristics of the throat pain? She has constant pain in the middle of his throat. This feels worse with swallowing. It radiates to the left ear. This is worsening over the past 2 months but has been present for about 6 months.
- Any masses in the neck? Yes, she notices a gradual increase in fullness of the neck on the left side.
- Has her voice been changing? She reports a raspy voice for the past several months. She was diagnosed with thrush initially, but did not improve with anti-fungal treatment. Her voice is not barely audible.
- Any difficulty breathing? Yes, she has been having worsening shortness of breath with exertion that is now present at rest as well. She now sleeps on multiple pillows and can lay flat only for short periods of time. She feels both her exertional and resting dyspnea have worsened over the past few weeks.
- Dysphagia to solids? Liquids? Both? She reports coughing when swallowing liquids.
- Weight loss? She has lost about 20 pounds in the past year unintentionally.
- Tobacco or alcohol use? 40 pack-year history of smoking, she reports quitting a few weeks ago.

Question: What additional aspects of the history are important?

- Any history of head and neck cancer? None personally or in the family.
- Any prior radiation exposure? No.
- Any recent hospitalizations? Yes, she was recently admitted for pneumonia at a community hospital. She is still on antibiotics for this.

Past Medical History

- Recent COPD diagnosis, on inhalers.
- Anxiety.
- Right side approach, anterior cervical discectomy and fusion.

Physical Examination

Appears her stated age, slightly cachectic. Vital signs are stable. She has mild audible biphasic stridor at rest but is comfortably seated on the bed. Her voice is very strained and raspy, and barely audible. She appears to be handling her secretions without difficulty.

Skin/scalp: no lesions.
Ears: within normal limits.
Nose: normal anterior rhinoscopy.
Cranial nerves: intact bilaterally.
Oral cavity: poor dentition, smells of smoke, no mucosal lesions.
Neck: normal laryngotracheal landmarks. She has a palpable enlarged left level IIA lymph node.

Fiberoptic scope examination demonstrates an ulcerative mass of the left true vocal fold extending to the right side (see Figure 17.1). There is no appreciable motion of the left true vocal fold. There is involvement of the left false vocal fold and

CASE 17   (continued)

arytenoid. The subglottis appears obscured due to the mass and is poorly visible due to the vocal fold immobility.

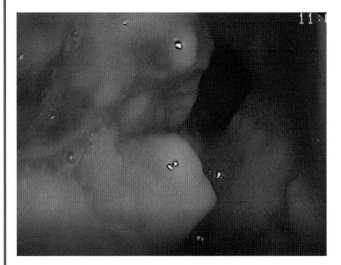

FIGURE 17.1   Fiberoptic scope examination indicating an ulcerative mass of the left true vocal fold extending to the right side.

Management

Question: Which of the following would be appropriate next steps in the evaluation and management of this patient? (Choose all that apply.)

- CT scan of the neck with IV contrast: **yes**/no.

This is an appropriate initial step for evaluation of this patient's laryngeal mass. This particular patient was recently hospitalized and underwent a CT scan of the neck at that time.

CT scan of the neck with contrast is performed and demonstrates a glottic tumor with obstruction of the airway (see Figure 17.2). There is destruction of the inner cortex of the thyroid cartilage and evidence of subglottic spread of the tumor, however no obvious extralaryngeal spread. In addition, there is a pathologic 2 cm left level IIA lymph node.

- CT scan of the chest with IV contrast: **yes**/no.

This is reasonable to perform in addition to the CT scan of the neck. Again, presuming a neoplastic diagnosis, the chest imaging will provide information regarding the possibility of pulmonary metastasis, as well as assess for primary lung tumors given the patient's smoking history. Again, this imaging study was performed during her recent hospitalization and is available to view. There are no lung masses.

- MRI of the neck with contrast: yes/**no**.

Given the workup done to this point, MRI of the neck would not offer additional information or change management.

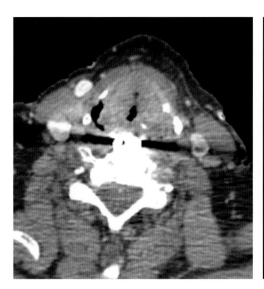 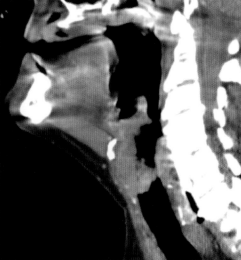

FIGURE 17.2   CT scan of the neck with contrast demonstrates a glottic tumor with obstruction of the airway. The white arrow in the paramedian sagittal view indicates subglottic spread of the tumor.

(Continued)

CASE 17   (continued)

In addition, this patient may not be able to tolerate the examination in his current state given her difficulty lying flat.

- Tissue diagnosis: **yes**/no.

At this point, the most likely diagnosis is neoplastic, and tissue sampling is needed to confirm this. The recommended route is biopsy of the mass via laryngoscopy. An additional option is an FNA biopsy of the nodal disease especially if intubation for general anesthetic is not safe or feasible, and the patient would not tolerate an awake flexible laryngoscopic biopsy. This patient underwent a prior direct laryngoscopy and biopsy with another provider a month ago that demonstrated SCC.

- MBS: **yes**/no.

Given her weight loss, recent pneumonia, and complaint of choking with liquids, this is important to determine risk of aspiration and the degree of laryngeal dysfunction. This patient underwent a prior MBS, which indicated severe penetration and aspiration of liquids.

A thorough discussion is held with this patient and her family regarding treatment and they would like more time to fully consider her options. Her referring doctor had arranged for a gastrostomy to be placed at her community hospital later the same week, given the degree of swallowing dysfunction.

On the day of the gastrostomy tube placement, you are called by the other hospital. She was provided sedation and the tube was successfully placed. However, she developed worsening obstructive breathing, anxiety and confusion, and stridor. Her blood gas indicated hypercarbia and acidosis. She is deemed stable for transfer and arrives to your ICU. Upon arrival she is noted to be have a tripod position, severe stridor, and persistent acidosis. This appears to be a decompensation of her ongoing airway obstruction.

Question: This patient requires a secured airway. What is your plan?

- Awake tracheostomy: **yes**/no.

In the setting of acute decompensation due to an obstructing laryngeal mass, a surgical airway is indicated. If the patient can lay reasonable supine, with mild sedation, awake tracheostomy is a safe approach. The goal is to place the airway incision distal enough to avoid tumor disruption of the subglottic component, but high enough that a stoma may be created without excess tension if laryngectomy is performed. Unfortunately, pretreatment tracheostomy placement is an independent predictor of poor disease-free survival. The exact mechanism for this is unclear. However, this must be accepted if a surgical airway is considered necessary. It is not expected that the cause of airway obstruction, the tumor, be addressed in the acute setting.

- Rapid sequence intubation with tracheostomy: yes/**no**.

Rapid sequence intubation is not advisable as orotracheal intubation may be impeded by the fixed obstruction, and if bag-masking is not possible, the airway may be lost.

- Awake fiberoptic intubation with tracheostomy: yes/**no**.

Awake fiberoptic intubation is reasonable but the passage of the flexible scope and endotracheal tube may be impeded by the tumor.

Question: Awake tracheostomy with direct laryngoscopy and biopsy is performed and the patient is medically stabilized. Repeat biopsies are performed of the mass and a diagnosis of SCC is confirmed. What is her current staging?

Answer: cT3N1M0.

The patient has a fixed left true vocal fold but no gross extralaryngeal spread and would this be T-stage 3. She has a single 2 cm left-sided abnormal lymph node and would thus be N-stage 1. She is group stage III.

Question: Given her stage and laryngeal function, what is the most appropriate treatment for this patient?

- Concurrent chemoradiation: yes/**no**.

Given the severe degree of laryngeal dysfunction in this patient, though anatomic preservation could be achieved, function preservation would be unlikely.

- Partial laryngectomy with adjuvant radiation: yes/**no**.

Partial laryngectomy is not possible given the degree of tumor burden.

- Total laryngectomy with nodal dissection and adjuvant therapy: **yes**/no.

She should be counseled to proceed with total laryngectomy.

Nonsurgical approaches, either upfront definitive concurrent chemoradiation, or induction chemotherapy followed by chemoradiation, are often undertaken as a means of "laryngeal preservation." However, studies in addition to RTOG 91-11 suggest that when comparing site- and stage-matched controls, locoregional control is inferior with upfront chemoradiation, although overall survival is not affected when these patients are treated with prompt surgical salvage for persistent or recurrent locoregional disease. Further, demographic studies have shown a decline in relative survival for patients with advanced-stage glottic cancer, early stage supraglottic cancers, and cT3N0 supraglottic cancers correlating with an increase in the use of nonsurgical upfront approaches. On a practical level, however, these demographic data may not be convincing to an individual patient who desires organ preservation and the patient has the option of upfront concurrent chemoradiation therapy. Here, due to the current status of laryngeal function, a nonsurgical approach would not be appropriate.

A total laryngectomy with bilateral neck dissection and left hemi-thyroidectomy is performed. There is a large left-sided glottis mass with extension to the subglottic region (see Figure 17.3). The entirety of the tracheostomy tract is excised en bloc with the extirpative procedure.

Question: The patient undergoes total laryngectomy with bilateral neck dissection. Additional pathologic

CASE 17   (continued)

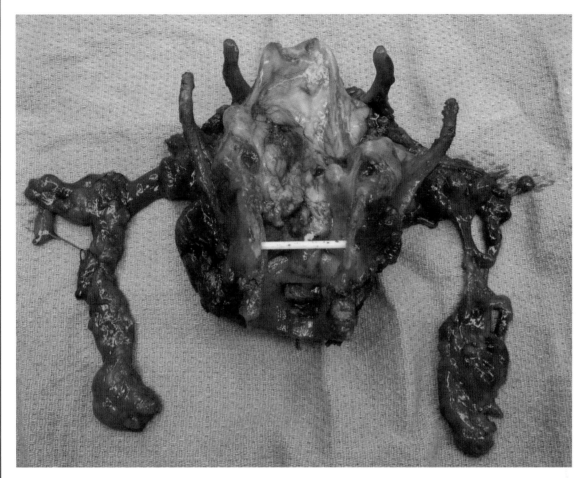

FIGURE 17.3   Laryngectomy and bilateral neck dissection specimen.

nodes are noted in the specimen and the final patholog-ic stage is **pT3N2b. There is no extranodal extension of tumor. The margins are negative. There is no apparent perineural invasion or lymphovascular invasion. What is the appropriate counseling for this patient?**

- Proceed with adjuvant chemoradiation to reduce the risk of distant metastases: yes/**no**.
  There is no indication for chemotherapy in the adjuvant setting for this patient, which is generally reserved for unresectable positive margins or extrano-dal extension.

- Proceed with adjuvant radiation to increase locoregional control: **yes**/no.
  This patient has multiple adverse pathologic features indicating the need for adjuvant radiotherapy includ-ing pT3 status and multiple involved lymph nodes. Observation alone would engender a high risk of loco-regional failure.

Key Points

- Advanced glottic cancer generally requires multimodal-ity therapy, either chemoradiation or surgery with adju-vant therapy.
- Laryngeal preservation is an option but is only worthwhile when there is intact laryngeal function prior to treatment. Those patients with severe dysphagia and aspiration, air-way obstruction, and loss of voice should be strongly con-sidered for upfront total laryngectomy.

- In general, cancer of the glottis infrequently metastasizes to regional nodal basins, especially in early stage disease. Elective nodal management should be considered for ad-vanced tumors and those involving the supraglottic and subglottic subsites.
- Tracheostomy prior to treatment is associated with worse survival, especially in the recurrent setting, but may be necessary for treatment of airway obstruction.

CASE 18

Chase Heaton

History of Present Illness

A 51-year-old male presents with about 6 months of hoarseness, worsening over the past 3 months.

Question: What additional questions would you want to ask in the initial evaluation?

- Any throat pain? No pain in the throat.
- Any masses in the neck? No, he does not note any neck masses.
- Any difficulty breathing? Yes, she has been having worsening shortness of breath with exertion that is now present at rest as well. She now sleeps on multiple pillows but can lay flat for short periods of time. She feels both the exertional and resting dyspnea have worsened over the past few weeks.
- Dysphagia to solids? Liquids? Both? No significant problems swallowing.
- Weight loss? No notable weight loss.
- Tobacco or alcohol use? 30 pack-year history of smoking, current half-pack-per-day smoker.

Question: What additional aspects of the history are important?

- Any history of head and neck cancer? None personally or in the family.
- Any prior radiation exposure? Patient denies.

Past Medical History

- Progression multiple sclerosis, currently not receiving any treatment.
- Osteoarthritis of the knees.

Physical Examination

Appears his stated age. Vital signs are stable. No stridor. Voice is very strained and raspy.

Skin/scalp: no lesions.

Ears: within normal limits.

Nose: normal anterior rhinoscopy.

Cranial nerves: intact bilaterally.

Oral cavity: poor dentition, smells of smoke, no mucosal lesions.

Neck: normal laryngotracheal landmarks. No palpable neck masses.

Fiberoptic nasolaryngoscopy is performed and demonstrates the presence of an exophytic mass of the right true vocal fold, with involvement of the anterior commissure and anterior aspect of the left true vocal fold (see Figure 18.1). The subglottic is not involved. There is intact symmetric vocal fold motion.

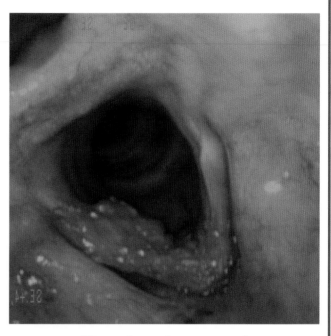

FIGURE 18.1 Fiberoptic nasolaryngoscopy demonstrating right glottic tumor.

Management

Question: Which of the following would be appropriate next steps in the evaluation and management of this patient? (Choose all that apply.)

- CT scan of the neck with IV contrast: **yes**/no.
  This is an appropriate initial step for evaluation of this patient's laryngeal mass.

- CT scan of the chest with IV contrast: **yes**/no.
  Presuming a malignancy of the glottis, this is appropriate for completion of staging as well as screening for synchronous tumors of the lungs given the smoking history.

- Whole-body PET/CT scan: yes/**no**.
  Presuming a malignancy of the glottis, this appears to be early stage disease. PET scan is not inappropriate, but not requisite at this time.

- MBS: **yes**/no.
  The patient does not have any swallowing complaints, and has no evidence of aspiration. MBS is not needed for the workup at this time, although may be helpful for pretreatment counseling by the speech and swallowing specialists.

- Tissue diagnosis: **yes**/no.
  A biopsy of the mass is needed to confirm malignancy and proceed with treatment. This is done under general anesthesia with direct laryngoscopy.

CASE 18   (continued)

The patient's CT neck does not indicate any cartilaginous involvement of the larynx. There are no masses or abnormal lymph nodes in the neck. A CT of the chest demonstrates moderate emphysematous changes without masses or nodules. The biopsy of the right true vocal fold indicates well differentiated SCC.

Question: What is the TNM stage of this patient's glottic SCC?

Answer: cT1bN0M0.

Both vocal folds are involved, but with intact bilateral vocal fold motion. This would indicate T1b status. The tumor is limited to the glottis with no evidence of supra- or subglottic extension, or weakness of the vocal fold, which would indicate cT2 staging. There is no vocal fold paralysis, involvement of the paraglottic space, or of the inner lamina of the thyroid cartilage, which would indicate cT3 status. Extralaryngeal involvement would upstage to cT4 status.

Question: What treatment would you recommend?

- Transoral laser resection: yes/**no**.

While transoral laser resection is a great treatment option for many early stage glottic cancers, this patient's tumor is not ideally suited to this modality. The extension of the tumor across the anterior commissure and onto the contralateral cord would likely result in anterior glottic webbing and a poor vocal outcome.

- Open partial laryngectomy: **yes**/no.

An open supracricoid laryngectomy can be considered in patients with patients with early stage glottic tumors if the subglottis is spared and there is preserved function of at least one cricoarytenoid unit. The location of this patient's tumor would be amenable to such an approach, however it would be important to evaluate pulmonary function given the risk of long-term microaspiration.

- Total laryngectomy: yes/**no**.

A total laryngectomy would offer a very high rate of locoregional and cure, however given that a high rate of cure is also achievable with less morbid modalities, this would be a poor choice for primary treatment.

- Definitive radiation therapy: **yes**/no.

This tumor is ideally suited to primary radiation therapy given the preserved function of the vocal cords, relatively superficial nature of the tumor and extension to the bilateral true vocal cords.

The patient completes definitive upfront laryngeal irradiation. One month after completion of radiation, he has worsening throat pain with new referred otalgia and declining voice quality. His radiation oncologist orders a CT scan of the neck.

A CT scan of the neck demonstrates an enhancing mass involving the right glottis with extension to the subglottic region (see Figure 18.2). There is no lymphadenopathy.

Given the concerning CT scan findings, the patient undergoes nasolaryngoscopy, which indicates fixation of the right true vocal fold. Subsequent direct laryngoscopy and biopsy of the suspicious area indicates persistent SCC of the right glottis with subglottic extension. The patient is counseled on and proceeds with total laryngectomy and elective nodal dissection.

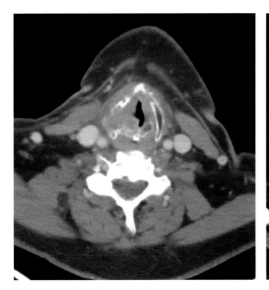 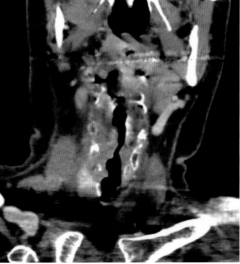

FIGURE 18.2   CT scan of the neck indicating an enhancing mass involving the right glottis with extension to the subglottic region.

(Continued)

CASE 18   (continued)

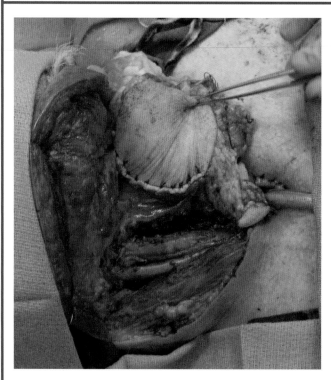

FIGURE 18.3   Intraoperative photograph demonstrating the radial forearm free flap reconstruction of the pharyngeal defect.

A radial forearm free flap is used to reconstruct the pharyngeal defect (see Figure 18.3). A relatively low incision on the trachea was performed due to subglottic extension, and to avoid excess neck skin tension on the stoma, the free flap is fabricated with a second skin island that is used for superior peri-stomal reconstruction as well as peri-operative flap monitoring.

Question: The patient undergoes resection including total laryngectomy, with use of a radial forearm free flap for closure of the pharynx, and a separate skin paddle use for peri-stomal reconstruction and flap monitoring purposes. On postoperative day 12, the patient develops a pharyngocutaneous fistula with purulence and salivary expression from the neck wound. Which of the following would not be appropriate?

- Correction of modifiable wound healing factors, NPO status, and antibiotics via feeding tube: **yes**/no.
- Flow diversion of the fistula with negative pressure wound therapy (NPWT): **yes**/no.
- Hyperbaric oxygen treatments: **yes**/no.

All modifiable wound healing factors should be addressed including thyroid function, nutritional deficiencies, and tobacco use. Ideally, these factors are optimized prior to surgery, but this may not be possible due to concerns of tumor progression. The immediate management of the fistula includes reduction of flow with NPO status, and antibiotics to address co-infection. Diversion of the fistula flow away from the tracheostoma and the great vessels is critical. NPWT has been shown to be effective with this, but placement of the device can be technically difficult. Hyperbaric oxygen administration can be helpful in wound healing after radiation.

- Immediate salvage reconstruction with regional flap options: yes/**no**.

Immediate salvage reconstruction is not generally offered, as the majority of fistulae close with conservative measures, but should be considered for large fistula with high flow, or due to inability to divert away from the airway and/or great vessels.

Key Points

- Salvage surgery can be needed for persistent or recurrent disease after upfront nonsurgical treatment of laryngeal cancer. This is associated with a high rate of wound healing and infectious complications such as pharyngocutaneous fistula.
- The use of vascularized tissue, either inset into the pharyngeal defect or as a muscle-only on-lay flap, can reduce the rate of wound healing issues.
- Pharyngocutaneous fistula after total laryngectomy can usually be successfully managed with conservative measures; immediate operative repair is infrequently necessary.
- The benefits of primary versus secondary tracheoesophageal puncture (TEP) and prosthetic placement is debatable and should be an individualized decision. Those at risk of wound complications may benefit from secondary procedures.

CASE 19

Laureano A. Giraldez-Rodriguez

History of Present Illness

A 68-year-old male presents with hoarseness. He was evaluated by a general otolaryngologist and then referred to you for further treatment of a suspicious laryngeal lesion. He was treated with steroids and his voice improved but eventually became more raspy.

Question: What additional questions would you want to ask in the initial evaluation?

- For how long has he had hoarseness? Three months, and has been worsening.
- Has this happened before? No previous voice concerns.
- Does the patient have a history of smoking? What type of tobacco and for how long? He smoked in the past but quit 20 years ago. He previously smoked a half-pack per day for 20 years.
- Any neck masses? Patient denies.
- Ear pain? Patient denies.
- Difficulty swallowing solids or liquids? Patient denies.
- Weight loss? Patient denies.
- Shortness of breath? Patient denies.

Question: What additional aspect of the history are important?

- Any history of head and neck cancer? He denies this for himself and any of his family members.
- Any prior radiation exposure? Patient denies.

Past Medical History

- He has no other medical conditions.
- Takes multivitamin every day.

Physical Examination

He appears his stated age. Vital signs are normal. He is breathing comfortably without stridor, but with a raspy and strained voice.

Skin/scalp: no lesions.
Ears: within normal limits.
Nose: normal anterior rhinoscopy.
Cranial nerves: intact bilaterally.
Oral cavity: poor dentition, smells of smoke, no mucosal lesions.
Neck: enlarged right level II lymph node, nontender, firm, mobile. No masses on the left.

Management

Question: Which of the following would be appropriate next steps in the evaluation and management of this patient? (Choose all that apply.)

- Flexible laryngoscopy with videostroboscopy: **yes**/no.

This is a good next step in the evaluation of a patient with hoarseness even if performed recently by the referring physician. Stroboscopy is very helpful to assess for submucosal involvement of any lesions and to verify vocal fold function. In this patient, flexible videostroboscopy shows an irregular lesion of the right vocal fold with surrounding erythema and ulcerated center in the midmembranous vocal fold that does not involve the anterior commissure nor the vocal process. The pliability of the mucosal wave is slightly reduced

- Narrow band imaging (NBI) of the larynx: **yes**/no.

NBI can be used to assess the extent of the lesion in the vocal fold. The lesion is limited to the epithelium of the glottis and does not extends beyond the inferior and superior arcuate lines of the vocal folds.

- CT scan of the neck with IV contrast: **yes**/no.

This is an appropriate initial step for evaluation of this patient's laryngeal mass, to assess for the extent of the primary tumor and for regional adenopathy. In this patient, no neck masses were seen, there is no involvement of the laryngeal framework, and there is no asymmetry in the thickness of the vocal folds by the imaging.

- In-office laryngeal biopsy: **yes**/no.

Biopsy of laryngeal tumors can be performed in the office with flexible laryngoscopic visualization, using either a curved cupped forceps or a working channel on the scope. Multiple studies have shown this to be effective for providing a timely diagnosis without the need for general anesthesia. Examination under anesthesia with direct laryngoscopy is the gold standard however, especially when complete tumor mapping and visualization is not possible in the office. An in-office biopsy of this patient's tumor indicates well differentiated SCC.

Question: You see the patient back in the office to discuss treatment options. Which of the following treatment options would be appropriate for this patient?

- Single modality radiotherapy: **yes**/no.
- Transoral laser microsurgery (**TLM**): **yes**/no.

For stage I and stage II glottic cancer single modality therapy, either surgery alone or radiotherapy alone is recommended. Treatment of this disease with either of these modalities is generally associated with excellent 5-year locoregional control rates, greater than 90% in several series.

- Chemoradiotherapy: yes/**no**.

There is no indication for the addition of chemotherapy for early stage larynx cancer.

- Open partial laryngectomy: yes/**no**.

The decision of modality can depend on the patient's fitness for surgery, operative exposure of the tumor, and institutional experience. Open partial laryngectomy for early

(*Continued*)

CASE 19 (continued)

glottic cancers is feasible, but is associated with significantly increased morbidity compared to TLM including dysphagia, need for tracheostomy, and prolonged hospitalization, and as such has largely fallen out of favor.

Question: The patient is inclined to pursue primary surgical resection with TLM. In considering whether to proceed with surgery, what are some important consideration(s)?

- Paralyzed vocal fold with involvement of cricoarytenoid joint: **yes**/no.
  Vocal fold paralysis and invasion of the arytenoid would upstage to T3 status, and the need to resect the cricoarytenoid unit is generally considered a contraindication to TLM. Subglottic extension can be addressed with a TLM approach

- Anterior commissure involvement: **yes**/no.
  Although involvement of the anterior commissure is not an absolute contraindication for TLM, there is known to be a decrease in local control rates with surgery alone when this finding is present. The mechanism is thought be difficulty with exposure leading to incomplete removal. In addition, there is a chance for understaging of the tumor if there is unrecognized involvement of the Broyle's ligament, which would upstage to T4 potentially. In addition, resection of the anterior commissure can lead to webbing or scar formation, requiring revision procedures, and decreasing voice quality in the long term.

- Impaired vocal fold mobility: **yes**/no.
  Decreased vocal fold mobility is still in keeping with a T2 tumor, but may indicate the need for a more extensive resection with removal of the vocal muscle.

Question: What is the stage of this patient's glottic SCC?
Answer: cT1aN0M0.

This unilateral lesion without extension to an adjacent site or to the contralateral true vocal fold is categorized as T1a. T1b lesions extend to involve both vocal folds. T2 can represent extension to an adjacent site or impaired but not fixed TVF mobility. T3 lesions result from extension to the paraglottic/pre-epiglottic fat, minor cartilage erosion, or true vocal fold fixation.

Question: Describe the European Laryngological Society classification of cordectomy

- Type I – only the mucosa.
- Types II–IV – varying depths of vocal ligament and vocalis muscle.
- Type V – entire cord with ligament, muscle, and perichondrium.
  The more involved the resection, the poorer the voice outcomes. In generally, radiation in considered to provide superior vocal outcomes compared to surgery, especially when

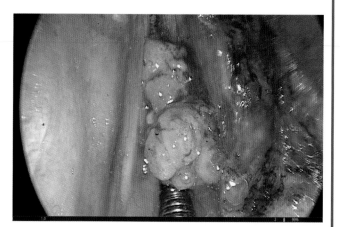

FIGURE 19.1 Intraoperative photo demonstrating an exophytic lesion of the right true vocal fold. The right false vocal fold has been excised to allow for exposure of the lateral extent of the tumor.

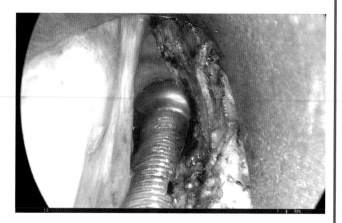

FIGURE 19.2 Intraoperative photo demonstrating the surgical field following complete tumor resection using the CO2 laser.

considering more advanced resections. Some studies have shown vocal equipoise for very superficial tumors, and those tumors arising from the middle of the vocal fold. The decision to treat with radiation versus TLM is a nuanced one. Given equivocal oncologic results, the advocates of radiotherapy cite superior voice outcomes over surgery, whereas the advocates of upfront surgery cite the speed of treatment, lower cost, avoidance of radiation-related tissue toxicities, and ability to preserve salvage treatment options.

This patient elected to proceed with TLM. This was performed with negative margins and the patient enjoyed an acceptable postoperative voice outcome (see Figures 19.1 and 19.2).

Key Points

- Early glottic cancer is generally approached with single-modality treatment, with equivalent oncologic outcomes between surgery and radiotherapy.
- Treatment is associated with excellent oncologic results, with some reports of greater than 90% locoregional control over 5 years.
- Voice outcomes are reportedly superior for radiotherapy compared to surgery, especially for a lesion requiring resection of the vocal ligament or vocalis muscle. The decision for surgery versus radiotherapy is a multifaceted and nuanced one.
- TLM is a surgical modality that can afford excellent results with hastened recovery. Involvement of the cricoid, vocal fixation, or extralaryngeal spread are contraindications to this modality.

CASE 20

Rizwan Aslam

History of Present Illness

A 59-year-old female presents to the emergency department with acute onset of dyspnea. She is accompanied by a family member who relates a history of progressive dyspnea, with significant worsening of her symptoms in the past 24 hours.

Question: What additional questions would you want to ask in the initial evaluation?

For how long has she had hoarseness? Several weeks, and has been worsening.

- Does the patient have a history of smoking? The patient smokes one pack per day.
- Any alcohol use? Consumes two to three drinks daily.
- Any neck masses? No.
- Ear pain? No.
- Difficulty swallowing solids or liquids? Yes, she is having pain with swallowing.
- Weight loss? Yes, 15 pounds over the past several weeks.

Question: What additional aspect of the history are important?

- Any history of head and neck cancer? She denies this.
- She has no other medical conditions.
- She does not take any prescription medications.

Physical Examination

She appears her stated age. She is slightly tachycardic and slightly tachypneic. She is able to maintain SpO2 >95% on room air. She has audible biphasic stridor; she has a raspy and strained voice.

Skin/scalp: no lesions.
Ears: within normal limits.
Nose: normal anterior rhinoscopy.
Cranial nerves: intact bilaterally.
Oral cavity: poor dentition, no mucosal lesions.

Neck: no masses are palpable. Laryngotracheal landmarks are midline and otherwise normal.

Management

Question: Which of the following would be appropriate next steps in the evaluation and management of this patient? (Choose all that apply.)

- Flexible laryngoscopy: **yes**/no.

You perform a bedside flexible laryngoscopy that demonstrates bilateral vocal cord mobility. The immediate subglottic larynx reveals a smooth partially obstructive lesion just inferior to the true vocal folds emanating from the right side (see Figure 20.1).

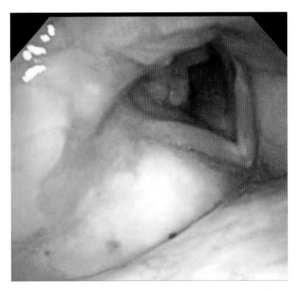

FIGURE 20.1   Flexible nasolaryngoscopic view of the glottis demonstrating the subglottic tumor with obstruction of the airway.

(Continued)

CASE 20 (continued)

- Plain films of the neck: yes/**no**.

Many types of high tracheal and subglottic obstructive pathology can be evaluated with a plain film. Plain films may provide additional information regarding the degree of obstruction, but in this case are unlikely to provide direction for definitive management.

- CT scan of the neck with IV contrast: **yes**/no.

This is an appropriate step for further evaluation of this patient's subglottic mass. In this case, it is critical to determine if the patient is able to maintain her airway and ventilation while laying supine for the scan. Fortunately, she was able to tolerate the supine position and underwent the CT scan (see Figures 20.2 and 20.3).

Question: The patient is observed after the CT scan and continues to have progressive symptoms of airway compromise. How would you manage this patient's impending airway obstruction?

- Awake fiberoptic intubation: **yes**/no.

Awake fiberoptic intubation is generally safe as spontaneous respiration is preserved. In this case, the flexible scope itself may not pass beyond the mass, let alone the endotracheal tube over the scope diameter.

- Cricothyroidotomy: yes/**no**.

Cricothyroidotomy would allow access to the airway, however, if neoplasm is suspected, this approach may grossly violate the tumor.

- Awake tracheostomy: **yes**/no.

Awake tracheostomy is the safest method of securing the airway.

- Rapid sequence intubation with video-laryngoscope: yes/**no**.

Rapid sequence intubation is not recommended due to the high risk of losing the airway once the patient is paralyzed and is found to not respond to bag-mask ventilation.

You perform an uneventful awake tracheostomy and secure her airway. A laryngoscopy is performed at the time and biopsy of the subglottic confirms your suspicion of a SCC.

Question: On laryngoscopy, the tumor is found to be limited to the subglottis, with no apparent involvement of the vocal folds. What is the T stage of this tumor?

Answer: T1.

T staging for subglottic tumors is as follows:

T1 – Tumor limited to the subglottis.

T2 – Tumor extends to vocal cord(s) with normal or impaired mobility.

T3 – Tumor limited to larynx with vocal cord fixation and/or inner cortex of the thyroid cartilage.

T4a – Moderately advanced local disease with invasion of cricoid or thyroid cartilage and/or invades tissues beyond the larynx (e.g., trachea, soft tissues of neck including deep extrinsic muscles of the tongue, strap muscles, thyroid, or esophagus).

T4b – Very advanced local disease with invasion of prevertebral space, encases carotid artery, or invades mediastinal structures.

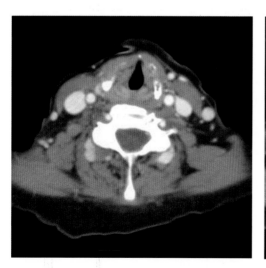 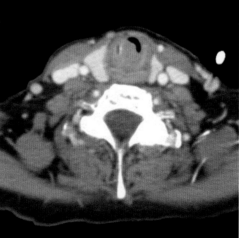

FIGURE 20.2   Axial cuts of the CT scan of the neck with contrast indicates a normal glottis. There is an enhancing mass of the subglottis emanating from the right side with >80% cross-sectional obstruction. There are no abnormal lymph nodes, no involvement of the thyroid or cricoid cartilages, and no extralaryngeal extension.

CASE 20   (continued)

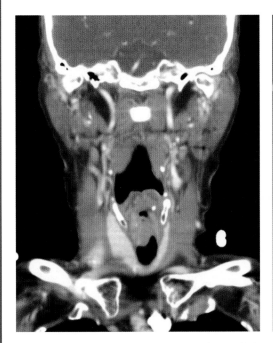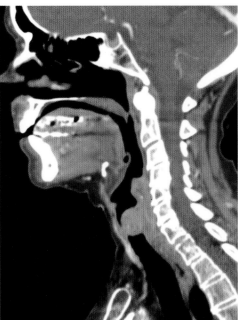

FIGURE 20.3   Coronal and sagittal views of the mass demonstrate high-grade obstruction of the airway.

A staging CT of the chest is performed and does not demonstrate any concern for distant metastatic spread.

You meet with the patient and her family as she recovers from her procedure to discuss treatment options. The treatment of subglottic cancer takes into account some specific clinic-pathologic attributes including predilection for submucosal spread, metastatic potential to the paralaryngeal and paratracheal lymph nodes, invasion of the thyroid gland, and potential for cartilaginous destruction. In addition, most cases of subglottic cancer present in advanced stages due to insidious growth patterns. Our patient became symptomatic from airway obstruction and she presented at an early stage.

Question: What would you counsel patient are appropriate treatment options?

- Total laryngectomy with lateral and paratracheal lymph node dissection: **yes**/no.
  Total laryngectomy, with appropriate nodal dissection and thyroidectomy, would be appropriate in most cases. Appropriate nodal dissection should include dissection of both the lateral neck lymph node compartments and then central neck lymph node compartments.

- Wide field radiotherapy: **yes**/no.
  Single modality radiotherapy would also be an appropriate option.

- Concurrent chemoradiotherapy: yes/**no**.
  There is no specific indication for the addition of chemotherapy, but this may be considered in select patients.

- Narrow field radiotherapy: yes/**no**.
  Narrow field radiation would be inappropriate as it is critical to provide treatment of the paratracheal and lateral neck nodal basins.

Question: This patient choses to undergo upfront radiotherapy. How would you counsel this patient regarding her expected oncology outcome?

Answer: Recent studies have indicated 5-year relative survival rates as follows: stage I at 65%, stage II at 56%, stage III at 47%, and stage IV at 32%. These are comparable to supraglottic tumor survival rates across stages. Early stage glottic tumor patients fare much better. There is no significant difference in survival between treatment modalities: disease-specific survival was 64.4% for patients receiving surgery alone, 56.7% for patients treated with radiotherapy alone, and 55.1% for patients receiving combined surgery and radiotherapy; with no statistically significant difference between groups. Stomal recurrence is a feared complication, and the rates of this can be high. Risk factors for stomal recurrence include: paratracheal nodal involvement, advanced T stage at presentation, performance of a tracheostomy prior to treatment, positive tracheal resection margins, and thyroid gland invasion.

(Continued)

CASE 21

Bharat Yarlagadda

History of Present Illness

A 74-year-old male is referred to your clinic for evaluation of a left-sided laryngeal tumor. He noted the development of a neck mass 6–8 weeks ago. Prior workup by the referring otolaryngologist has found the neck mass to be due to a laryngeal tumor.

Question: What additional questions would you want to ask in the initial evaluation?

- Any pain? No, the patient denies pain.
- Voice change and/or breathing difficulty? He denies any subjective voice changes or breathing problems.
- Dysphagia to solids? Liquids? Both? No, swallowing is normal.
- Weight loss? His weight is stable.
- Tobacco or alcohol use? He has a remote smoking history in his teens for a few years. He drinks alcohol rarely at social functions.

Question: What additional aspects of the history are important?

- Any history of head and neck cancer? He denies this for himself and any of his family members.
- Any prior radiation exposure? Patient denies.
- Any prior cancer history? Patient denies.

Past Medical History

- Coronary artery disease s/p CABG 8 years ago.
- Hypertension.
- Hypercholesterolemia.
- Walks for several miles daily with his dog.

Physical Examination

Appears his stated age, well nourished, and in no distress. Vital signs are normal. He is breathing comfortably without stridor. His voice is slightly strained and raspy.

Skin/scalp: no lesions.
Ears: within normal limits.
Nose: normal anterior rhinoscopy.
Cranial nerves: intact bilaterally.
Oral cavity: good dentition. No lesions or masses.
Neck: 4 cm mass, firm, nontender, left neck, anterior aspect of level II adjacent to the thyroid cartilage. No other neck masses.

Fiberoptic nasolaryngoscopy reveals the presence of a submucosal mass of the larynx occupying the medial aspect of the left pyriform sinus (see Figure 21.1). The mucosa is intact. The left vocal fold demonstrates appreciable motion but abduction appears limited due to the presence of the mass. There is appropriate glottic closure and a normal mucosal wave to phonation on stroboscopy.

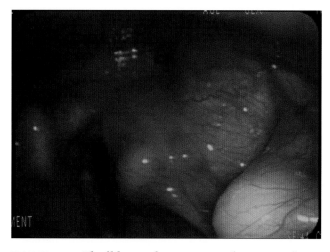

FIGURE 21.1 Flexible nasolaryngoscopy demonstrating the presence of a submucosal mass of the larynx.

Management

Question: Which of the following would be appropriate next steps in the evaluation and management of this patient? (Choose all that apply.)

CASE 21   (continued)

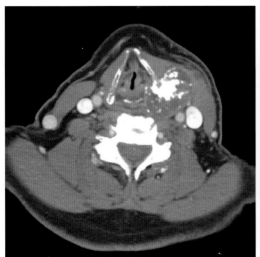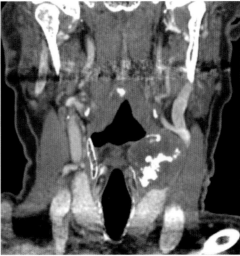

FIGURE 21.2   A CT scan of the neck with contrast indicates the presence of a 4 cm mass emanating from the anterior-lateral aspect of the thyroid cartilage.

- CT scan of the neck with IV contrast: **yes**/no.

This is an appropriate initial step for evaluation of this patient's laryngeal mass. One can presume a diagnosis of neoplasm based on this patient's medical history and presentation. The CT scan will provide information regarding extent of the laryngeal mass, and potential nodal disease.

A CT scan of the neck with contrast is performed and indicates the presence of a 4 cm mass emanating from the anterior-lateral aspect of the thyroid cartilage (see Figure 21.2). It is well circumscribed and demonstrates a "dots and commas" pattern of speckled calcification. There is no cervical lymphadenopathy. There is no narrowing of the airway.

- CT scan of the chest with IV contrast: **yes**/no.

This is reasonable to perform in addition to the CT scan of the neck. Again, presuming a neoplastic diagnosis, the chest imaging will provide information regarding the possibility of pulmonary metastasis. The chest CT in this patient was normal.

- Examination under anesthesia (EUA) via direct laryngoscopy: yes/**no**.

Based on the imaging findings and the presence of intact mucosa, the differential diagnosis can be narrowed and will include tumors of the laryngeal framework. However, tissue diagnosis may be helpful. Transmucosal biopsies can be performed, but deep bites are needed to ensure diagnostic specimen. Violation of the mucosa may affect surgical treatment and resection in the future, however.

- 18F-FDG PET/CT scan: yes/**no**.

Although reasonable, this patient has already undergone cross sectional imaging of the neck and chest with no evidence of metastatic disease. PET/CT scan would not add significantly to the workup or management at this point.

- MBS: yes/**no**.

This patient is not having any symptoms of dysphagia and there are no clinical signs of aspiration. MBS would not add to the management in this case.

Question: This patient underwent a percutaneous needle biopsy that indicated a chondrosarcoma (see Figure 21.3). Describe some typical clinicopathologic features of laryngeal chondrosarcomas.

- Low-grade or well differentiated, chondrosarcoma is the most common.
- Typically occurs in areas of ossification.
- Frequently invades adjacent tissues.

Low-grade tumors comprise the majority of laryngeal chondrosarcomas. Grade 2 lesions are less common, and grade 3 lesions are relatively rare. These tumors arise in areas of laryngeal ossification, such as the posterior inner plate of the cricoid signet. Direct extension or infiltration of adjacent cartilaginous units of the larynx is not typically seen, but adjacent cartilages can be affected due to mass effect with extremely large tumors. The tumor tissue will, however, invade the adjacent normal cartilage of the laryngeal unit of origin, and also can often invade the adjacent soft tissues of the neck. Interestingly, overlying laryngeal mucosa is infrequently involved.

Question: In summary, this patient has a low-grade (grade 1) chondrosarcoma of the left thyroid lamina with intact laryngeal function. What treatment would you recommend?

(Continued)

CASE 21   (continued)

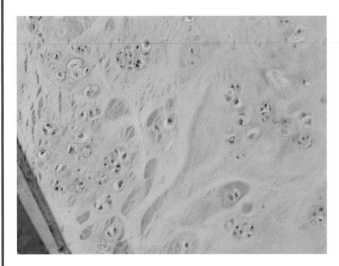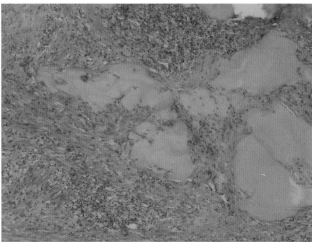

FIGURE 21.3 High-power H&E stain of a laryngeal chondrosarcoma (left) shows hypercellular chondroid stroma with binucleated chondrocytes. Low-power field (right) demonstrates invasion of the chondromyxoid stroma into the adjacent soft tissues.

- Partial laryngectomy: **yes**/no.

Surgery is the treatment of choice for laryngeal chondrosarcoma. Conservative resection with a reasonable margin of normal cartilage and adjacent soft tissue is recommended if possible. Partial laryngectomy can be performed via laryngofissure, thyrotomy, or endoscopic approaches. Unlike our patient, most cases involve the cricoid cartilage.

- Total laryngectomy and bilateral neck dissection: yes/**no**.

Total laryngectomy may be indicated in advanced cases. If the morbidity of laryngectomy is unacceptable to the patient, repeated endoscopic resections of the cricoid component have been shown to produce acceptable quality of life and oncologic control. Nodal dissection is not needed as regional metastatic spread is not associated with this pathology.

- Radiation: yes/**no**.

Upfront radiation, with or without chemotherapy, is ineffective for this pathology

Patient underwent partial laryngectomy with thyroid cartilage resection and preservation of the entire left cricoarytenoid unit (see Figure 21.4). This is performed via external approach with the use of a high-speed bur to perform thyrotomy. The inner perichondrium of the left thyroid lamina is preserved. The mucosa is not violated. The mass is released with disarticulation of the cricothyroid joint after identification of the recurrent laryngeal nerve.

Question: The patient does well after surgery, and returns to baseline swallowing and speech function. Where is he most likely to experience recurrence?

Answer: The most common pattern of failure is local recurrence.

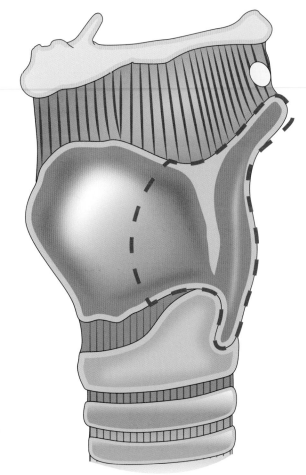

FIGURE 21.4 This schematic indicates the resection of this patient's tumor.

CASE 21   (continued)

When treated appropriately, laryngeal chondrosarcoma is associated with excellent survival outcomes. Large series indicate 5-year disease-specific survival of up to 91.4%. The most common pattern of failure is local recurrence. Distant metastatic disease is very rare; the literature describes approximately 2% chance. Distant disease may be associated with higher-grade lesions. Some studies have indicated that local recurrence is more likely with higher-grade lesions as well; other studies have not found any impact on recurrence related to tumor grade or which cartilage was involved. Overall recurrence can be as high as 35%, but recurrence is not actually associated with an increase in disease-specific mortality.

Key Points

- Laryngeal chondrosarcoma is an uncommon tumor with a low rate for regional or distant metastatic spread.
- Most tumors are low grade and arise from the cricoid cartilage.
- Treatment is surgical with conservative excision via partial laryngectomy or endoscopic resection when feasible, or total laryngectomy when necessary.
- Laryngeal chondrosarcoma has a propensity for local recurrence, but these cases can be salvaged with excellent 5-year disease-free survival rates.

Multiple Choice Questions

1. A patient with cT2 supraglottic cancer requests partial laryngectomy. Which is **not** considered a contraindication to the performance of upfront partial laryngectomy?

   a. Paraglottic space tumor involvement.

   b. Severe COPD with abnormal pulmonary function testing.

   c. Vocal fold fixation.

   d. Matted cervical lymphadenopathy.

   Answer: a. Upfront partial laryngeal surgery can be performed via open approach through a neck incision and pharyngotomy or cricothyrotomy, transoral approach with laser microsurgery, or transoral robotic approach. Gross extralaryngeal spread, such as involvement of the strap muscles, the thyroid gland, base of tongue, or pharynx, would not be amenable to partial laryngectomy. The pre-epiglottic space and para-glottic spaces can be cleared, however. Patients with severe underlying pulmonary disease, especially when resection may impair swallowing, may have a relative contraindication to partial laryngectomy due to the likelihood of severe aspiration postoperatively. Vocal fold fixation has traditionally been an indication for total rather than partial laryngectomy, although sound results have been reported with the performance of a vertical partial laryngectomy in selected patients. Matted lymphadenopathy, or the overt presence of extranodal extension of tumor, is generally an indication for concurrent chemoradiation. This would be offered as an upfront nonsurgical approach to address both the laryngeal and nodal disease, with surgery for salvage as needed. Although encouraging results have been reported in many scenarios, partial laryngeal surgery demonstrates superior results when used as an upfront single modality in patients without the anticipated need for adjuvant therapies due to either local or regional disease factors.

2. You are performing a total laryngectomy on a patient with a T3N1 glottic laryngeal SCC. The tumor involves the left vocal cord with subglottic extension, and a single 2cm ipsilateral level III lymph node. How should the neck be managed in this patient?

   a. Left modified radical neck dissection, levels II–IV.

   b. Bilateral radical neck dissection, levels I–V.

   c. Left modified radical neck dissection, levels I–V.

   d. Bilateral selective neck dissection, levels II–IV.

   Answer: d. You recommend bilateral lateral neck dissections – a left therapeutic neck dissection levels II–IV, and a right elective neck dissection level II–IV. The risk of contralateral occult neck involvement in supraglottic laryngeal cancers with unilateral metastases is high (about 40%), particularly for more advanced lesions extending to or involving the midline larynx. The rate of occult disease is much lower for glottic tumors in general, but an elective contralateral nodal dissection is appropriate in this particular patient with transglottic spread and known ipsilateral nodal disease. Involvement of level I is rare for laryngeal cancers. A comprehensive left neck dissection (levels I–V) could be considered given the evidence of metastatic disease. In the context of planned adjuvant therapy, it is not clear if such an approach would provide improvement in disease control.

3. After salvage laryngectomy, which closure has the highest risk of wound dehiscence and pharyngocutaneous fistula?

   a. Primary tension-free mucosal closure.

   b. Primary tension-free mucosal closure with pectoralis muscle interposition flap.

   c. Free tissue reconstruction of the pharynx.

   d. Supraclavicular flap reconstruction.

   Answer: a. Total laryngectomy in the salvage setting is associated with a high rate of wound healing complications and fistula formation. The RTOG 91-11 data have indicated that 16% of laryngeal cancer patients treated with concurrent chemotherapy require salvage laryngectomy, and 72% remained free of disease within the postoperative follow-up period. This dataset indicates that up to 59% of salvage laryngectomy patients develop major or minor postoperative complications, with pharyngocutaneous fistula occur. The use of either vascularized free tissue or pectoralis flap reconstruction reduces the incidence of fistula formation in the salvage setting. Even if tension-free primary mucosal closure is possible, studies have indicated a decrease in fistula formation when vascularized pectoralis muscle is placed on the suture line in an overlay fashion.

4. You see a patient after laryngectomy who wishes to proceed with voice rehabilitation with TEP and prosthetic placement. Which of the following is true regarding TEP?

   a. Secondary TEP and prosthetic placement has higher rates of infections.

   b. Secondary TEP procedures have a superior speech fluency and earlier speech acquisition.

   c. Intelligible speech is similar between those who underwent primary pharyngeal closure compared to vascularized flap inset reconstruction of the pharynx.

   d. Electrolarynx use and esophageal speech acquisition are mandatory prior to TEP.

   Answer: c. Primary TEP and prosthetic placement at the time of laryngectomy has been associated with an increased risk of wound complications and delay in healing. However, this has not been associated with a significant increase in measurable adverse outcomes or morbidity. Studies have shown that primary TEP procedures may lead to earlier speech acquisition, but in general fluency, use of the device, and complications are equivocal between approaches. TEP voice quality and fluency is determined by multiple factors including patient motivation, extent of pharyngeal resection, and reconstruction methods. The use of an jejunal conduit for reconstruction, for instance, reduces speech quality. Greater mucosal preservation during surgery may result in increased voice quality, but this is not definitively proven. Routine use of the electrolarynx and esophageal speech may predict improved speech acquisition with TEP, but this is not mandatory prior to the procedures.

5. Which of the following lasers cannot be used for resection of invasive SCC of the larynx?

   a. CO_2 laser.

   b. 532-nm KTP laser.

   c. Photodynamic therapy.

   d. 585- or 595-nm pulsed dye laser.

   Answer: c. The most widely used laser for TLM is the CO_2 laser. This is delivered either via a micromanipulator coupled to the microscope, or with a flexible hollow tube. The KTP laser is also used, has reported excellent hemostatic properties, but an increased depth of tissue penetration and injury. The pulsed dye laser is generally used for premalignant lesions, but some studies demonstrate favorable outcomes for treatment of invasive disease as well. Photodynamic therapy is a means of introducing a photosensitizing agent and then applying light to the lesion. There are reports of success with some premalignant lesions, but is not a routine method treating invasive cancer.

6. What are the boundaries of the subglottic larynx?

   a. Superior glottis to the upper margin of the cricoid cartilage.

   b. Lower boundary of the glottis to the lower margin of the cricoid.

   c. Lower boundary of the glottis to the upper margin of the cricoid.

   d. Upper margin of the cricoid through the first tracheal ring.

   Answer: b. The subglottis extends from the lower boundary of the glottis to the lower margin of the cricoid cartilage.

7. Which of the following is true regarding laryngeal chondrosarcoma?

   a. This pathology most commonly affects the thyroid cartilage.

   b. Females are more commonly affected than males.

   c. This is the most common sarcoma of the larynx.

   d. Radiation exposure is a risk factor for development of this.

   Answer: c. Laryngeal chondrosarcoma is a rare entity, and makes up approximately 1% of laryngeal malignancies. This disease disproportionately affects males more than females, almost 4 : 1, with a mean age of presentation in the 7th decade of life in large series. Although rare overall, this is the most common type of sarcoma affecting the larynx. The etiology is unknown, but it thought to be due to ischemic change resulting in malignant degeneration of a precursor lesion such as benign chondroma. Radiation exposure to the head and neck can also result in a secondary sarcoma, but is not specifically associated with chondrosarcoma.

Suggested Reading

Basheeth, N., O'Leary, G., and Sheahan, P. (2013). Elective neck dissection for no neck during salvage total laryngectomy: findings, complications, and oncological outcome. *JAMA Otolaryngol. Head Neck Surg.* 139: 790–796.

Bennett, M.H., Feldmeier, J., Hampson, N.B. et al. (2016). Hyperbaric oxygen therapy for late radiation tissue injury. *Cochrane Database Syst. Rev.* 4: CD005005.

Birkeland, A.C., Rosko, A.J., Issa, M.R. et al. (2016). Occult nodal disease prevalence and distribution in recurrent laryngeal cancer requiring salvage laryngectomy. *Otolaryngol. Head Neck Surg.* 154 (3): 473–479.

Birkeland, A.C., Rosko, A.J., Beesley, L. et al. (2017). Preoperative tracheostomy is associated with poor disease-free survival in recurrent laryngeal cancer. *Otolaryngol. Head Neck Surg.* 157 (3): 432–438.

Chin, O.Y., Dubal, P.M., Sheikh, A.B. et al. (2017). Laryngeal chondrosarcoma: a systematic review of 592 cases. *Laryngoscope* 127 (2): 430–439.

Clayman, G.L., Weber, R.S., Guillamondegui, O. et al. (1995). Laryngeal preservation for advanced laryngeal and hypopharyngeal cancers. *Arch. Otolaryngol. Head Neck Surg.* 121 (2): 219–223.

Coskun, H., Mendenhall, W.M., Ronaldo, A. et al. (2019). Prognosis of subglottic carcinoma: is it really worse? *Head Neck* 41 (2): 511–521.

Dubal, P.M., Svider, P.F., Kanumuri, V.V. et al. (2014). Laryngeal chondrosarcoma: a population-based analysis. *Laryngoscope* 124: 1877–1881.

Farrag, T.Y., Lin, F.R., Cummings, C.W. et al. (2006). Neck management in patients undergoing postradiotherapy salvage laryngeal surgery for recurrent/persistent laryngeal cancer. *Laryngoscope* 116: 1864–1866.

Forastiere, A.A., Goepfert, H., Maor, M. et al. (2003). Concurrent chemotherapy and radiotherapy for organ preservation in advanced laryngeal cancer. *N. Engl. J. Med.* 349 (22): 2091–2098.

Gitomer, S.A., Hutcheson, K.A., Christianson, B.L. et al. (2016). Influence of timing, radiation, and reconstruction on complications and speech outcomes with tracheoesophageal puncture. *Head Neck* 38 (12): 1765–1771.

Greulich, M.T., Parker, N.P., Lee, P. et al. (2015). Voice outcomes following radiation versus laser microsurgery for T1 glottic carcinoma: systematic review and meta-analysis. *Otolaryngol. Head Neck Surg.* 152 (5): 811–819.

Hoffman, H.T., Porter, K., Karnell, L.H. et al. (2006). Laryngeal cancer in the United States: changes in demographics, patterns of care, and survival. *Laryngoscope* 116 (9 Pt 2 Suppl. 111): 1–13.

Koss, S.L., Russell, M.D., Leem, T.H. et al. (2014). Occult nodal disease in patients with failed laryngeal preservation undergoing surgical salvage. *Laryngoscope* 124: 421–428.

Kowalski, L., Rinaldo, A., Robbins, K.T. et al. (2003). Stomal recurrence: pathophysiology, treatment and prevention. *Acta Otolaryngol.* 123: 421–432.

Marchiano, E., Patel, D.M., Patel, T.D. et al. (2016). Subglottic squamous cell carcinoma: a population-based study of 889 cases. *Otolaryngol. Head Neck Surg.* 154: 315–321.

Microvascular Committee of the AAO-HNS (2019). Salvage laryngectomy and laryngopharyngectomy: multicenter review of outcomes associated with a reconstructive approach. *Head Neck* 41 (1): 16–29.

Mo, H.L., Li, J., Yang, X. et al. (2017). Transoral laser microsurgery versus radiotherapy for T1 glottic carcinoma: a systematic review and meta-analysis. *Lasers Med. Sci.* 32 (2): 461–467.

Paisley, S., Warde, P.R., O'Sullivan, B. et al. (2002). Results of radiotherapy for primary subglottic squamous cell carcinoma. *Int. J. Radiat. Oncol. Biol. Phys.* 52: 1245–1250.

Panwar, A., Militsakh, O., Lindau, R. et al. (2018). Impact of primary tracheoesophageal puncture on outcomes after total laryngectomy. *Otolaryngol. Head Neck Surg.* 158 (1): 103–109.

Patel, U.A., Moore, B.A., Wax, M. et al. (2013). Impact of pharyngeal closure technique on fistula after salvage laryngectomy. *JAMA Otolaryngol. Head Neck Surg.* 139 (11): 1156–1162.

Patel, U.A., Moore, B.A., Wax, M. et al. (2013). Impact of pharyngeal closure technique on fistula after salvage laryngectomy. *JAMA Otolaryngol. Head Neck Surg.* 139 (11): 1156–1162.

Piazza, C., Del Bon, F., Grazioli, P. et al. (2014). Organ preservation surgery for low- and intermediate-grade laryngeal chondrosarcomas: analysis of 16 cases. *Laryngoscope* 124 (4): 907–912.

Potochny, E.M. and Huber, A.R. (2014). Laryngeal chondrosarcoma. *Head Neck Pathol.* 8 (1): 114–116.

Remacle, M., Eckel, H.E., Antonelli, A. et al. (2000). Endoscopic cordectomy: a proposal for a classification by the Working Committee, European Laryngological Society. *Eur. Arch. Otorhinolaryngol.* 257: 227–231.

Rödel, R.M.W., Steiner, W., Müller, R.M. et al. (2009). Endoscopic laser surgery of early glottic cancer: involvement of the anterior commissure. *Head Neck* 31: 583–592.

Weber, R.S., Berkey, B.A., Forastiere, A. et al. (2003). Outcome of salvage total laryngectomy following organ preservation therapy: the Radiation Therapy Oncology Group Trial 91-11. *Arch. Otolaryngol. Head Neck Surg.* 129 (1): 44–49.

Wolf, G., Hong, K., Fisher, S. et al. (1991). Induction chemotherapy plus radiation compared with surgery plus radiation in patients with advanced laryngeal cancer: the Department of Veterans Affairs Laryngeal Cancer Study Group. *N. Engl. J. Med.* 324: 1685–1690.

SECTION 5

Hypopharynx

Tanya Fancy

CASE 22

Rizwan Aslam

History of Present Illness

A 65-year-old male presents to the clinic for evaluation of throat discomfort and throat clearing. He has a history of gastric cancer and underwent partial gastrectomy over a year ago. He states that it took several months to recover from surgery and adjuvant therapy. A gastroenterologist is following him, and a mass in his pharynx was noted on his recent esophagogastroduodenoscopy (EGD). He has diabetes and hypertension. Prior surgeries include hernia repair, partial gastrectomy, jejunostomy feeding tube. Currently, he is taking hydrochlorothiazide, low-dose aspirin, and antihistamine medications. He has a significant history of alcohol use but is now sober, and a 40+ pack-year smoking history, and only recently quit.

Question: What are the other important points in history that you would like to know?

Answer: Asking about voice changes or hoarseness is important because a vocal cord paralysis could be a symptom of a locally advanced tumor. Asking about dyspnea, dysphagia, or odynophagia and weight loss are important. Inquiring about any neck masses is another important point since regionally metastatic disease is a common initial finding in patients with head and neck cancers.

He does not report any voice changes, difficulty swallowing, or weight loss. He had not noticed any neck masses.

Physical Examination

Except for mild dysphonia, his examination is within normal limits.

Question: What is the next step in assessment?

Answer: Fiberoptic flexible laryngoscopy is a critical component of initial evaluation and is required in almost all head and neck patients. Hypopharyngeal cancers are insidious processes, and early tumors may be challenging to identify. Performing a Valsalva Maneuver can allow visualization of tumors involving the hypopharynx. One should assess for the following: obliteration of the pyriform fossae, pooling of secretions in the pyriform fossae, edema of the arytenoids, fixation of the cricoarytenoid joints or true vocal cords.

On fiberoptic nasolaryngoscopy, an exophytic posterior pharyngeal wall lesion is seen. The vocal cords appear to have normal mobility and are free of disease.

Question: What would you recommend next?

Answer: In this patient, there are enough findings to recommend further imaging. Computed tomography (CT) scan is the most useful initial study of choice. CT scan is a useful modality for assessing deep tumor spread (pre-epiglottic, paraglottic space, laryngeal cartilage invasion, direct extension such as toward the prevertebral muscles or carotid), and the presence of lymphadenopathy. While magnetic resonance imaging (MRI) may be practical in detecting earlier invasion into surrounding structures such as the thyroid cartilage, it is typically not utilized in the initial portion of the evaluation. In general, positron emission tomography (PET)/CT is indicated for advanced disease but may be beneficial in identifying pathologic lymphadenopathy and distant staging. PET/CT is often used to complete staging, even in early cancers treated with radiation +/− chemotherapy. In this patient, adding PET to CT rarely changes the management. A chest CT is adequate in assessing the most common site of distant metastases. Though

(Continued)

Essential Cases in Head and Neck Oncology, First Edition. Edited by Michael G. Moore, Arnaud F. Bewley, and Babak Givi.
© 2022 American Head and Neck Society. Published 2022 by John Wiley & Sons Ltd.

CASE 22   (continued)

ultrasound can be useful in looking for evidence of lateral neck disease, it will have limited ability to delineate the primary tumor.

A neck and chest CT was obtained. The patient was noted to have thickening of the posterior pharyngeal wall without any signs of deep invasion into surrounding structures, including the posterior pharyngeal wall. There are no pathologic lymph nodes. A CT scan of the chest did not show any evidence of distant metastases.

Question: What would you recommend next?

Answer: Direct laryngoscopy and exam under anesthesia would provide the best information on the tumor's extent and allow obtaining a biopsy sample. Direct laryngoscopy is required in most hypopharyngeal tumors. If a patient is not a suitable candidate for general anesthesia or obtaining a tissue sample is possible in the clinic, this could be omitted. However, especially if surgical treatment is considered, it is best to have all of the information on the patient's anatomy and the extent of the tumor beforehand.

Direct laryngoscopy reveals a friable exophytic lesion involving the posterior pharyngeal wall. You approximate the size of the lesion to be 2.5 cm. The lesion appears limited to the posterior pharyngeal wall without any extension into additional subsites. The biopsy is consistent with moderately differentiated squamous cell carcinoma.

Question: What is the stage of this disease?

Answer: According to the updated 2018 AJCC guidelines, if a tumor has grown into more than one part of the hypopharynx, or it has grown into a nearby area, or it is larger than two but no larger than 4 cm across and has not affected the vocal cords, has not spread to nearby lymph nodes, and does not demonstrate distant disease, it would be categorized as cT2N0M0, stage II.

Question: What are the treatment options for this patient's disease?

Answer: According to the National Comprehensive Cancer Network (NCCN) guidelines, the patient is eligible for single modality surgery (with risk-based adjuvant therapy pending final pathology). Surgical approaches to the primary tumor include: transoral laser microsurgery, transoral robotic surgery, or open transcervical approach through a lateral or suprahyoid pharyngotomy. The management of the nodal basins is critical in the treatment of hypopharyngeal cancer. There is a high incidence of occult cervical node metastasis (30–50%) in clinically node-negative hypopharyngeal cancer patients. Either elective neck dissection or radiation therapy (RT) should be included as part of the initial treatment. Bilateral prophylactic neck dissections are often considered, given the rich lymphatic drainage of this subsite. Bilateral prophylactic nodal radiation should be offered in the setting of definitive radiation. Careful consideration must be given to addressing the retropharyngeal

nodes, which are present in up to 15% of cases of tumors involving the posterior pharyngeal wall. The most commonly involved lymph nodes in the clinical N0 neck are levels II and III.

A total pharyngectomy with or without laryngectomy would not be indicated in this patient with limited disease.

An alternative to surgery would be single modality treatment with radiation and surgery reserved for salvage in the setting of recurrence. Multimodality therapy is considered for advanced stage tumors, either due to the presence of nodal disease or a T3/4 primary tumor. Therefore, concurrent chemoradiotherapy is not indicated for this patient.

The patient is reluctant to proceed with any intervention that would be "deforming" and is not willing to undergo chemoradiation therapy. He does not want any open procedures, including tracheostomy. After your discussions, the patient elects to proceed with transoral robotic surgery and neck dissection (Figures 22.1 and 22.2).

After transoral robotic pharyngeal resection with concurrent neck dissection is performed, the patient recovers

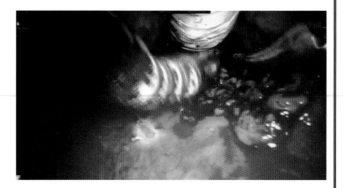

FIGURE 22.1   Intraoperative photo before transoral robotic removal of a posterior pharyngeal wall tumor of the hypopharynx.

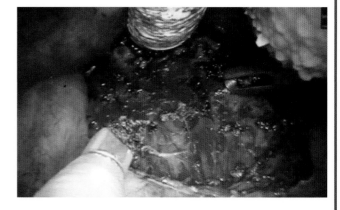

FIGURE 22.2   Intraoperative photo after transoral robotic removal of a posterior pharyngeal wall tumor of the hypopharynx.

CASE 22   (continued)

well without the need for a feeding tube or tracheostomy. The final pathology report shows a 2.2 cm tumor, completely excised with negative margins and no lymphovascular or perineural invasion. All of the dissected nodes are negative for carcinoma. The final stage is pT2N0M0, stage II.

Question: What would you recommend next? What are the indications for recommending adjuvant therapy?

Answer: Patients with lymphovascular invasion, perineural invasion, or N2 or N3 nodal involvement on the neck dissection specimen would benefit from adjuvant radiation. Consideration must also be given to the treatment of close margins. Concurrent chemoradiation should be offered in patients with positive margins or extracapsular extension. None of these indications exist in this patient. Therefore, observation is reasonable.

Question: What is the recommended surveillance routine for this patient?

Answer: The NCCN recommends a history and physical exam every 1–3 months in the first year post-treatment, every 2–4 months in the second year, every 4–6 months in years 3–5, and every 6–12 months beyond 5 years. Close consultation with speech and nutrition services is paramount in the patient's overall quality of life.

Key Points

- Hypopharyngeal cancers are more common in men and are strongly associated with a history of heavy tobacco use.
- The majority of hypopharyngeal cancers arise in the pyriform sinus (65–80%).
- Early stage tumors (I and II) can be treated with single modality treatment with surgery or radiation only.
- The incidence of occult regional metastatic spread is high (30–50%), and the bilateral, regional lymphatic basins should be addressed with surgery or radiation.
- The overall survival (OS) for these tumors is low relative to other types of head and neck cancer, with only 40–50% of patients alive at 5 years.

CASE 23

Chad Zender

History of Present Illness

A 65-year-old man presents with a 3–4-month history of a left neck mass, which he discovered while rubbing his neck. He is not sure if the mass is stable in size or growing. There is no pain associated with the mass.

He also reports mild left ear pain. No fevers, chills, night sweats. No history of prior skin cancer or head and neck malignancy. He has a history of hypertension, hyperlipidemia, abdominal aortic aneurysm (repaired 8 years ago), and hyperhomocysteinemia.

He is a current one-pack-per-day cigarette smoker. He reports 45 years of heavy drinking; he quit 2–3 years ago but has started to have one drink on social occasions.

His mother and father both died due to lung cancer in their 70s.

Question: What additional questions would you want to ask?

Answer: Asking about voice changes, dysphagia, odynophagia, dyspnea, and weight loss are important whenever a neck mass is present. These symptoms could lead the physician toward specific sites in the head and neck and direct the physical exam. Asking about the presence of trismus is another important question that could be easily overlooked.

He does not report any other symptoms.

Physical Examination

A 4 cm round, firm, nontender, mobile, left level III mass is palpated without any overlying skin changes.

Fiberoptic nasolaryngoscopy is performed. The nasal cavity and nasopharynx are normal. There are no lesions of the base of the tongue. The larynx shows supraglottic edema involving the arytenoids and epiglottis. There is a mass involving the left pyriform sinus (see Figure 23.1). The airway was patent, and the true vocal fold moved freely on the right with some restriction of abduction of the left true vocal fold.

Management

Question: What would you recommend next?

Answer: There is enough clinical suspicion for an upper aerodigestive tract malignancy. Therefore, imaging is prudent to further delineate the extent of the abnormal findings. CT scan is the most useful initial study. CT scan allows for assessment of deep tumor spread (pre-epiglottic, paraglottic space, laryngeal cartilage invasion, direct extension such as toward the prevertebral muscles or carotid), and the presence of lymphadenopathy.

(Continued)

CASE 23 (continued)

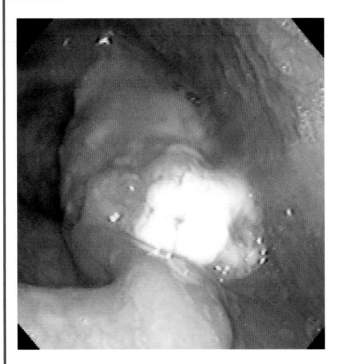

FIGURE 23.1 **Transnasal flexible endoscopy indicates the presence of a mass effacing the left pyriform sinus.**

MRI may be practical in detecting invasion into surrounding soft-tissue structures and may serve as a complement to CT. However, due to motion artifact with swallowing and respiration and the higher cost, it is usually not the imaging modality of first choice.

A CT of the neck is performed (see Figure 23.2).

Question: What would you recommend next?

Answer: The clinical diagnosis at this point is most consistent with advanced hypopharyngeal cancer. Therefore, obtaining tissue for pathologic confirmation and complete staging is the next step.

Exam under anesthesia and direct laryngoscopy and esophagoscopy (at minimum cervical esophagoscopy) and possibly bronchoscopy, would be the optimal way of obtaining a tissue diagnosis as it would provide ample tissue from the primary tumor, allow the opportunity for the surgeon to evaluate the extent of the primary disease, and rule out any concurrent second primary tumors that would alter the course of treatment.

Whole-body FDG PET/CT in this case, after establishing pathologic diagnosis, considering the advanced stage is appropriate and could be complementary to exam under anesthesia. PET/CT is especially helpful in detecting secondary lung primaries in this patient with significant smoking history (see Figure 23.3).

If the resources are not available for a timely examination under anesthesia and biopsy of the primary tumor, a fine needle aspiration (FNA) of the neck mass could establish a pathologic diagnosis. However, interpreting the histologic characteristics of the tumor is difficult on FNA. Excisional or incisional biopsies are not recommended.

Direct laryngoscopy shows a 4.1 cm mass involving the left pyriform sinus, without evidence of involvement of

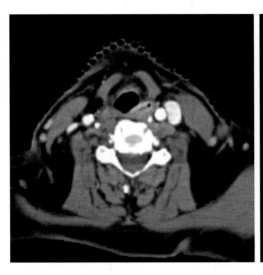
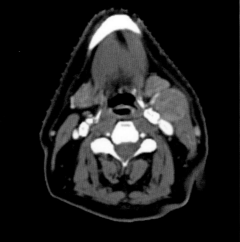

FIGURE 23.2 **In these axial cuts of a contrast-enhanced CT of the neck, there is an enhancing mucosally based mass of the left pyriform sinus. There is pathologic ipsilateral lymphadenopathy with a single 3.5 cm node. There is no cartilaginous destruction or extension to the central neck soft tissues or muscles.**

CASE 23 (continued)

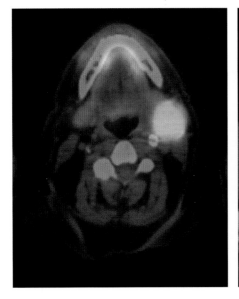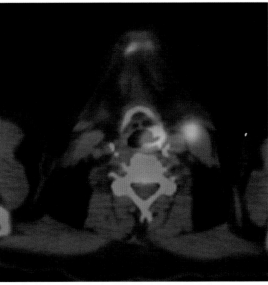

FIGURE 23.3 FDG PET/CT indicates uptake involving the left pyriform sinus mass and a single left cervical lymph node. There is no contralateral neck activity and no evidence of distant metastatic disease.

other subsites. The biopsy is consistent with squamous cell carcinoma.

Question: What is the stage of the disease (based on AJCC 8th Edition)?

Answer: The stage is T3N2aM0, stage IVA. T stage is 3 based on size >4cm and fixation of the hemilarynx. N stage 2A based on a single node >3cm and <6cm. M0 given no evidence of distant metastatic disease. The overall stage is IVA.

Question: What treatment would you recommend?

Answer: A multidisciplinary assessment and discussion of treatment in this advanced case is the most prudent way to proceed. Studies comparing definitive chemoradiation to surgery plus adjuvant radiation show similar outcomes in regards to survival. Surgical treatment, in this case, would require total laryngectomy and partial pharyngectomy and neck dissection and adjuvant radiotherapy or chemoradiotherapy, depending on the pathologic features. Since he has a functioning larynx and does not have significant functional morbidity at this time, an organ preservation strategy is usually recommended. Therefore, definitive concurrent chemoradiotherapy, preferably with a platinum-based agent, is recommended.

Key Points

- PET/CT imaging is important in patients with advanced hypopharyngeal cancer, given the high rate of regional metastatic spread and risk for distant failure.
- In appropriately selected patients, laryngeal preservation with definitive chemoradiation has equivalent survival to laryngopharyngectomy with adjuvant radiation.
- Pretreatment dysphagia is associated with worse disease-free survival (DFS) and OS in the early post-treatment period.
- PET/CT scans performed before 12 weeks post-treatment have a higher false-positive rate and may lead to unnecessary interventions.

CASE 24

Bharat Yarlagadda and Chase Heaton

History of Present Illness

A 74-year-old man is referred to you with a 6-month history of worsening dysphagia. He has a history of cT1N0 squamous cell carcinoma of the epiglottis, which was treated 4 years ago with single modality definitive dosing radiation with bilateral nodal coverage.

His past medical history also includes hypertension and depression. He has a 40 pack-year history of smoking and quit about 5 months ago. He continued to smoke through, and after, treatment of his initial laryngeal cancer. He is a former heavy alcohol user, now abstinent.

Question: What additional questions would you want to ask?

Answer: This patient is at risk for a recurrence or second primary or sequela of treatment. Therefore, asking about voice changes or hoarseness, difficulty breathing or dyspnea, aspiration episodes, new neck masses, and weight loss are important.

He does not have any other symptoms and had not noticed a neck mass.

Physical Examination

No abnormal effort of breathing, voice is slightly muffled, but there is no stridor. No lesions or masses are visible or palpable in the oral cavity and oropharynx.

Neck exam shows fibrotic changes consistent with postradiotherapy sequela, no palpable masses, laryngotracheal landmarks appear normal. Cranial nerves are grossly intact, including facial sensation, facial motion, tongue motion, and shoulder shrug.

Fiberoptic laryngoscopy is performed. The nasal cavity and nasopharynx are normal. There are no lesions of the base of the tongue. The larynx shows supraglottic edema involving the arytenoids and epiglottis. The vocal folds appear and move normally. There is an exophytic mass with retained secretions and debris of the left pyriform sinus. The postcricoid mucosa appears edematous.

Question: What would you recommend next?

Answer: The scenario is highly suspicious for a recurrence or second primary. Imaging of the neck or even a PET/CT in this patient with a history of malignancy is justified. In most scenarios, a dedicated neck CT with fine cuts is needed to delineate the extent of the tumor in the neck, in addition to the CT images from the PET.

Due to the history of progressive dysphagia, a barium swallow could also be obtained to assess the swallowing function.

You order a contrast-enhanced CT scan of the patient's neck (see Figure 24.1).

PET/CT scan has been performed, which indicates a left pyriform sinus tumor extending to the postcricoid region. There is no evidence of distant metastatic disease. A barium swallow indicates the hold up of liquids, solids, and pills and the esophageal inlet.

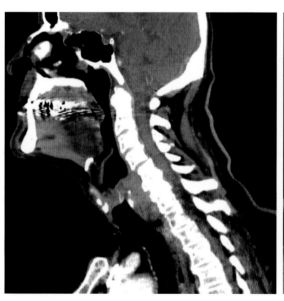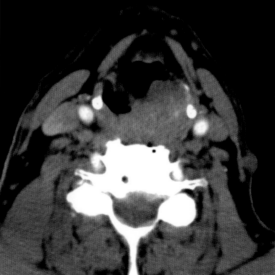

FIGURE 24.1   CT scan of the neck with contrast indicates a mass of the left pyriform sinus, postcricoid region, with extension to the cervical esophagus.

CASE 24 (continued)

Question: What would you recommend next?

Answer: Direct laryngoscopy and examination under anesthesia is the best way to obtain an adequate tissue biopsy and identify the extent of the tumor and its relationship to other structures. If an examination under anesthesia is planned, it is important to perform direct laryngoscopy, esophagoscopy, and at minimum a tracheoscopy to assess the entire upper aerodigestive tract.

Upon endoscopy, a mass of the left pyriform sinus with extension to the apex of the pyriform sinus, involving the postcricoid mucosa, and abutting the left arytenoid and aryepiglottic fold is identified. A cervical esophagoscope cannot be passed beyond the mass. A biopsy is performed, and histology indicates squamous cell carcinoma.

Question: If the maximal dimension of the primary tumor is 4.2 cm, what is the patient's stage and what would be the most appropriate next steps in management of this patient?

Answer: cT3N0M0 left hypopharynx cancer. The best approach is a multidisciplinary review for this patient who has a history of radiation. Due to recent radiation, another round of definitive high dose radiation is not practical. Therefore, the only option is surgical-based treatments. At this time, there are no definitive chemotherapy agents for squamous cell carcinomas of the upper aerodigestive tract.

Question: What type of surgery (to what extent) would you recommend?

Answer: Total laryngectomy is indicated due to tumor involvement of the left arytenoid, history of prior radiation, and anticipated aspiration with laryngeal preservation. Further, the involvement of the postcricoid mucosa might necessitate a total pharyngectomy or a near-total pharyngectomy. Laryngeal preservation approaches have been reported in the setting of partial pharyngectomy surgery. However, the risk, especially in the postradiation setting, is that of continuous aspiration postoperatively with resultant pneumonias, which can be life-threatening. As such, for most procedures with an appreciable loss of pharynx, laryngectomy is indicated for aerodigestive separation, particularly if a total or near-total pharyngectomy is possible. Although there is no evidence of neck disease, due to the extent of tumor and high risk of occult metastasis in hypopharyngeal tumors, bilateral neck dissection is indicated.

He is counseled on and wishes to proceed with surgical therapy, which includes total laryngectomy, pharyngectomy, bilateral neck dissection. The surgery is performed with appropriate removal of tumor with what appear to be clear margins assessed grossly during surgery and with frozen section.

Question: What do you recommend for reconstruction of the defect, if any?

Answer: The goals of reconstruction following laryngopharyngectomy are to provide alimentary tract continuity and restore speech and swallowing function, preferably in a single stage with low morbidity and operative mortality. While options such as cervical skin (i.e., Wookey flap, deltopectoral flap), gastric pull-up, or pectoralis major flaps have been used for reconstruction of laryngopharyngeal defects, the high success rate, low morbidity, superior functional outcomes, and myriad reconstructive options offered by microvascular free tissue transfer (specifically the radial forearm and anterolateral thigh) have made free flaps the preferred reconstructive option of choice for most surgeons (see Table 24.1).

Table 24.1 Pharyngeal reconstructive techniques.

Method of reconstruction	Advantages	Disadvantages
Cervical skin (Wookey flap, deltopectoral flap, etc.)	Local, pedicled skin flaps	-Multistage reconstruction -Open pharyngostoma necessary -Skin often irradiated -Morbidity, prolonged NPO
Pectoralis rotational flap	-Myogenous or myocutaneous options -Outside of the radiation field -Consistent vascular pedicle	-Bulky, difficult to tube for complete laryngopharyngeal recon -Donor site morbidity
Visceral tube (gastric/esophageal pull-up and jejunal free flap)	-Tubed structure -Mucosal lined -Low fistula rate -Outside of the radiation field	-Abdominal surgery, donor site morbidity -Wet, "cavernous" voice -Regurgitation, dysmotility, slow transit with swallow
Microvascular free tissue transfer (radial forearm and anterolateral thigh)	-Minimal donor site morbidity -Thin, pliable skin for tubing -Low fistula rate -Comparable tracheoesophageal puncture (TEP) voice to laryngectomy without reconstruction -Outside of the radiation field	-OR complexity/time -Need for free tissue monitoring postoperatively

(Continued)

CASE 24 (continued)

Question: The patient undergoes a laryngopharyngectomy with bilateral neck dissection, esophageal preservation, and tubed forearm flap reconstruction. Approximately 6 months after surgery, the patient complains of increasing soft-solid and liquid dysphagia and regurgitation. A barium swallow is obtained and indicates a stricture of the neo-pharynx (see Figure 24.2), corresponding to the anastomosis of the flap reconstruction with the esophagus. What is the next appropriate step?

Answer: Assessment for recurrence is always appropriate, but it is unlikely that a recurrent tumor would result in a short segment high-grade stricture, as pictured in Figure 24.2. The problem is likely a postsurgical stricture at the anastomosis between the free flap and the esophagus. Dietary modifications such as a liquid diet can be used but are unacceptable to some patients and may result in malnutrition. Dilation is often a first step as it has the potential to restore oral intake across a range of food consistencies. In the setting of severe stenosis, dilation can be performed over a guidewire. Retrograde wire placement through the gastrostomy can be utilized when there is difficulty identifying a lumen via an anterograde approach. Serial dilations are often required to sustain the benefit. Secondary reconstruction via incision of the stricture with interposition of additional tissue such as a pectoralis myocutaneous flap is an option if serial dilation fails. Several measures are described in the literature to prevent the formation of stricture at the esophageal anastomosis. This includes flaying or "fishmouthing" of the proximal esophagus and the use of a salivary bypass tube as a stent at the anastomosis. The reported success of these methods varies.

Question: Do you recommend or attempt any voice restoration for this patient?

Answer: TEP placement is successfully performed and reported with standard laryngectomy closure, patch reconstruction, tubed reconstruction, and GI mucosal conduit placement. The presence of GI mucosa can result in altered and "wet" voice quality.

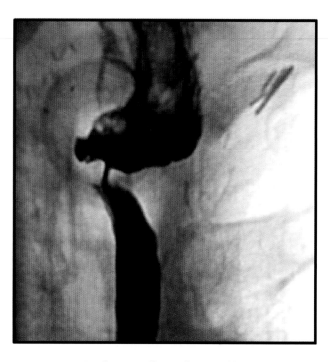

FIGURE 24.2 Barium swallow after total laryngopharyngectomy with free flap reconstruction indicating a narrow segment high-grade stricture.

The preference of primary (at the time of laryngopharyngectomy) versus secondary (as a second procedure after wound healing accomplished) TEP placement is debated in the literature. Earlier return to phonation has been shown with primary TEP, although some studies suggest an increase in wound healing complications and pharyngocutaneous fistula. Therefore, this patient is a candidate for TEP placement. Depending on the experience of the treating team, a secondary TEP might be the safest option.

Key Points

- For most primary surgical resections where there is an anticipated significant loss of pharyngeal mucosa, laryngectomy is indicated for aerodigestive separation, particularly if total pharyngectomy is anticipated.
- Nonirradiated tissue is paramount to restore the alimentary tract and prevent fistula in salvage surgery for hypopharyngeal cancer.
- Serial dilation is often a safe and effective first step in addressing strictures that develop at the anastomosis site between the neopharynx and esophagus.
- Production of esophageal speech and patient motivation are excellent predictors of success with the use of TEP.

Multiple Choice Questions

1. Which statement is true regarding the epidemiology of hypopharyngeal carcinomas?

   a. More common in women than men.

   b. Known genetic risk factors exist in the development of hypopharynx cancer.

   c. It is more common in younger patients.

   d. Hypopharyngeal cancers are more common than larynx cancer.

Answer: b. Hypopharyngeal carcinoma tends to be more common in men in their sixth decade. It accounts for 6% of all head and neck cancers. In North America and Europe, the main etiologies of hypopharyngeal carcinoma are tobacco usage and alcohol. In addition, environmental factors and occupational exposure are associated with the development of hypopharyngeal carcinoma, including asbestos and iron compound fumes. Nutritional deficiencies have also been linked to the development of this cancer, including Vitamin C and iron. Plummer-Vinson syndrome is a rare condition with genetic and nutritional etiologies; the constellation of findings include oral mucosal atrophy, odynophagia, angular cheilosis, esophageal webs, and a predisposition to the development of hypopharyngeal and esophageal squamous cell carcinoma.

2. Which of the following is the most common location for tumors involving the hypopharynx?

   a. Posterior pharyngeal wall.

   b. Aryepiglottic folds.

   c. Postcricoid space.

   d. Pyriform sinus.

Answer: d. Tumors involving the pyriform sinus make up 65–80% of all hypopharyngeal carcinomas, while the posterior pharyngeal wall and the postcricoid space make up 10–20% and 5–15%, respectively. The posterior pharyngeal wall, is contained by the following boundaries: the level of the cricoarytenoid joints, the level of the vallecula, and the constrictor muscles with overlying mucosa.

3. Which of the following statements regarding nonsurgical treatment for locally advanced hypopharyngeal cancer is true?

   a. In appropriately selected patients, laryngeal preservation with definitive chemoradiation is clearly inferior to laryngopharyngectomy with adjuvant radiation with regards to OS.

   b. Laryngeal preservation with definitive chemoradiation always results in poor functional outcomes.

   c. In appropriately selected patients, laryngeal preservation with definitive chemoradiation is oncologically equivalent to laryngopharyngectomy with adjuvant radiation.

   d. In appropriately selected patients, hypopharyngeal cancer treated with definitive chemoradiation almost never results in laryngeal preservation.

Answer: c. Studies comparing upfront chemoradiation to surgery plus adjuvant radiation show similar outcomes in regards to survival, although some studies show a trend toward improved survival in surgically treated patients. This illustrates the need for careful selection and further studies but demonstrates that laryngeal preservation is possible in these patients.

4. Which of the following is true regarding a patient's pretreatment swallowing function and clinical outcomes?

   a. Pretreatment swallowing function has no impact on a patient's early post-treatment survival.

   b. Pretreatment dysphagia is associated with worse DFS and OS in the early post-treatment period.

   c. There are currently no methods to accurately assess a patient's swallowing pretreatment.

   d. Post-treatment dysphagia is associated with worse DFS and OS in the early post-treatment period.

Answer: b. The presence of pretreatment dysphagia appears to have a significant impact on outcomes in head and neck cancer patients. The MD Anderson Dysphagia Inventory (MDADI) helps identify these at-risk patients and appears to be more sensitive than fiberoptic endoscopic evaluation of swallowing (**FEES**) alone.

5. Optimal timing of the post-treatment PET/CT scan in a patient treated with definitive chemoradiation for advanced hypopharyngeal cancer is which of the following?

   a. 4 weeks.

   b. 8 weeks.

   c. 12 weeks.

   d. 16 weeks.

Answer: c. PET/CT scans performed before 12 weeks post-treatment have a higher false-positive rate and may lead to unnecessary interventions. In the setting of continued improvements in clinical findings, a 12-week post-treatment PET/CT is preferred.

6. What finding during physical exam of the head and neck might suggest that a laryngopharyngeal tumor is not resectable?

   a. Bilateral cervical lymphadenopathy on multiple levels.

   b. Inability to pass an esophagoscope beyond the tumor at the time of endoscopy.

   c. Fixation of the larynx to the posterior neck.

   d. Loss of the laryngeal "click" on manipulation of the larynx.

Answer: c. Fixation of the larynx would suggest tumor infiltration into the prevertebral fascia. Firm bilateral lymphadenopathy, while a concerning finding, would still be something that could be addressed with surgery as long as no distant metastatic disease is present. The inability to pass an esophagoscope means that the distal extent of the tumor is not known and that preparation for a completion esophagectomy may be needed, pending additional imaging workup. The loss of the laryngeal crepitus or click is common after radiation due to the edema in the retropharyngeal space. It does not suggest tumor involvement.

7. What is the preferred reconstructive option for a patient who has undergone total laryngectomy and total pharyngectomy, with esophagectomy, in a previously irradiated surgical field?

    a. Colonic interposition.

    b. Gastric pull-up and pharyngeal anastomosis.

    c. Tubed fasciocutaneous free flap reconstruction.

    d. Free jejunal flap.

Answer: b. Nonirradiated tissue is paramount to restore the alimentary tract and prevent fistula. The primary methods of reconstruction for this type of defect include free tissue (jejunum, radial forearm, or anterolateral thigh) and esophageal/gastric pull-up. All have been used successfully. The advantages and disadvantages of free tissue transfer are described in the table. Size limits of the skin paddle for the radial forearm and anterolateral thigh free flap may preclude the use of these reconstructive methods for larger resections, especially with esophagectomy. Moreover, an anastomosis below the thoracic inlet is not only technically difficult, but any leak that might result would put the patient at high risk for mediastinitis. Esophageal/gastric pull-up has the advantage of having only one anastomosis site; however, the operative mortality and postoperative morbidity are typically higher. This remains the preferred method of reconstruction at some institutions. Free jejunum may be used for short or long esophageal defects, has a relatively small operative burden, and often has an acceptable morbidity profile. This is the preferred mode of reconstruction at some institutions.

Suggested Reading

Chakravarty, P.D., AEL, M.M., Banigo, A. et al. (2018). Primary versus secondary tracheoesophageal puncture: systematic review and meta-analysis. *J. Laryngol. Otol.* 132 (1): 14–21.

Haerle, S.K., Strobel, K., Hany, T.F. et al. (2010). 18F-FDG-PET/CT versus panendoscopy for the detection of synchronous second primary tumors in patients with head and neck squamous cell carcinoma. *Head Neck* 32 (3): 319–325.

Harris, B.N., Biron, V.L., Donald, P. et al. (2015). Primary surgery vs chemoradiation treatment of advanced-stage hypopharyngeal squamous cell carcinoma. *JAMA Otolaryngol. Head Neck Surg.* 141 (7): 636–640.

Juloor, A., Koyfman, S.A., Geiger, J.L. et al. (2018). Definitive chemoradiation in locally advanced squamous cell carcinoma of the hypopharynx: long-term outcomes and toxicity. *Anticancer Res.* 38 (6): 3543–3549.

Kato, H., Watanabe, H., Iizuka, T. et al. (1987). Primary esophageal reconstruction after resection of the cancer in the hypopharynx or cervical esophagus: comparison of free forearm skin tube flap, free jejunal transplantation and pull-through esophagectomy. *Jpn. J. Clin. Oncol.* 17 (3): 255–261.

Lewin, J.S., Barringer, D.A., May, A.H. et al. (2005). Functional outcomes after circumferential pharyngoesophageal reconstruction. *Laryngoscope* 115: 1266–1271.

Yang, C.J., Roh, J.L., Choi, K.H. et al. (2015). Pretreatment dysphagia inventory and videofluorographic swallowing study as prognostic indicators of early survival outcomes in head and neck cancer. *Cancer* 121 (10): 1588–1598.

Yu, P., Hanasono, M.H., Skoracki, R.J. et al. (2010). Pharyngoesophageal reconstruction with the anterolateral thigh flap after total laryngopharyngectomy. *Cancer* 116 (7): 1718–1724.

SECTION 6

Thyroid

Rusha Patel

CASE 25

Chad Zender

History of Present Illness

A 64-year-old female was referred for a right thyroid nodule found incidentally on a computed tomography (CT) scan for a lung nodule. She has had a sensation of pressure on the right side of her neck but is otherwise asymptomatic.

Question: What additional signs or symptoms would you like to know about?

Answer: Asking about dysphagia or odynophagia is important. Any changes in voice or hoarseness need to be investigated. For any thyroid or neck masses, asking about shortness of breath, weight loss, fevers, or night sweats, and hemoptysis is necessary.

This patient does not report any of these symptoms.

Question: Which of the below aspects of the patient's medical history are important with regard to thyroid nodules? (Choose all that apply.)

Any history of radiation therapy: **yes**/no. Important to ask as prior radiation therapy increases the risk of thyroid malignancy.

Any family history of thyroid disease: **yes**/no. Also important as certain cancers are associated with familial syndromes. Most notably, MEN2a and 2b are associated with medullary thyroid cancer. Gardner's syndrome is an autosomal dominant condition where well-differentiated thyroid cancer can be paired with polyposis of the colon as well as skull osteomas, epidermoid cysts, and fibromas. Outside of these syndromes, Familial Medullary and Papillary Thyroid Cancers have also been described. A single first degree relative with a thyroid cancer may be due to chance. However, three or more first degree relatives with thyroid cancer may indicate a familial syndrome and would warrant further work up by medical genetics.

Any environmental exposure to radioactive materials (such as proximity to nuclear plants or areas of endemic high radioactivity): **yes**/no. This is an important point that needs to be asked as such exposure has been shown to be related to increased risk of development of thyroid cancer.

She does not have any history of radiation or environmental exposure or a family history of thyroid disease.

Physical Examination

The full head and neck exam is within normal limits. No thyromegaly or palpable thyroid nodules are identified. No other neck masses are found. Mirror laryngoscopy shows normal, bilateral vocal cord movement.

Management

Question: What would be the next step in the workup for this incidental thyroid nodule?

Answer: According to the American Thyroid Association (ATA) guidelines in the management of thyroid nodules, the first steps are thyroid ultrasound and thyroid function tests.

The patient had thyroid function labs done prior to evaluation and these were normal. She also had an ultrasound of the thyroid performed, with the following findings: A 3.5 cm hypoechoic nodule, wider than tall, with clear borders in the right thyroid lobe. No evidence of extrathyroidal extension (ETE) is seen. No nodules on the left lobe are seen. No central or lateral adenopathy (see Figure 25.1).

(Continued)

Essential Cases in Head and Neck Oncology, First Edition. Edited by Michael G. Moore, Arnaud F. Bewley, and Babak Givi.
© 2022 American Head and Neck Society. Published 2022 by John Wiley & Sons Ltd.

CASE 25 (continued)

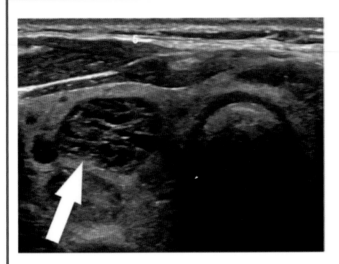

FIGURE 25.1 This transverse image from a thyroid ultrasound shows the right thyroid nodule in question (white arrow).

Question: What would you recommend next in the evaluation of this patient?

Answer: The nodule is larger than 1.5cm, hypoechoic, and solid with a TI-RADS criteria score of 4. Although not highly suspicious, it does meet the criteria for fine needle aspiration (FNA).

An ultrasound-guided FNA was performed. A picture and description of the result is provided below (see Figure 25.2).

Question: Based on this information, what is the most likely classification of this nodule?

Answer: Follicular lesion of undetermined significance (FLUS) (Bethesda III). The follicular cells have round to oval nuclei that lack nuclear features diagnostic of papillary thyroid carcinoma (PTC). These findings meet diagnostic criteria for Bethesda category 3 FLUS.

Question: What would you recommend next to this patient?

Answer: Based on 2017 classifications, Bethesda 3 lesions or FLUSs carry a 5–15% risk of malignancy. A hemithyroidectomy is a reasonable treatment option for this patient.

Question: What are the recommendations during surgery to reduce the risk of recurrent laryngeal nerve injury?

Answer: According to ATA visual identification of the recurrent laryngeal nerve is required in all cases. Steps should be taken to preserve the external branch of the superior laryngeal nerve during the dissection of the superior pole. Intraoperative neural stimulation could be considered (with or without monitoring). The evidence that routine use of the nerve monitor reduces the risk of recurrent laryngeal nerve injury is weak at this point.

Patient undergoes a hemithyroidectomy. The case was uncomplicated and the surgeon identifies and preserves the recurrent laryngeal nerve during the operation. The final pathologic description is shown below (see Figure 25.3).

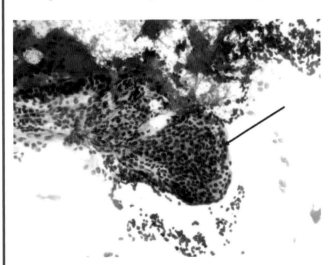

FIGURE 25.2 On FNA biopsy, smears contain scattered three-dimensional sheets and crowded clusters of follicular cells (arrow) in a background of blood and only scant colloid. The follicular cells have round to oval nuclei. No Orphan Annie eye nuclear inclusions or psammoma bodies are seen (Papanicolaou stain, 200×).

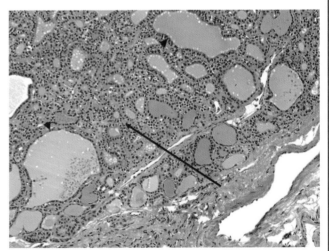

FIGURE 25.3 Sections from the hemithyroidectomy specimen show a partially encapsulated dominant nodule with a mixed microfollicular (arrow) and macrofollicular (arrowheads) growth pattern. No Orphan Annie eye nuclear inclusions or psammoma bodies are seen (H&E, 100×).

CASE 25 (continued)

Question: What is the best classification for this nodule?

Answer: Nuclear features of PTC are absent. These features are diagnostic of an adenomatous (hyperplastic) nodule. There is no evidence of necrosis or dedifferentiation that warrants the diagnosis of anaplastic thyroid carcinoma. The specimen does not have any features of medullary thyroid carcinoma (Round, plasmacytoid, polygonal or spindle cells in nests, cords or follicles).

Question: Postoperatively, the patient notes hoarseness but is otherwise well. Flexible laryngoscopy was performed, showing an immobile right true vocal cord. What would you recommend?

Answer: Although the nerve was identified and preserved during the operation, this is consistent with recurrent laryngeal nerve injury. Data does suggest that the use of nimodipine, a calcium channel blocker, for 12 weeks has been shown to improve the rate of recovery in patients with recurrent laryngeal nerve paresis. The majority of injuries are temporary, and a full recovery is expected in most cases when the nerve is physically intact. In this case, if the symptoms are not too burdensome, a period of conservative management is justified. However, if hoarseness or aspiration symptoms are significant, temporary bridging interventions, such as vocal cord injection, could be considered. If there is no recovery after 6 months or longer, consideration of more permanent interventions, such as medialization thyroplasty, is justified.

Key Points

- The initial workup of incidentally identified thyroid nodules should include an ultrasound and thyroid function tests.
- Low-dose radiation to the head and neck and a first-degree relative with thyroid cancer are risk factors for the development of well-differentiated thyroid cancer.
- The TI-RADs ultrasound grading scale for nodules can use ultrasonic characteristics to risk-stratify which nodules can be observed and which require further workup (FNA).
- The 2017 Bethesda system of classifying thyroid nodules assigns a risk of malignancy based on FNA results.
- Papillary carcinoma has characteristic Orphan Annie eye nuclear inclusions and psammoma bodies on histologic review.
- Nerve integrity monitoring has a role in thyroid surgery, and its use in reoperative surgery has shown a significant reduction in transient recurrent nerve palsy.

CASE 26

Bharat Yarlagadda

History of Present Illness

A 37-year-old male presents for a routine physical examination with his primary care physician. A low, right-sided neck mass was palpated. His primary care physician was suspicious of a thyroid abnormality and referred the patient to you.

Question: If you are suspicious of a thyroid pathology, what other points in history are important?

- Has the patient experienced dysphagia, voice change, or weight loss? **yes**/no. These are important questions to ask about when thyroid mass is in the differential.
- Does the patient have a family history of thyroid disease? **yes**/no
- Has the patient been exposed to radiation? **yes**/no. Radiation exposure can increase the risk of developing thyroid pathology.
- This patient has no other symptoms and has no thyroid disease history in his family or radiation exposure.

Physical Examination

A complete physical examination is conducted, including fiberoptic nasolaryngoscopy. The examination is within normal limits except for an approximately 2 cm palpable mass referable to the right thyroid lobe. No other masses are evident.

Fiberoptic nasolaryngoscopy is performed and shows normal anatomy and normal bilateral vocal cord mobility.

Question: What is the recommended initial workup?

Answer: The initial recommended workup includes a thyroid ultrasound and thyroid function tests.

His recent thyroid-stimulating hormone (**TSH**) was normal at 1.54 mU/L. Thyroid ultrasound was obtained (see Figure 26.1).

Question: What would you recommend next?

Answer: Considering this is a solid nodule, greater than 2 cm, an FNA is justified, preferably with image guidance.

FNA is done. The cytology report indicates the following: Cellular specimen with atypical follicular cells suspicious for papillary carcinoma of thyroid. Note: The differential also includes the noninvasive follicular thyroid neoplasm with papillary-like nuclear features.

Question: What is an appropriate recommendation for this patient?

CASE 26 (continued)

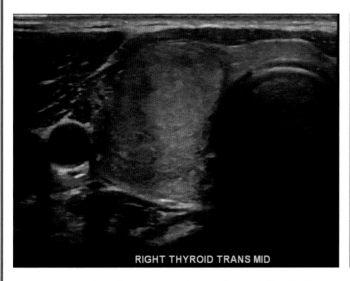 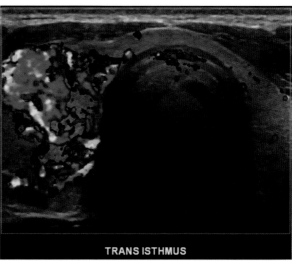

RIGHT THYROID TRANS MID

TRANS ISTHMUS

FIGURE 26.1 Thyroid ultrasound is performed that indicates a right lobe solid nodule measuring 2.1×2×2 cm, with peripheral and central flow on color Doppler. There are no calcifications. There are no apparent abnormal lymph nodes either in the central neck or bilateral lateral neck compartments. There are no nodules noted on the left side.

Answer: Right thyroid lobectomy. According to the 2017 Bethesda system for reporting thyroid cytopathology, the risk of malignancy with the above categorization of "suspicious" is 50–75%. Upon resection, thyroid nodules with this cytologic category may be diagnosed as a noninvasive follicular thyroid neoplasm with papillary-like features. If this is considered benign, the risk of malignancy of a "suspicious" cytology is in the 45–60% range. For this cytology, the recommendations are to either proceed with thyroid lobectomy or total thyroidectomy. Observation is not recommended in this case, considering the size and the risk of papillary thyroid cancer.

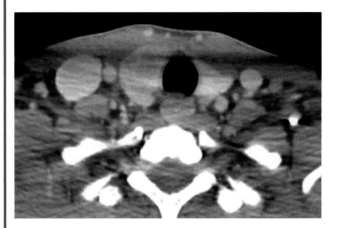

FIGURE 26.2 A contrast-enhanced CT scan of the neck confirms the presence of a heterogeneous 2 cm right thyroid nodule with no evidence of central or lateral neck lymphadenopathy.

In this patient, a contrast-enhanced CT of the neck was performed (see Figure 26.2). While a neck CT is not recommended in many patients with well-differentiated thyroid cancer, it can be helpful in aggressive malignancies to evaluate the adjacent airway and esophagus and also to outline the extent of pathologic lymphadenopathy.

Management

The patient proceeds with right thyroid lobectomy and possible total thyroidectomy. Intraoperative nerve monitoring is used. During the surgical approach, the vagus nerve is identified, and stimulates appropriately as a positive control for the nerve monitor function. The right lobe is mobilized and the recurrent laryngeal nerve is identified. It stimulates appropriately upon identification. Nerve dissection is performed as the nerve closely approximates the ligament of Berry. The lobe is dissected away and the gland ligated at the isthmus. At this point, neither the recurrent nerve or the vagus nerve produces an appropriate response with stimulation. Visibly, there does not appear to be injury to the recurrent nerve.

Question: What is the most appropriate next intraoperative step?

Answer: If loss of stimulation is noted during surgery without evidence of transection, an algorithm must be used to troubleshoot. A positive control should be established early in the surgery with vagus nerve identification and stimulation with an appropriate response. An initial maneuver to address loss of stimulation is palpation of the posterior cricoarytenoid muscle (PCA) with vagal stimulation. If a PCA twitch is achieved, the endotracheal tube may need repositioning. The contralateral vagus nerve

CASE 26   (continued)

can be identified and stimulated to assist with troubleshooting. If laryngeal motion is absent with both ipsilateral and contralateral vagal stimulation, one must assess for issues such as neuromuscular blockade, and /or appropriate grounding and connections on the nerve monitor and stimulator. If contralateral vagal stimulation produces a response, a true ipsilateral neural injury must be considered. If a true nerve injury is noted, it is appropriate to terminate the procedure to assess for glottic function rather than proceeding with contralateral lobectomy and risk bilateral vocal fold paresis. For patients with suspected intraoperative bilateral recurrent laryngeal nerve injury, airway management must take priority. This may involve a controlled trial of extubation, prolonged intubation, or in severe cases a tracheostomy.

In this patient, the procedure is terminated, the wound is closed, and the patient awakens and recovers. Postoperatively he is found to have a hoarse voice with fiberoptic scope examination indicating no apparent motion of the right true vocal fold. He has no swallowing difficulty clinically and is not immediately bothered by the dysphonia. He is discharged home and is seen for follow-up.

The patient's voice steadily improved, and there was appreciable but slightly reduced motion of the right true vocal fold noted on flexible nasolaryngoscopy approximately 2 weeks postoperatively.

Question: What would you recommend for the management of the vocal cord paresis?

Answer: Conservative management in this patient who has no aspiration and shows evidence of improvement is justified. The rate of recovery from nontransection injury varies in the literature. Full recovery can be as high as 67%. Recovery can occur within days to weeks, with 80% of recovery occurring within 6 months of injury. The use of calcium channel blockers may improve the rate of recovery of paresis and should be considered in patients that lack contraindications.

Before the 6 month interval, the role of medialization via injection depends on the patient's speech and swallowing status. Permanent medialization via implant should be delayed until at least 6 months injury. In these instances, a laryngeal electromyography (EMG) may be helpful to assess for potential nerve recovery.

The pathology report shows: Multifocal PTC, follicular variant, largest foci is 2.4 cm. The tumor extends into peri thyroid soft tissue but does not invade the muscle. Tumor is unencapsulated, and suspicious foci of lymphovascular invasion (LVI) are seen. Margins of resection are free of tumor. No lymph nodes in the specimen. TNM stage: pT3, pNX, pMX.

Question: What would you recommend next?

Answer: This patient has demonstrated multiple adverse pathologic risk features on the lobectomy specimen that include multifocality, ETE, and size of tumor greater than 1 cm. Completion thyroidectomy is recommended, in most scenarios, for this patient due to the risk of multifocal disease in the contralateral lobe despite the lack of sonographically evident nodules.

The National Comprehensive Cancer Network indicates that thyroid lobectomy alone is adequate for circumstances of papillary carcinoma <4 cm without radiation exposure, no other risk features, no extrathyroidal or vascular invasion, and unifocal disease.

Question: What is the recommended timing for completion thyroidectomy?

Answer: The optimal timing for completion thyroidectomy is debatable. Most authors advocate waiting 6–8 weeks from initial surgery to allow for improvement in the immediate postoperative inflammatory changes. In this instance, it also would be recommended to wait until recovery of the vocal fold mobility is seen. If the immobility persists longer than 6 months, suggesting a permanent injury, consideration may also be given to a two-step ablation of the contralateral lobe using radioactive iodine (RAI) in an effort to avoid the risk of bilateral true vocal fold immobility.

Question: Would you recommend central compartment neck dissection in this patient?

Answer: Performance of central neck dissection for clinically negative compartment is a debated topic. Large recent studies have shown the oncologic safety of observing the clinically negative central neck, with very low rates of central neck nodal failure. Therefore, in the absence of clinical evidence of disease, most experts recommend observation.

Key Points

- The 2017 Bethesda classification includes a consideration of the diagnosis of NIFPT. This can help in further risk stratification of thyroid nodules and should be clarified by pathology.
- Intraoperative nerve monitoring should be used as a guide for determining nerve injury. If injury is detected, consideration should be given to delaying the contralateral side.
- Vocal cord paralysis is considered permanent after 6–12 months. Immediate postoperative management includes steroid treatment and calcium channel blockers; however, there is not definitive evidence of improved outcomes with these medications.
- Indications for completion thyroidectomy after a diagnosis of papillary thyroid cancer includes tumor >4 cm, extrathyroidal invasion, multifocal disease, or evidence of regionally metastatic disease.
- For patients with suspected intraoperative bilateral recurrent laryngeal nerve injury, airway management must take priority. This may involve a controlled trial of extubation, prolonged intubation, or in severe cases a tracheostomy.

CASE 27

Luiz P. Kowalski

History of Present Illness

A 22-year-old woman was first diagnosed with thyroid nodules 6 years ago. After clinical evaluation and ultrasound in a community hospital, clinical follow-up was recommended. Two years ago, she developed enlarged bilateral slow-growing lymph nodes that were considered reactive. In the last 6 months the nodes have become more apparent but did not cause any other symptoms.

Question: What are the other important points in history that you would like to know?

- Does the patient have changes in voice, dysphagia, or odynophagia? **yes**/no. These are important questions to ask when working up a lower neck mass.
- Has the patient had exposure to radiation, either environmental or with medical treatments? **yes**/no. Radiation exposure can predispose to several malignancies, specifically those of the thyroid.
- Does the patient have a family history of thyroid disease? **yes**/no. A family history of thyroid disease could allude to similar pathology in the patient.
- Has the patient had any other noticeable lymphadenopathy? **yes**/no. Considering other systemic disease in select populations is important, including lymphoma, tuberculosis and metastatic disease.
- She has not noticed any changes in her voice or any difficulty in swallowing or weight loss. She has no family history of thyroid cancer or exposure to radiation.

Physical Examination

Neck palpation reveals bilateral levels II, III, and Vb lymph nodes. The largest one measuring 5 cm in size is in the right level II region (see Figure 27.1).

The thyroid is palpable with multiple mobile hard nodules, the largest one in the left lobe measures 3 cm.

The rest of the examination, including flexible laryngoscopy is normal.

Management

Question: What would you recommend next?

Answer: The probability of a neoplastic disease is high enough that imaging of the neck and FNA of the lymph nodes and thyroid nodules is recommended. The initial imaging of choice in this scenario is ultrasound.

Ultrasound shows multiple enlarged, hypoechoic lymph nodes without a fatty hilum (see Figure 27.2) in both sides of the neck. The thyroid shows multiple nodules with microcalcifications. There is no evidence of ETE on ultrasound. An

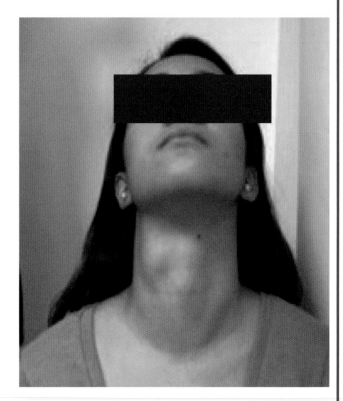

FIGURE 27.1   This photo shows the patient's prominent right neck mass seen on physical exam.

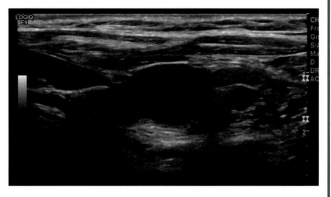

FIGURE 27.2   This transverse ultrasound image shows a hypoechoic lymph node without a fatty hilum.

FNA of one lymph node is performed and metastatic PTC was diagnosed.

Question: What would you recommend next?

Answer: The mainstay of treatment in PTC is surgery. In this patient, the treatment would require total thyroidectomy,

CASE 27 (continued)

central compartment neck dissection and bilateral neck dissection.

Question: What other tests or studies (if any) you would like to obtain before proceeding with surgery?

Answer: Considering the volume of the disease and the fact that it has been neglected for years, additional tests might be indicated here. Measuring Thyroglobulin is not routinely recommended, but in this case could establish a baseline for future surveillance. Additionally, a very high thyroglobulin level could warrant a further workup to rule out distant metastatic disease. However, even the presence of distant metastatic disease is not a contraindication for surgical treatment.

CT scan is recommended as an adjunct to ultrasound for patients with suspected advanced local or regional disease, including patients with multiple/bulky lymph nodes or invasive primary tumors. Obtaining a CT scan to delineate the anatomic details and ruling out tracheal invasion and better study the central compartment for operative planning might be helpful in this case.

Question: What type of neck dissection would you recommend?

Answer: In the presence of bilateral metastases, level II, III, IV, and Vb must be included in the dissection. Level I and Va are not usually involved, and can be spared in most patients. In almost all cases of lateral lymph node metastases it is essential that the central compartment (level VI) nodes are addressed and dissected.

The surgery is performed. The patient recovers without complications. Her voice is normal and she does not have hypocalcemia.

Final pathology report shows multifocal conventional thyroid papillary carcinoma with no ETE. The largest primary tumor was 3.8 cm in size. Bilateral lymph node metastases were confirmed from levels II to VI (largest with 5.5 cm) with extracapsular extension. Radioiodine scan was negative for distant disease.

Question: What is the stage of this disease?

Answer: T2N1bM0, younger than 55 years old, stage I. It is a T2 disease because the largest tumor is larger than 2 cm but smaller than 4 cm without ETE. The N stage is N1b because

there are lateral cervical nodes involved positive lymph nodes. The clinical stage is I because the patient is younger than 55 years and there is no distant metastases detected.

Question: According to ATA guidelines, what is the risk of recurrence for this patient?

Answer: This patient is in the high-risk group because of the presence of more than three positive lymph nodes and extranodal extension (ENE) (approximately 40% recurrence risk).

Question: What would you recommend next?

Answer: ATA guidelines recommend RAI in patients at high risk of structural recurrence. This generally includes patients with well-differentiated thyroid cancer >4 cm in size or gross nodal disease. In the same risk group, initial TSH suppression to below 0.1 mU/L is recommended. This patient has clear indications for recommending RAI therapy and TSH suppression.

Question: Patient received 175 mCi of RAI. The patient is followed with serial ultrasounds of the central and lateral neck, as well as thyroglobulin (Tg) levels and thyroglobulin antibody (Tg-ab). After 1 year of follow-up, her labs are Tg of 15 ng/mL and Tg-Ab <0.1 with a TSH of <0.1. Ultrasound shows postoperative changes in the thyroid bed and no clear evidence of recurrent disease in the neck. Whole-body iodine scan does not show any uptake. What could be considered next to rule out recurrent disease?

Answer: FDG-PET/CT. Patients who present with laboratory values concerning for recurrent disease should undergo imaging. Patients with a negative whole-body iodine scan, elevated Tg (>10 ng/mL), and negative Tg-Ab should undergo FDG-PET/CT. Certain well-differentiated thyroid cancers may lose iodine avidity over time; these tumors can be better detected with FDG-PET/CT. The sensitivity of FDG-PET/CT decreases in patients with a Tg level <10 ng/mL and, in this situation, should be avoided. Ultrasound can be an adjunct to FDG-PET/CT and may help identify small areas of nodal recurrence; however, ultrasound may miss retropharyngeal or retrocervical nodal recurrences.

Key Points

- A growing neck mass in an otherwise asymptomatic patient with thyroid nodules is likely to be metastatic thyroid cancer.
- Initial workup should include laryngoscopy. Ultrasound is recommended of the central and lateral neck to evaluate for nodal disease. CT should be considered for advanced/extensive disease.
- Level Vb must be included in the neck dissection for lateral neck disease in cases of metastatic thyroid cancer.
- Lymph nodes >3 cm, incomplete tumor resection, gross thyroidal extension, and distant metastatic disease all place a patient at high risk on the ATA risk stratification system.
- FDG-PET/CT should be considered in patients with Tg > 10 ng/mL and negative whole-body iodine imaging.

CASE 28

Arnaud Bewley and Michael G. Moore

History of Present Illness

A 33-year-old male presents to your office with a chief complaint of bilateral neck masses. He first noticed them a few months ago and they have slowly been enlarging since then.

What additional questions would you want to ask in the initial evaluation?

- Any other symptoms from it? Yes. Mild pain around the masses.
- Any fevers, chills, or night sweats? Patient denies.
- Any other adjacent lumps that have been noticed? Yes. He has had a vague fullness in each side of his lateral neck that has been slowly enlarging over this same period.
- Any change to his voice or swallowing? No voice change. Mild difficulty swallowing solid foods.
- Any throat pain or ear pain? Patient denies.
- Any prior skin tumors removed or history of head and neck cancer? Patient denies.
- Any weakness or twitching of the face? Patient denies.
- Any numbness of the face? Patient denies.
- Any change in hearing? Patient denies.
- Any tinnitus? Patient denies.
- Any difficulty opening and closing the mouth? Patient denies.

Question: What additional aspects of the history are important?

- Has he had any prior evaluation of the area? Patient denies.
- Any prior head and neck surgery or radiation? Patient denies.
- Any family history of neck masses or thyroid disease? Mother with thyroid cancer of an unknown type. Patient's sister had a pituitary adenoma removed in her 20s.
- Any history of tobacco use? Patient denies.
- Any history of regular alcohol use? Patient denies.
- Any heat or cold intolerance or known thyroid disease? Patient denies.
- Any palpitations or flushing? Patient denies.

Physical Examination

General: he is an adult male with a normal voice, breathing comfortably and in no distress.
  Ears: within normal limits, bilaterally.
  Anterior rhinoscopy is normal.
  Oral cavity exam shows no lesions. Normal salivary flow. No obvious stones.
  Oropharynx: no lesions. Soft palate elevates in the midline.
  Neck exam shows bilateral firm, mobile LAD from levels II–V (see Figure 28.1). All nodes are less than 6 cm in size. The thyroid is mildly enlarged and has firm nodularity bilaterally. It feels mobile from surrounding structures. No other palpable neck masses noted.

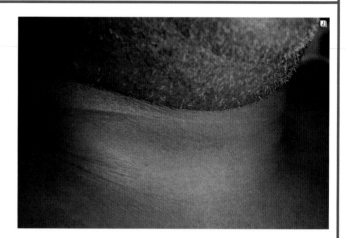

FIGURE 28.1   This photo shows an area of fullness in the right neck representing underlying lymphadenopathy.

Cranial nerves: II–XII grossly within normal limits.

Management

Question: What else would you consider as part of your initial evaluation? (Choose all that apply.)

- Fiberoptic exam? **Yes**/no. There were no obvious mucosal lesions. The anatomy of the nasopharynx, oropharynx, hypopharynx and larynx appeared normal and the sensation and motion of the larynx were intact.
- Office ultrasound? **Yes**/no. Office ultrasound demonstrates the following:
  Right side: Diffusely enlarged lymph nodes within levels II–V, with the largest being a 3.3 cm node in level IV.
  Left side: Multiple enlarged lymph nodes in levels II–V with the largest being a 2.5 cm node in level IV.
  The thyroid has multiple hypoechoic nodules.
  You perform an FNA biopsy of the thyroid mass in your office under ultrasound guidance.
- Thyroid function test: **Yes**/No. This is always a reasonable consideration for any patient being evaluated for a thyroid nodule. In this instance, the TSH and free T3 and free T4 were normal.

Question: Which of the following would be the most appropriate next step in the evaluation of this patient?

- Excisional lymph node biopsy: yes/**no**. For patients with presumed regionally metastatic cancer of the thyroid or aerodigestive tract, tissue diagnosis should be obtained with an FNA. Excisional biopsies should only be performed with FNA shows no cancer and there is a concern for underlying lymphoma.
- CT of the neck, chest, and abdomen with IV contrast: **yes**/no. This is a young patient with significant bilateral cervical lymphadenopathy along with concerning thyroid

CASE 28   (continued)

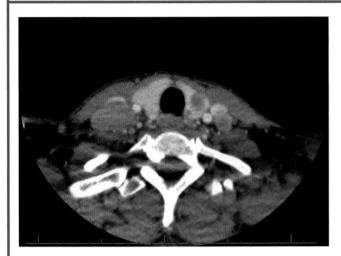

FIGURE 28.2   **This is an axial CT scan of the neck with IV contrast demonstrating bilateral pathologic lymphadenopathy as well as a left-sided thyroid nodule.**

nodules. The differential diagnosis is most consistent with a thyroid malignancy, likely medullary thyroid cancer. The next appropriate step would therefore be to continue the staging workup by evaluating the neck, chest, and abdomen with a CT with IV contrast (see Figure 28.2).

Question: With the leading diagnosis in this patient being metastatic medullary thyroid cancer, what would be additional next steps to consider in the evaluation of this patient?

Answer: In this patient with regionally advanced medullary thyroid cancer, the next step is to complete their staging with assessment of the serum calcitonin to evaluate the overall disease burden. Additionally, it is also important to consider the potential presence of an underlying genetic mutation and/or a familial syndrome. For medullary thyroid cancer, the most frequently implicated gene affected is the RET oncogene, with the type of mutation often predicting clinical behavior.

Medullary thyroid cancer can be sporadic or occur in the contest of familial medullary thyroid cancer, or as a component of familial multiple endocrine neoplasia syndromes 2A and 2B. In MEN 2A, medullary thyroid cancer is also associated with pheochromocytomas and hyperparathyroidism, while in MEN 2B patients are predisposed to MTC and pheochromocytomas, without hyperparathyroidism. In addition to checking a serum intact PTH, 24-hour urine catecholamines and metanephrines should also be sent.

The patient's calcitonin level was found to be 3110 and there was no observed RET mutation or evidence of pheochromocytoma. Calcium and PTH levels were normal. The patient was offered primary surgery.

Question: Which of the following should be discussed with the patient as a risk from the surgery? (Choose all that apply.)

- Tumor recurrence: **yes**/no. Given the extent of disease, this patient would be at risk for local, regional and distant recurrence.
- Dry mouth: yes/**no**. This may occur if adjuvant radiation is employed but not from the primary surgery.
- Change in speech: **yes**/no. A low risk of injury to cranial nerve XII exists with neck dissection, but this would not be a likely outcome.
- Change in voice: **yes**/no. This patient has a normal preoperative fiberoptic laryngoscopy suggesting intact vagal and recurrent laryngeal nerve function. Due to the extent of lateral and central neck disease, there is the potential for paresis or paralysis of the nerve with surgery.
- Development of first-bite syndrome: yes/**no**. This complication is more likely when significant surgery is required on the superior aspect of the carotid arterial system. A modified radical or lateral neck dissection is not likely to result in this complication, which is thought to be caused by disruption of the sympathetic input to the parotid glands.
- Need for further treatment: **yes**/no. With the extent of local and regional disease, consideration should be made for possible adjuvant external beam radiation therapy (EBRT).
- Shoulder weakness: **yes**/no. This is a risk of any lateral or modified radical neck dissection due to dissection around the spinal accessory nerve.
- Hypocalcemia: **yes**/no. This is a significant risk in this patient given the extent of primary and adjacent central neck disease. For patients undergoing bilateral surgery, the risk of transient and permanent hypoparathyroidism ranges from 19 to 38% and 0 to 3%, respectively. Assessment of intraoperative or postoperative PTH levels as well as corrected serum calcium should be performed, providing supplementation as needed.
- Chyle fistula: **yes**/no. With extensive nodal disease, especially low in the neck, there is the potential for injury to the thoracic duct and/or other dilated accessory lymphatic channels. The patient is scheduled for a total thyroidectomy, bilateral central neck dissection, and bilateral extended lateral neck dissection levels II–Vb.

Question: At the time of the surgery and central neck dissection, both inferior parathyroid glands are involved with nodal disease. The right superior parathyroid appears dusky in appearance while the left superior parathyroid gland appears normal. What would be the most appropriate course of action?

Answer: Reimplantation of the right superior parathyroid gland in the ipsilateral sternocleidomastoid muscle. In this patient with aggressive cancer, it would not be advisable to

(Continued)

CASE 28 (continued)

reimplant the inferior parathyroid glands as they are involved with disease. Similarly, it is typically not recommended to re-implant tissue from a field involved with cancer to a distant site. As a result, forearm reimplantation would not be recommended here. While MTC and hyperparathyroidism can be linked in patients with MEN 2A, this patient does not carry this diagnosis and as a result, it would not be recommended to remove the glands. If a parathyroid gland appears healthy in situ, it should ideally be left in place. If it appears dusky, it is recommended to morselize it and implant it in an adjacent muscle pocket as a free graft to optimize the chance of recovery of function.

During the right central neck dissection the right recurrent laryngeal nerve is noted to be grossly involved with tumor (see Figure 28.3). Despite intact stimulation at the onset of the case, manipulation of the involved nerve and dissection of the surrounding tumor results in loss of nerve conduction as measured by your nerve monitor. The tumor is otherwise free from the trachea and esophagus. The contralateral lobe of the thyroid has been successfully removed and contralateral nerve function is confirmed to be intact.

Question: What would be the most appropriate course of action?

Answer: Sacrifice of the nerve with the goal of gross total resection. For papillary and follicular carcinoma, the ATA and NCCN recommend preserving an involved nerve and debulking to microscopic disease. These recommendations rely on the efficacy of the RAI in ablating small volume remnants of disease while maximizing the chance of a complete functional

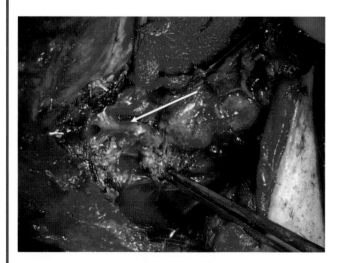

FIGURE 28.3 This intraoperative image shows the right recurrent laryngeal nerve that is anatomically intact but with obvious pathologic change related to the patient's medullary thyroid cancer.

recovery. However, adjuvant therapy for medullary relies on EBRT and these tumors are unfortunately not particularly radiosensitive. Gross residual disease left in the neck after surgery can be difficult to cure and as such all efforts should be made to obtain a gross total resection even if requiring sacrifice of one recurrent nerve. Primary anastomosis with a nerve graft or an ansa cervicalis neurorrhaphy should be considered at the time of the surgery.

Question: The patient undergoes a successful total thyroidectomy, bilateral central neck dissection, bilateral level II–V selective neck dissection and reimplantation of the right superior parathyroid gland. Postoperatively, they are noted to have a PTH of 2 pg/mL in the recovery room. Their corrected serum calcium is 8.9. They have no peri-oral or hand numbness or tingling. No muscle cramping. What would be the most appropriate course of action?

Answer: Institute oral calcium and vitamin D supplementation. In this patient, they have postoperative hypoparathyroidism. With a level less than 15 pg/mL (some studies use 10 or 12), it is recommended by the ATA to institute oral calcium and calcitriol supplementation and/or to start serial serum calcium measurements until calcium stability has been confirmed. It is important to note that while hypoparathyroidism can be observed almost immediately after surgery (half-life of parathyroid hormone is around 3–5 minutes) hypocalcemia will have a much more delayed presentation. As a result, it is important to observe the calcium trend to confirm stability at least 12–24 hours after surgery. Efforts should be made to avoid IV calcium unless symptoms are observed or the hypocalcemia is severe as this may delay the parathyroid hormone level recovery. Oral supplementation does not result in such suppression.

Question: You see the patient 2 months after surgery and he is recovering well – his voice and swallowing are rehabilitated with a vocal cord medialization procedure. You send the patient for a serum calcitonin and CEA. The calcitonin level comes back at 500 and the CEA is also elevated. What would be the most appropriate next step?

Answer: Cross-section imaging of the neck, chest, and abdomen with contrast-enhanced CT. Postoperative calcitonin levels above 150 pg/mL are highly associated with the presence of persistent locoregional or distant disease and should prompt a complete imaging workup with a full-body CT scan or positron emission tomography (PET)/CT. Imaging of the liver should use a four-phase liver protocol. Persistent locoregional disease should be evaluated with re-resection. Unresectable or distant disease can be observed if asymptomatic or treated with systemic therapy.

Key Points

- An initial diagnosis of medullary thyroid cancer should prompt a hormonal and genetic workup including metanephrines, serum PTH and calcitonin, as well as RET protooncogene testing.
- The mainstay of medullary thyroid cancer is surgery. This should include prophylactic central neck dissection and lateral neck surgery for nodal disease.
- Patients should be cautioned about the potential need to remove critical structures that are involved with tumor.
- Serum calcitonin levels are a reliable tumor marker in medullary thyroid cancer. Levels >150 pg/mL after treatment suggest metastatic disease.

CASE 29

Antoine Eskander

History of Present Illness

A 64-year-old Caucasian male presents to the emergency department with a recent growth in the left neck.

Question: What additional aspects of the history would be important?

- Does the patient have dysphagia? **yes**/no. This is an important question in working up a new neck mass.
- Has the mass grown since the patient noticed it? **yes**/no. A history of rapid growth could correlate to malignancy.
- Has the patient had any weight loss? yes/no. Asking about weight loss can help differentiate between benign and malignant etiologies.
- Has the patient had radiation before? **yes**/no. Radiation exposure can predispose to thyroid malignancy.
- Has the patient noticed a change in voice? **yes**/no. Asking about voice changes is always prudent when asking about a neck mass.
- The patient noticed the mass 3 weeks ago and feels that it has grown rapidly since then. He has had some dysphagia to solids but not liquids. He has unintentionally lose 10 pounds in the last month. He has not noticed any voice changes and has no history of radiation exposure.

Physical Examination

General: appears well without distress.
Neck: large mass, measuring about 6 cm in size in left level IV/VI. No overlying skin changes. The mass is fixed to the adjacent airway.
Larynx: normal voice. Larynx is mobile on exam.
Fiberoptic nasolaryngoscopy: normal vocal fold mobility and no mucosal abnormalities.

Management

A CT scan of the neck without contrast (see Figure 29.1) demonstrates a mass centered on the left thyroid lobe. Maximum

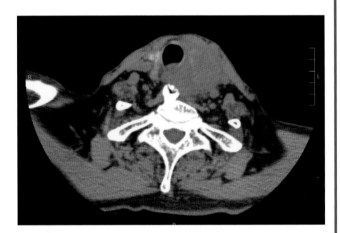

FIGURE 29.1   This is an axial CT scan of the neck without IV contrast showing a large tumor of the left thyroid gland with loss of the fat plane with the adjacent esophagus.

measurements are 4.7 cm AP by 5.2 cm transverse by 6.2 cm craniocaudal. There is heterogeneous attenuation within the mass, as well as several calcifications. There is loss of a fat plane and suspected infiltration of the esophagus. No clear extension of the mass into the tracheal lumen.

An FNA biopsy is performed of the mass and demonstrates cells with large round nuclei and prominent central nucleoli in a background of inflammation. The pathologist report shows a poorly differentiated neoplasm.

Question:Which would be an appropriate next step in the management of this patient? (Choose all that apply.)

- Core needle biopsy: **yes**/no. This can provide more information on morphology and architecture for a diagnosis. The leading diagnoses in consideration here are anaplastic thyroid cancer or poorly differentiated cancer.

(Continued)

CASE 29 (continued)

While lymphoma is still being considered, immunostaining may allow for an FNA to rule it out.
- Open biopsy: **yes**/no. An open thyroid biopsy can often help provide a large piece of tissue for testing and diagnosis. If this is considered, it should only be performed in a way that would still allow for en bloc resection of the entire biopsy tract if further surgery is planned.
- Thyroidectomy: yes/**no**. Given the extent of involvement, further information on the diagnosis in this patient is needed prior to going down the route of thyroidectomy.

You arrange for a core biopsy and this confirms thyroid origin. Pathology overview favors an anaplastic thyroid cancer after immunohistochemical evaluation.

Question: Which of the following would help in the management of this patient?
- Whole-body imaging: **yes**/no. Whole-body imaging should be performed to evaluate for distant disease.
- Esophagoscopy/bronchoscopy: **yes**/no. Patients with suspected invasion of tumor into the trachea or esophagus should undergo endoscopic evaluation to determine resectability.

PET/CT including imaging of the chest demonstrates disease localized only to the neck. After multidisciplinary consultation, the tumor is deemed to be resectable.

Question: Given the imaging information above, how would you classify the T-category?

Answer: T4a. The imaging demonstrates invasion into the esophagus, but no evidence as of yet that it has invaded the prevertebral fascia (and information earlier in the case suggests that the mass/larynx are mobile). According to the AJCC 8th Edition Staging Manual, this would be a T4a tumor.

Question: What clinical situations preclude surgical treatment of anaplastic thyroid cancer?

Answer: In the setting of a growing neck mass with impending airway compromise, treatment should only be delayed if there are imminent life-threatening effects from metastatic disease. This includes spinal cord compression, brain herniation, or pulmonary hemorrhage from metastatic disease.

Surgical treatment of anaplastic thyroid cancer must be weighed with surgical morbidity. The initial workup should include whole body cross-sectional imaging and high-definition ultrasound evaluation nodal basins. In patients who present with symptoms of airway and/or esophageal involvement, endoscopy of the aerodigestive tract should be performed.

If locoregional disease is present and a grossly negative margin (R0/R1 resection) can be achieved, surgical resection should be considered. R0/R1 resection can prolong disease-free survival and may improve overall survival in the right setting. The majority of anaplastic thyroid cancer patients will present with ETE, which may involve the trachea, esophagus,

or prevertebral region. Nodal disease may involve cranial nerves, mediastinal structures, and/or the carotid artery. Neither ETE nor the presence of nodal disease should in itself preclude surgical treatment, but the morbidity needs to be weighed with the overall low survival of anaplastic thyroid cancer. Extensive resections involving total laryngectomy/esophagectomy or resection of critical structures should typically be avoided.

In patients with systemic disease, resection of the primary tumor for palliation should be considered to avoid current or eventual airway or esophageal obstruction. However, debulking procedures (R2 resection) are not routinely recommended since these are unlikely to result in local control and do not improve survival.

All patients with a diagnosis of anaplastic thyroid cancer should be offered evaluation with a multidisciplinary team of radiation oncologists, medical oncologists, and surgeons. In addition to imaging, initial presurgical evaluation should include a review of concurrent medical comorbidities, as well as evaluation of the airway. Elective tracheostomy is not routinely recommended in patients without symptoms of airway compromise. Tracheostomy placement results in an increased burden of care that may be otherwise avoided, even in patients with advanced disease. Patients who present with airway compromise should be managed in the operating room with preoperative intubation if possible. Tracheostomy in these situations may require tumor debulking and should not be attempted in an uncontrolled setting.

Question: If the patient is not a surgical candidate because the disease is unresectable what treatment would you offer?

Answer: Patients who are to receive radiation for unresectable thyroid cancer or in the postoperative setting should, where available, be treated with IMRT; however, treatment should not be delayed because of lack of availability of IMRT. The use of cytotoxic chemotherapy involving some combination of taxane (paclitaxel or docetaxel), and/or anthracyclines (doxorubicin) and/or platin (cisplatin or carboplatin) therapy should be considered in combination with radiation therapy or altered fractionated radiotherapy in good performance status patients with nonmetastatic ATC who desire aggressive therapy.

Clinical trials, where available, should be offered to patients with advanced disease. Additional molecular testing of tumor specimens for therapeutic targets (ex. BRAF) should also be considered.

Question: For the case in question, the patient underwent esophagoscopy and bronchoscopy, which showed no translumenal tumor invasion into either structure. Surgery was performed consisting of total thyroidectomy, central neck dissection and ipsilateral recurrent laryngeal nerve sacrifice. Final pathology shows an incidentally resected anaplastic thyroid cancer

CASE 29   (continued)

within a background of a largely classical variant papillary thyroid cancer. How should this patient be followed in the future?

Answer: This was a largely well-differentiated cancer with a small focus of anaplastic thyroid cancer that was completely resected (R0). Therefore serum Tg is still indicated but will not help prognosticate the anaplastic component of the cancer, which does not produce Tg. Due to the advanced nature of the well-differentiated component, a postsurgical RAI scan (and subsequent therapeutic RAI therapy, as directed based on the final pathology) will be indicated.

Following initial staging and therapy, patients without evidence for persistent structural disease desiring ongoing aggressive management should have cross-sectional imaging of the brain, neck (and/or ultrasound), chest, abdomen, and pelvis at 1- to 3-month intervals for 6–12 months, then at 4- to 6-month intervals for a minimum of 1 additional year.

[18]FDG PET scanning should be considered about 3–6 months after initial therapy in patients with no clinical evidence of disease to identify small volume disease that may require a change in the management plan. Furthermore, [18]FDG PET scanning should also be considered at 3- to 6-month intervals in patients with persistent structural disease as a guide to the response to therapy and to identify new sites of disease that may necessitate a change in the management plan.

While neither serum Tg measurements nor RAI scanning or therapy are recommended in the initial management of ATC, in this instance, it would be helpful in the management and surveillance for the well-differentiated portion of the cancer.

Key Points

- Anaplastic thyroid cancer can arise from a benign nodule or well-differentiated thyroid cancer through a series of mutations.
- Patients with anaplastic thyroid cancer often present with advanced-stage disease. Initial evaluation should include systemic imaging as well as a determination of goals of care.
- Surgery for anaplastic thyroid cancer should be balanced with surgical morbidity and patient goals.
- Airway management in patients with anaplastic thyroid cancer remains controversial for asymptomatic patients.
- Chemotherapeutics, radiation, and immunotherapy are all part of the multidisciplinary treatment of anaplastic thyroid cancer.

CASE 30

Dustin A. Silverman, Peter J. Kneuertz, Fadi A. Nabhan, and Stephen Kang

History of Present Illness

A 68-year-old Caucasian male with a history of hypertension and gastroesophageal reflux disease presents to the emergency department with shortness of breath. The patient notes progressive dyspnea with ambulation and cannot walk across the room more than 10 steps without pausing for air.

Question: What additional questions would you like to know about the patient's presenting symptoms?

- How long has the patient been having these symptoms?. He has been short of breath for over the course of a month and his symptoms are getting worse.
- Has the patient experienced a change in voice: He has not noticed a change.
- Has the patient had any difficulty eating?. Patient denies.
- Has the patient had any hemoptysis?. He has also been coughing up blood daily.

He has no history of cancer or prior irradiation. His past medical history is otherwise noncontributory.

Physical Examination

General: the patient appears comfortable without respiratory distress on room air. He is unable to lie flat without feeling an increase in his shortness of breath and must sit upright.
Voice: his voice is strong; however, there is an audible biphasic stridor that worsens upon ambulation.
Neck: the thyroid is nodular, diffusely enlarged, measures approximately 6.0 cm, and feels fixed to underlying structures. There are no overlying skin changes.

Question: Which of the following is the next best step in management? (Choose all that apply.)

- Flexible fiberoptic laryngoscopy: **yes**/no. As the patient is stable, bedside flexible fiberoptic laryngoscopy is required

(Continued)

CASE 30   (continued)

to fully evaluate the patient's larynx and upper airway. In addition to assessing for lesions that may explain the patient's hemoptysis, structural abnormalities that may explain the source of biphasic stridor may be quickly discerned and influence the need for urgent or emergent operative intervention.

- OR for emergent tracheostomy: yes/**no**. Evaluation of the larynx in a stable patient should be performed when able prior to airway intervention.
- CT angiogram: yes/**no**. While imaging modalities such as US, CT angiogram of the neck and chest, and other studies to assess for the presence of a pulmonary embolus, pseudoaneurysm, or angioinvasive mass are indicated, these may be obtained following a complete physical examination.

Management

Flexible fiberoptic laryngoscopy demonstrates mobile true vocal folds with subglottic narrowing and submucosal fullness of the anterior tracheal wall. No other masses, lesions, or obvious source of bleeding are appreciated.

CT of the neck with contrast is obtained and demonstrates a heterogeneous, irregular, and mildly enhancing mass measuring 6.1 × 3.3 × 2.8 cm (AP × transverse × craniocaudal) arising from the thyroid involving the left greater than right thyroid lobes and isthmus with invasion through the left lateral tracheal wall (see Figure 30.1). Resulting tracheal stenosis measuring 4 mm in minimal dimension at the level of the T2 vertebral body is visualized. Multiple central compartment lymph nodes are subcentimeter but appear suspicious for

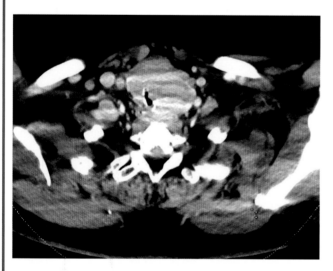

FIGURE 30.1   This axial CT scan of the neck with IV contrast shows a thyroid mass with narrowing of the trachea and associated intraluminal disease.

metastatic disease. No obvious esophageal infiltration is appreciated. FNA of the thyroid is completed and returns consistent with PTC.

When considering management options for this patient, additional diagnostic studies are obtained to rule out the presence of other cardiopulmonary etiologies that may be exacerbating the patient's dyspnea and worsening hemoptysis. CT chest, EKG, echocardiogram, and pulmonary embolism studies are unremarkable. Notably, imaging is negative for the presence of metastatic disease

Question: In cases where tracheal invasion is determined preoperatively, which of the following must be performed prior to completing surgical resection?

- Bronchoscopy: **yes**/no. In cases where airway invasion is known prior to definitive surgical resection, preoperative or intraoperative bronchoscopy (either flexible or rigid) is used to estimate intraluminal extent of invasion, degree of luminal compression, and determine resectability. Bronchoscopy may also be performed following reanastomosis for intraluminal evaluation of the trachea.
- Esophagoscopy: **yes**/no. Esophagoscopy is also recommended in cases of suspected or confirmed digestive tract involvement. This can be aided by esophageal ultrasound (EUS) to help define invasion. Photodocumentation may also be obtained.
- MRI: **yes**/no. Contrast-enhanced CT and MRI have both been demonstrated to be effective in diagnosing aerodigestive invasion, while US may also be used in experienced hands. Specifically, the preoperative use of cross-sectional imaging is recommended as an adjunct to US for patients with clinical suspicion for advanced disease
- Genetic testing: yes/**no**. Genetic testing is indicated in many settings, particularly in cases of medullary thyroid carcinoma or MEN syndrome; however, this would not be used to determine tracheal invasion.
- Sentinel lymph node biopsy: yes/**no**. Sentinel lymph node biopsy is not routinely used in cases of advanced thyroid carcinoma.

After multidisciplinary tumor board presentation and thorough discussion of treatment options, the patient elects to undergo oncologic surgical resection via a combined approach with a head and neck trained otolaryngologist and a thoracic surgeon.

Question: Which of the following surgical techniques may be considered for the treatment of advanced thyroid carcinoma with aerodigestive tract invasion? (Choose all that apply.)

- Shave resection: **yes**/no. Shave resection involves sharp separation of the thyroid gland from the tracheal wall with tangential resection or scraping of the tracheal surface to remove a thin layer of airway tissue for

CASE 30   (continued)

histopathologic analysis. This is performed in cases without gross intraluminal involvement. The goal of shave resection is to achieve long-term disease control after removing all gross disease; however, the risk of locoregional recurrence is the primary limitation to this technique. Due to the translumenal invasion seen on CT imaging, it would not be recommended in this patient.

- Window resection: **yes**/no. Window resection results in the creation of a local defect in the tracheal wall. It is recommended that only a small fraction of the tracheal circumference and no more than approximately 30% of the cricoid cartilage may be resected in an effort to avoid an unstable tracheal lumen. As much as 50% of the thyroid cartilage and external laryngeal framework may be resected without the need for complex reconstruction or tracheostomy. Primary reconstructive options for a window defect include a local muscle or myoperichondrial flap, but suture closure is rarely possible. Due to the broad amount of lateral trachea involved on the CT image, it would not be an appropriate option for this patient.

- Laryngotracheal sleeve resection: **yes**/no. The preferred method of tracheal and laryngotracheal sleeve resection consists of *en bloc* resection of the thyroid gland and attached trachea, although a discontinuous resec-

tion may also be performed. If more than one tracheal ring is to be excised, sleeve resection and reanastomosis is required. Advantages of this technique include a full-thickness tracheal specimen allowing for determination margin status and depth of invasion at the time of immediate airway reconstruction and reanastomosis.

- Total laryngectomy: **yes**/no. Total laryngectomy and cervical exenteration (e.g., combined removal of the larynx, pharynx, cervical esophagus, thyroid, and lymph nodes) are typically reserved for salvage cases where extensive invasive disease or locoregional recurrence following prior resection and/or radiation has occurred.

- Cervical exenteration: **yes**/no. The length of resected trachea dictates the need for either a cervical or mediastinal tracheostomy. Esophageal reconstruction is performed with a gastric, jejunal, or colonic transposition.

All of the surgical techniques may be appropriate and are selected based upon patients' individual disease extent, comorbidities, and treatment goals. Figure 30.2 helps explain the decision-making in these challenging cases.

The patient undergoes surgical resection including total thyroidectomy with mediastinal dissection, bilateral central neck dissection, and segmental tracheal resection with reanastomosis. Flexible fiberoptic bronchoscopy at the beginning of

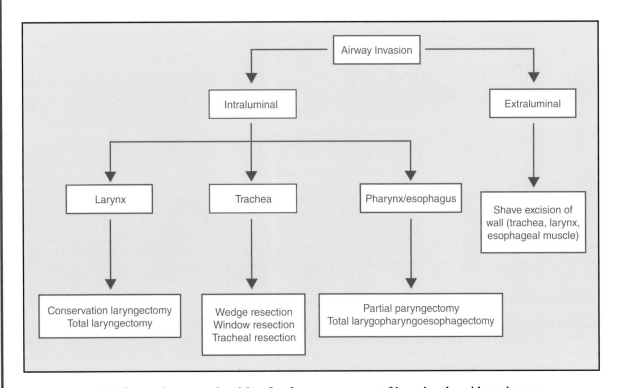

FIGURE 30.2   This figure shows an algorithm for the management of invasive thyroid carcinoma.

(Continued)

CASE 30   (continued)

the case shows that the tumor involves approximately 2 cm of the proximal trachea with direct invasion of the anterior tracheal wall. The patient is then safely intubated with a 6.0 cuffed endotracheal tube below the level of tumor infiltration. Esophagoscopy is negative for tumor infiltration.

Notably, the anterior branch of the left recurrent laryngeal nerve is found to be encased with tumor and unable to be dissected free without leaving gross residual disease behind. Frozen section biopsy is obtained and returns consistent with PTC. The anterior branch of the nerve is ultimately sacrificed and included *en bloc* with the main tumor specimen. Further dissection reveals that the tumor invades the trachea at the first tracheal ring.

After mobilization of the tumor, 3 cm of trachea is excised with gross total resection of the thyroid cancer. Tracheal anastomosis is performed (see Figure 30.3).

Postoperative flexible bronchoscopy 2 months following tracheal resection demonstrated the tracheal anastomosis with adequate healing (see Figure 30.4).

An inferiorly based left sternocleidomastoid pedicle flap is rotated medially to completely cover the tracheal anastomosis and provide additional reconstructive support. At the conclusion of the case, a tracheostomy is performed two rings below the

tracheal reconstruction and a 6.0 cuffed proximal extended XLT tracheostomy tube is placed. Flexible bronchoscopy 1 week and 2 months following surgery demonstrates excellent tracheal closure with appropriate healing. Final pathology reveals the following synoptic report for thyroid cancer:

> Procedure: total thyroidectomy and tracheostomy.
> Tumor location: thyroid.
> Tumor size: 6.5 cm.
> WHO histologic type: PTC with tall cell features.
> LVI: present.
> Perineural invasion (PNI): not identified.
> Encapsulated: no
> Tumor extent:
> > ETE: present.
> > Focality: unifocal.
> > Invasion of adjacent structures: present, trachea.

Margins:

> Main specimen margins: positive for carcinoma, left lobe soft-tissue margin.
> Additional separately submitted margins (frozen tissue specimens): not applicable.
> Additional resection margins (nonfrozen tissue): positive.

(a)　　　　　　　　　　(b)　　　　　　　　　　(c)

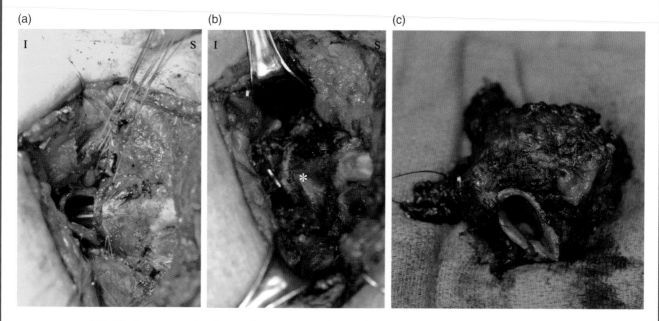

FIGURE 30.3   (a) This intraoperative image demonstrates the tracheal resection with stay sutures in place. The endotracheal tube is visualized through the anterior defect in the tracheal wall (I, inferior; S, superior). (b) This intraoperative photo is following tracheal reanastomosis with interrupted suture technique. The line of reanastomosis is visualized above the level of the thoracic inlet (asterisk). (c) Composite thyroid resection specimen with tracheal resection and left recurrent laryngeal nerve sacrifice.

CASE 30   (continued)

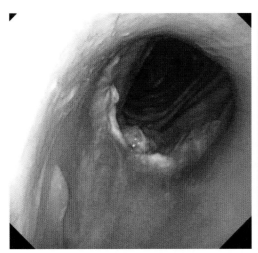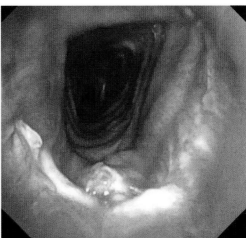

FIGURE 30.4   These 2-month bronchoscopic views at the level of the subglottis show a patent airway visualized to the carina and a suture line with appropriate healing and minimal granulation tissue.

Lymph nodes:
  Number examined: 8.
  Number involved: 8.
  Size of largest metastatic nodal deposit: 1.9 cm.
  ENE: present.

Postoperatively, the patient is considered for adjuvant therapy and discusses his options with the oncology team's endocrinologist.

Question: Based on this patient's pathology report, what is the final TNM staging?

Answer: T4aN1aMX. According to the AJCC 8th Edition definitions for TNM staging, T4a disease includes tumors of any size with gross ETE with invasion of the subcutaneous soft tissues, larynx, trachea, esophagus, or recurrent laryngeal nerve(s). T4b disease includes tumors of any size with ETE and invasion of the prevertebral fascia or encasement of the carotid artery and/or mediastinal vessels. In contrast to the AJCC 7th Edition staging, minor ETE has been removed from the definition of T3 disease, with updated T3a and T3b subdivisions. T3a is defined as tumors >4 cm limited to the thyroid while T3b disease includes tumors of any size with gross ETE invading only strap musculature. This patient classifies as T4aN1a with tracheal invasion of the 6.5 cm PTC through the anterior tracheal wall.

Question: In cases of advanced thyroid carcinoma with aerodigestive invasion, what is the recommended adjuvant treatment following surgical resection? (Choose all that apply.)

- RAI: **yes**/no. The mainstay of postoperative adjuvant therapy remains RAI with TSH suppression; however, patients with locally invasive thyroid carcinoma are more likely to have aggressive histologic variants that may not fully or effectively concentrate RAI.
- EBRT: **yes**/no. Patients with increased risk for residual microscopic disease or significant local aerodigestive invasion, EBRT should be considered. EBRT has been associated with improved locoregional control in differentiated thyroid cancer in several series. As controversy remains, the decision for adjuvant EBRT should be jointly discussed via a multidisciplinary approach between surgeons, radiation oncologists, and endocrinologists.
- Kinase inhibitor therapy: yes/**no**. Kinase inhibitor therapy should be considered in patients with RAI-refractory differentiated thyroid carcinoma with metastatic, symptomatic, imminently threatening, or rapidly progressive disease not amenable to local control with surgical resection or other treatment modalities.
- Systemic cytotoxic chemotherapy: yes/**no**. Cytotoxic chemotherapies are less effective in treating advanced thyroid cancer, but may provide clinical benefit in cases of metastatic disease. Salvage resection may be considered in cases of locoregional recurrence.

Three months following surgery, the patient undergoes a pretherapy RAI scan that demonstrates focal uptake within the resected thyroid bed without distant foci of increased activity to suggest nodal or metastatic disease. He subsequently completes 150 mCi of I^{131} therapy without complication. He is decannulated without difficulty. He additionally underwent in-office left true vocal fold augmentation for his left vocal fold paralysis following intraoperative sacrifice of the left recurrent laryngeal nerve with marked improvement in voice clarity.

(Continued)

Key Points

- The primary treatment of advanced differentiated thyroid cancer is surgery. The main adjuvant treatments are RAI and external beam radiation.
- Initial airway management is based on patient symptoms and should include flexible laryngoscopy in a stable patient.
- Metastatic disease is not a contraindication to control of neck disease.
- The extent of surgical resection is dependent on disease burden and patient situation. Resection that results in persistent gross or microscopic disease is acceptable in certain situations, though has a higher rate of locoregional recurrence.

Multiple Choice Questions

1. Which of the following increases a patient's risk of having well-differentiated thyroid cancer?

   a. Family history of thyroid cancer in a first-degree relative.

   b. Smoking history.

   c. History of radiation therapy for acne as a child.

   d. All of the above.

   e. a and c.

   Answer: e. Individuals with a history of low-dose radiation therapy and a first-degree relative with well-differentiated thyroid cancer are at increased risk for thyroid malignancy.

2. Which of the following features are associated with the *LOWEST* risk of malignancy in a nodule on ultrasound?

   a. Hypoechogenicity.

   b. Spongiform.

   c. Microcalcifications.

   d. Irregular borders.

   Answer: b. Spongiform lesions have a low risk of malignancy (<3%). The ATA and the American College of Radiology (ACR) have both determined systems to risk-stratify thyroid nodules based on ultrasound imaging characteristics. While there is some variation between systems, both agree that spongiform lesions have a low risk of malignancy. The TI-RADS system favors ultrasound follow-up for benign nodules, while the ATA guidelines recommend FNA for large but benign-appearing nodules. Comparisons between the two systems is ongoing, but overall both systems perform well at the evaluation of benign versus suspicious thyroid nodules.

3. You perform a total thyroidectomy on a patient for papillary thyroid cancer. The patient had a straightforward intubation, and a neuromonitoring endotracheal tube is used. The tumor partially encases the right recurrent laryngeal nerve. You are able to preserve the nerve and have an adequate electrical response. You proceed with the contralateral thyroid dissection; nerve stimulation on this side shows a weak response. Which of the following is the next best step in airway management for this patient?

   a. Tracheostomy.

   b. Finish the case and extubate as usual.

   c. Place an airway exchange catheter.

   d. Leave the patient intubated.

   Answer: c. Every effort should be taken by the surgeon to prevent airway compromise from bilateral recurrent laryngeal nerve injury. In advanced cases, EMG activity of the recurrent laryngeal nerve may be preserved but at a low amplitude. In cases where bilateral paresis is suspected, the surgeon and anesthesia team should have an airway plan in place. Tracheostomy should be reserved for patients in whom respiratory distress occurs due to bilateral true vocal fold immobility. For a patient with an uncomplicated intubation, standard extubation with close observation or extubation over an airway exchange catheter with concurrent flexible laryngoscopy can help with both oxygenation and airway evaluation. Prolonged intubation is an option but does not allow for evaluation of vocal cord mobility.

4. Which of the following statements is true?

   a. Anaplastic thyroid cancer is more common in the pediatric population.

   b. Anaplastic cancers can develop from long-standing papillary thyroid cancers or from poorly differentiated thyroid tumors.

   c. Anaplastic thyroid cancer is never managed with surgery.

   d. External beam radiation is a mainstay of therapy.

   Answer: b. The distinction between poorly differentiated and anaplastic cancers can be challenging and in reality is a continuum from well-differentiated papillary thyroid cancer to anaplastic cancers. The below figure shows a histopathology example of a patient with anaplastic thyroid cancer that developed from a well-differentiated thyroid cancer.

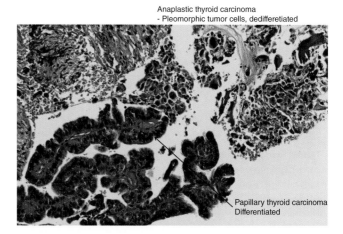

This H&E slide shows an anaplastic thyroid carcinoma arising in a setting of papillary thyroid cancer. **Source: Wolters Kluwer Health.**

5. When should a goals-of-care discussion occur with patients who have the diagnosis of anaplastic thyroid cancer?

   a. Only if impending airway compromise.

   b. If patient requests the discussion.

   c. Prior to initiating definitive management.

   d. At the time of diagnosis.

   Answer: d. Goals-of-life discussions should occur early in patients with anaplastic thyroid cancer because of the high mortality rate, the rapidity of disease of progression, and poor prognosis.

6. In patients presenting with laryngotracheal invasion secondary to a thyroid malignancy, which of the following symptoms is most commonly observed?

   a. Pain.

   b. Hemoptysis.

   c. Dyspnea.

   d. b and c.

   e. Asymptomatic.

   Answer: d. Symptoms tend to underestimate the depth of airway invasion and may only be present in a small subset of patients with the most advanced stages of invasion. In several series of tracheal resection with tumors invading the trachea, both hemoptysis and dyspnea as a result of airway obstruction were more commonly observed, with rates ranging from approximately 10–80% and 5–90%, respectively. Symptomatology may vary depending on the degree and location of invasion. Voice changes may also be observed. Although rare, some patients may present in an asymptomatic manner, especially in the early stages of invasion. The presence of obstructive airway symptoms and hemoptysis should heighten awareness for infiltrative disease.

7. Which of the following statements is true regarding the surgical treatment of patients with advanced-stage well-differentiated thyroid cancer?

   a. All patients with aerodigestive tract invasion should undergo neoadjuvant treatment prior to surgery.

   b. Patients should be immediately referred for supportive care and hospice consultation.

   c. The presence of metastatic disease is not an absolute contraindication to surgical resection.

   d. RAI treatment should be offered prior to surgical resection.

   Answer: c. According to 2015 ATA guidelines, surgery in the presence of aerodigestive tract involvement is recommended in combination with adjuvant RAI and/or EBRT. While surgical resection may offer a chance for cure, it is also recommended for regional neck palliation in patients with impending asphyxiation or significant hemoptysis even in the presence of distant metastatic disease. Removal of the thyroid also allows for the use of RAI to treat distant metastatic disease.

8. Upon performing a total thyroidectomy in a patient with known PTC with cervical nodal metastases, the surgeon discovers that the thyroid appears fixed to the airway with invasion through the tracheal wall. This was neither suspected nor identified upon preoperative evaluation. What is the next best step in management?

   a. Perform tracheal sleeve resection.

   b. Leave gross residual disease at the level of the trachea.

   c. Identify and stimulate bilateral recurrent laryngeal nerves.

   d. Obtain a frozen section to confirm malignant disease.

   e. Abort the case.

   Answer: d. In cases of thyroid malignancy with aerodigestive invasion, a high proportion are discovered intra- rather than preoperatively. Tracheal invasion occurs most commonly via direct extension of the primary tumor through anterior or lateral tracheal wall. Spread from metastatic paratracheal lymph nodes may also occur. A confirmatory pathologic diagnosis should be obtained prior to determining the next surgical steps. Performing a shave resection or more extensive sleeve resection with reanastomosis of the trachea may be indicated; however, the first step would be to confirm the presence of malignant invasive disease intraoperatively. Attempts to resect gross residual disease should be performed to decrease the risk of locoregional recurrence. Identification and preservation of bilateral recurrent laryngeal nerves should occur in all total thyroidectomy cases, when feasible.

9. Which of the following statements regarding laryngotracheal resection for differentiated thyroid carcinoma is false?

   a. As much as 50% of the external laryngeal framework may be resected.

   b. Shave procedures are associated with lower survival compared to radical resection.

   c. The presence of macroscopic disease following resection portends an increased risk of locoregional recurrence.

   d. Laryngotracheal invasion is an independent predictor of death.

   e. Tracheal resection totaling 5–6 cm may be primarily anastomosed without tracheal or laryngeal mobilization.

   Answer: b. While controversial, several retrospective series have found no difference in survival between shave resection and radical resection when all gross disease is completely resected; however, higher rates of locoregional recurrence and decreased survival have been observed in patients with incomplete resection and residual macroscopic disease. As much as 30% of the cricoid and 50% of the thyroid cartilage may be resected without the need for complex reconstruction or tracheostomy. Laryngotracheal invasion is an independent predictor of death in these patients, with airway obstruction as the primary cause of death in as many as 50% of cases. The amount of trachea that may be safely resected prior to mobilization is approximately 6 cm, although this may vary and requires the ability for neck flexion. Additional length and mobilization may be achieved with several techniques including supralaryngeal release, release of suprahyoid musculature, division of the thyrohyoid membrane, and sternotomy with hilar mobilization.

Suggested Reading

Alexander, E.K., Kennedy, G.C., Balock, Z.W. et al. (2012). Preoperative diagnosis of benign thyroid nodules with indeterminate cytology. *N. Engl. J. Med.* 367 (8): 705–715.

Cayo, A.K., Yen, T.W.F., Misustin, S.M. et al. (2012). Predicting the need for calcium and calcitriol supplementation after total thyroidectomy: results of a prospective, randomized study. *Surgery* 152: 1059–1067.

Chen, J., Tward, J.D., Shrieve, D.C., and Hitchcock, Y.J. (2008). Surgery and radiotherapy improves survival in patients with anaplastic thyroid carcinoma: analysis of the surveillance, epidemiology, and end results 1983–2002. *Am. J. Clin. Oncol.* 31: 460–464.

Cibas, E.S. and Ali, S.Z. (2017). The 2017 Bethesda system for reporting thyroid cytopathology. *Thyroid* 27 (11): 1341–1346.

Gaissert, H.A., Honings, J., Grillo, H.C. et al. (2007). Segmental laryngotracheal and tracheal resection for invasive thyroid carcinoma. *Ann. Thorac. Surg.* 83 (6): 1952–1959.

Haugen, B.R., Alexander, E.K., Bible, K.C. et al. (2015, 2016). American Thyroid Association management guidelines for adult patients with thyroid nodules and differentiated thyroid cancer: the American Thyroid Association guidelines Task Force on Thyroid Nodules and Differentiated Thyroid Cancer. *Thyroid* 26 (1): 1–133.

Honings, J., Stephen, A.E., Marres, H.A., and Gaissert, H.A. (2010). The management of thyroid carcinoma invading the larynx or trachea. *Laryngoscope* 120 (4): 682–689.

Middleton, W.D., Teefy, S.A., Reading, C.C. et al. (2018). Comparison of performance characteristics of American College of Radiology TI-RADS, Korean Society of Thyroid Radiology TI-RADS, and American Thyroid Association Guidelines. *Am. J. Roentgenol.* 210 (5): 1148–1154.

Nikiforov, Y.E., Steward, D.L., Robinson-Smith, T.M. et al. (2009). Molecular testing for mutations in improving the fine-needle aspiration diagnosis of thyroid nodules. *J. Clin. Endocrinol. Metab.* 94 (6): 2092–2098.

Nixon, I.J., Ganly, I., Patel, S.G. et al. (2013). Observation of clinically negative central compartment lymph nodes in papillary thyroid carcinoma. *Surgery* 154 (6): 1166–1172.

Nixon, I.J., Simo, R., Newbold, K. et al. (2016). Management of invasive differentiated thyroid cancer. *Thyroid* 26 (9): 1156–1166.

Orloff, L.A., Wiseman, S.M., Bernet, V.J. et al. (2018). American Thyroid Association statement of postoperative hypoparathyroidism: diagnosis, prevention, and management in adults. *Thyroid* 28 (7): 830–841.

Price, D.L., Wong, R.J., and Randolph, G.W. (2008). Invasive thyroid cancer: management of the trachea and esophagus. *Otolaryngol. Clin. North Am.* 41 (6): 1155–1168, ix–x.

Randolph, G.W., Dralle, H., International Intraoperative Monitoring Study Group et al. (2011). Electrophysiologic recurrent laryngeal nerve monitoring during thyroid and parathyroid surgery: international standards guideline statement. *Laryngoscope* 121 (S1): 1–16.

Sachdeva, U.M. and Lanuti, M. (2018). Cervical exenteration. *Ann. Cardiothorac. Surg.* 7 (2): 217–226.

Smallridge, R.C., Ain, K.B., Asa, S.L. et al. (2012). American Thyroid Association Guidelines for management of patients with anaplastic thyroid. *Cancer* 22 (11): 1104–1139.

Song, J.S.A., Dmytriw, A.A., Yu, E. et al. (2018). Investigation of thyroid nodules: a practical algorithm and review of guidelines. *Head Neck* 40 (8): 1861–1873.

Tam, S., Amit, M., Boonsripitayanon, M. et al. (2017). Adjuvant external beam radiotherapy in locally advanced differentiated thyroid cancer. *JAMA Otolaryngol. Head Neck Surg.* 143 (12): 1244–1251.

Tessler, F.N., Middleton, W.D., Grant, E.G. et al. (2017). ACR thyroid imaging, reporting and data system (TI-RADS): white paper of the ACR TI-RADS Committee. *J. Am. Coll. Radiol.* 14 (5): 587–595.

Tuttle, R.M., Haugen, B., and Perrier, N.D. (2017). Updated American Joint Committee on Cancer/Tumor-Node-Metastasis Staging System for Differentiated and Anaplastic Thyroid Cancer (Eighth Edition): what changed and why? *Thyroid* 27 (6): 751–756.

Wang, L.F., Lee, K.W., Kuo, W.R. et al. (2006). The efficacy of intraoperative corticosteroids in recurrent laryngeal nerve palsy after thyroid surgery. *World J. Surg.* 30 (3): 299–303.

Wells, S.A. Jr., Asa, S.L., Dralle, H. et al. (2015). Revised American Thyroid Association guidelines for the management of medullary thyroid carcinoma. *Thyroid* 25 (6): 567–610. https://doi.org/10.1089/thy.2014.0335.

SECTION 7

Parathyroid

Liana Puscas

CASE 31

Raymond Chai

History of Present Illness

A 33-year-old female presents for an annual physical examination with her primary care physician, and routine blood work identifies a calcium level of 11.3 mg/dl. She reports no history of kidney stones, bone pain or prior fractures. There is no family history of high calcium, kidney stones, brain tumors, neck tumors, or abdominal tumors. Review of symptoms reveals mild recent fatigue and memory loss. She denies any prior head and neck surgery. No history of prior malignancy.

> **Past medical history:** significant for polycystic ovary syndrome.
> **Past surgical history:** none.
> **Medications:** fish oil, multivitamin, vitamin C.
> No known drug allergies.
> **Review of symptoms:** negative except for what was previously mentioned.

Physical Examination

Well-appearing female in no acute distress.
Normal function of cranial nerves II–XII.
Nasal and oral cavity examination are normal.
No palpable neck masses are identified.

Question: What additional biochemical studies should be ordered?

- Serum total Ca: **yes**/no: 11.3 mg/dl.
- Intact serum PTH: **yes**/no: 369 pg/ml.
- Serum creatinine (Cr): **yes**/no: 0.48 mg/dl.
- 25-hydroxyvitamin D (vitamin D): **yes**/no: 26.0 ng/ml.

This otherwise healthy patient is presenting with hypercalcemia and the primary diagnosis on your differential should be primary hyperparathyroidism. The diagnosis of primary hyperparathyroidism can be made with biochemical studies alone, which should include a serum Ca, PTH level, Cr, and vitamin D. The relative values of Ca and intact serum PTH are more important than the absolute values as relatively elevated values that are still within the normal range can still be consistent with the diagnosis. Serum Cr and vitamin D levels are important to check as other potential causes of hypercalcemia. It is important to remember that imaging has no use in confirming or excluding the diagnosis of primary hyperparathyroidism.

Question: What additional laboratory testing can be considered?

- 24-hour urine calcium: **yes**/no: 252 mg/d. 24-hour urine collection to evaluate for calcium excretion is not required to make the diagnosis of hyperparathyroidism but including it in the workup is recommended. If marked hypercalciuria is present (>400 mg/d), stone risk can be evaluated by a urinary biochemical stone risk profile. In addition, a 24-hour urine calcium is important in ruling out familial hypocalciuric hypercalcemia.
- Parathyroid hormone-related protein: yes/**no**. PTHrP can be secreted by certain malignancies resulting in hypercalcemia of malignancy. It has no role in the workup of patients with primary hyperparathyroidism.

(*Continued*)

Essential Cases in Head and Neck Oncology, First Edition. Edited by Michael G. Moore, Arnaud F. Bewley, and Babak Givi.
© 2022 American Head and Neck Society. Published 2022 by John Wiley & Sons Ltd.

CASE 31 (continued)

- Urine metanephrines: yes/**no**. These are useful in evaluating patients with suspected secreting paragangliomas. For example, they can be useful in evaluating a patient with suspected parathyroid hyperplasia secondary to MEN 2A given the potential for concurrent pheochromocytoma. Including these as part of initial workup of primary hyperparathyroidism is not recommended.

Question: What imaging studies would you recommend?

- Neck/thyroid ultrasound (US): **yes**/no. A dedicated thyroid and parathyroid US is an appropriate primary imaging modality with suspected parathyroid adenoma, both to potentially identify the location of the adenoma and to evaluate for any thyroid pathology that should be managed concurrently.

The patient undergoes a thyroid US and a representative image is shown in Figure 31.1, which demonstrates a 1.1×0.6×0.5 cm ovoid hypoechoic, hypovascular soft-tissue nodule that has no discernible echogenic fatty hilum located posterior to the lower pole of the right lobe. This finding is suggestive of a probable right inferior parathyroid adenoma.

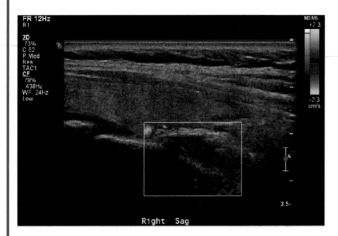

FIGURE 31.1 Thyroid US demonstrating a 1.1×0.6×0.5 cm ovid hypoechoic, hypovascular soft-tissue nodule posterior to the lower pole of the right thyroid lobe.

- Sestamibi parathyroid scan: **yes**/no. A sestamibi scan is also an accepted primary imaging modality for evaluating the potential location of a parathyroid adenoma. This patient did not undergo sestamibi scan.
- Four-dimensional (4D) CT angio: **yes**/no. A 4D computed tomography scan is also a well-established imaging modality for evaluating parathyroid pathology. It relies on the differential contrast wash-out between thyroid and parathyroid tissue.

This patient underwent a 4D CT and representative images are shown in Figure 31.2a–c, depicting an elongated

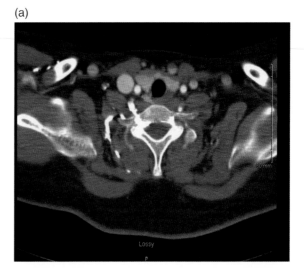

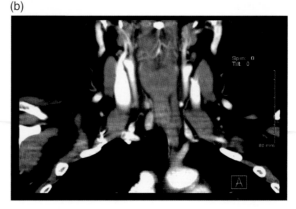

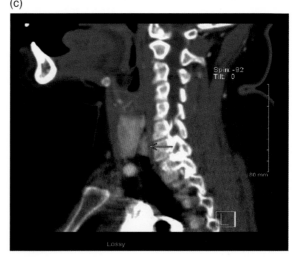

FIGURE 31.2 4D CT scan views demonstrating an elongated nodule posterior to the inferior right thyroid lobe: (a) axial, (b) coronal, and (c) sagittal.

CASE 31 (continued)

nodule posterior to the inferior right thyroid lobe measuring 2.3 cm craniocaudad x 0.6 cm x 0.6 cm, showing robust arterial phase enhancement and rapid washout on venous phase; findings consistent with parathyroid adenoma.

- Dual-energy x-ray absorptiometry (DEXA) scan: **yes**/no. A DEXA examination should be performed for all patients with primary hyperparathyroidism to screen for clinically relevant osteopenia or osteoporosis. Bone mineral density is measured at the lumbar spine, hip and distal radius.

This patient undergoes a DEXA scan, which shows a left femoral neck T score of −1.2, left hip T score of −1.0, and left radius T score of −0.7.

Question: You see the patient back in the office to review results of her imaging and discuss potential surgery. What are accepted indications for parathyroidectomy?

- Symptomatic: **yes**/no. Symptomatic patients typically derive clear benefits from curative parathyroidectomy. Observation and medical therapy are less effective and less cost-effective.
- Serum calcium levels greater than 1 mg/dl above the upper limit of normal: **yes**/no. Parathyroidectomy is indicated when the serum calcium level is greater than 1 mg/dl above normal. This is true regardless of whether objective symptoms are present or absent.
- Objective evidence of renal involvement: **yes**/no. Renal involvement includes silent nephrolithiasis on renal imaging, nephrocalcinosis, hypercalciuria (24-hour urine calcium level >400 mg/dl) or impaired renal function.
- Osteoporosis, fragility fracture, or evidence of vertebral compression fracture: **yes**/no. Primary hyperparathyroidism causes a decrease in bone mineral density, primarily in the cortical bone sites such as the distal third of

the radius. This improves following parathyroidectomy and fracture rate decreases. T score <−2.5 at any site is an indication for surgery.
- Age of 50 years or younger: **yes**/no. Young patients require prolonged monitoring and are more likely to develop symptomatic disease over time. In addition, many patients considered to by asymptomatic report improvement in quality-of-life indexes after parathyroidectomy.

Question: Given this patient's young age (33), a decision is made to proceed with parathyroidectomy. Intraoperatively, an obvious normal right inferior parathyroid gland is identified in the normal position abutting the lower pole of the right thyroid gland. An obvious adenoma is not immediately identified. Given the imaging results, where is the most likely location of the missed adenoma?

Answer: Deep to the right recurrent laryngeal nerve (overly descended superior parathyroid adenoma):

Given the localizing imaging results, the most likely location is deep to the right recurrent laryngeal nerve within the right tracheoesophageal groove. This corresponds to an overly descended superior parathyroid adenoma. This phenomenon is known to be frequently encountered during primary parathyroid surgery and is a significant factor in persistent disease and reoperative surgery.

Further exploration reveals an obvious parathyroid adenoma deep to the right recurrent laryngeal nerve near the inferior right thyroid lobe. The mass is weighed at 620 mg and confirmed as hypercellular parathyroid tissue on frozen section. Baseline preincision PTH of 380 pg/ml drops to 32.7 pg/ml 10 minutes postresection, indicating successful biochemical exploration. Neck exploration is stopped and the incision is closed. The patient remains eucalcemic 3 years after surgery.

Key Points

- A diagnosis of primary hyperparathyroidism can be made with biochemical studies alone and does not require image confirmation of an adenoma.
- 24-hour urine calcium should be checked in patients being evaluated for primary hyperparathyroidism to rule out familial hypocalciuric hypercalcemia.
- Neck US should be performed in patients being considered for parathyroidectomy both to evaluate for potential adenoma location and to evaluate for concurrent thyroid disease.
- Parathyroidectomy surgery should be considered in all symptomatic patients, those with serum Ca >1 mg/dl above normal and in those <50 years old.
- Additional indications for parathyroidectomy include renal involvement with silent nephrolithiasis on renal imaging, nephrocalcinosis, hypercalciuria (24-hour urine calcium level >400 mg/dl), or impaired renal function, as well as osteoporosis, fragility fracture, or evidence of vertebral compression fracture.

CASE 32

Tanya Fancy

History of Present Illness

A 42-year-old female is referred to you by her endocrinologist for evaluation of hypercalcemia. She has a prior history of renal calculi (three episodes). Bloodwork is as follows:

- Intact PTH 145 pg/ml (range 14–64 pg/ml).
- Serum calcium 10.9 mg/dl (range 8.6–10.4 mg/dl)
- 24-hour urinary calcium 305 mg (range 50–200 mg/day)
- Phosphorus 1.9 mg/dl (range 2.5–4.7 mg/dl)
- Cr 0.8.

  Past medical history: hypertension.
  Past surgical history: endoscopic resection of pituitary adenoma at age 25.
  Medications: amlodipine, atorvastatin.
  No known drug allergies.

Physical Examination

Well-appearing female in no acute distress.
Normal function of cranial nerves II–XII.
Nasal and oral cavity examination are normal.
No palpable neck masses are identified.

Question: Based on this patient's biochemical studies, you diagnose her with primary hyperparathyroidism. You discuss surgery with the patient and she is agreeable. What would be the next best step in management?

- Parathyroid exploration with RLN monitoring: yes/**no**. This patient's biochemical abnormalities are consistent with a diagnosis of primary hyperparathyroidism. However, prior to proceeding with surgical management, imaging studies should be obtained to identify the potential location of the adenoma.
- US: **yes**/no. Neck US can potentially identify the location of the adenoma and assist with surgical planning. On US, parathyroid glands typically appear as oval, hypoechoic nodules with internal vascularity at the periphery of the thyroid gland. US can also identify any concurrent thyroid pathology that may warrant evaluation prior to parathyroid surgery.
- Nuclear medicine scanning with sestamibi: **yes**/no. Nuclear medicine scanning with a sestamibi scan can also be used in defining the location of the adenoma. Tc99m sestamibi is absorbed faster by hyperfunctioning glands than by normal glands.
- Parathyroid fine needle aspiration (FNA): yes/**no**. This is typically not recommended except in unusual or difficult cases.
- 4D CT angio of the neck: **yes**/no. 4D CT angio of the neck is also a useful imaging modality for identifying the location of a parathyroid adenoma, particularly when an US and sestamibi are nonlocalizing.

You elect to proceed with US and sestamibi nuclear medicine scans and results are as follows:

US: Thyroid is small but uniform in echogenicity. Multiple bilateral nodules and cysts less than 5 mm identified as described in the body of the report, one may consider follow up US in 1 year. No enlarged parathyroid glands appreciated.

Sestamibi scan: No focal accumulation of tracer within the neck, negative study for parathyroid adenoma.

Question: Which of the following information would be appropriate as part of the counseling of this patient?

- It is very common for parathyroid adenomas to not localize on imaging: yes/**no**. This is not true. With dual modality imaging, most (85–92%) patients with primary hyperparathyroidism have a potential location for their adenoma identified. It is important to remember that imaging results should not be used to select patients for surgical referral. Patients with negative imaging results remain candidates for parathyroidectomy. In fact, imaging should only be performed after the decision has been made to proceed with parathyroidectomy.
- Additional diagnostic/radiologic testing is necessary prior to pursuing surgery: yes/**no**. Additional diagnostic/radiologic testing is not necessary; however, it could be considered. This is a clinical scenario where a 4D CT angio of the neck may demonstrate an adenoma not previously detected.

Your radiologist suggests a 4D CT angio of the neck. The results are as follows:

There are two arterially enhancing nodular foci adjacent to the thyroid that are lower density than the thyroid gland (see Figure 32.1). The lesion on the right measures 3 × 3 × 7 mm and is posterior to the midpole of the thyroid. The lesion on the left measures 3 × 5 × 12 mm and is immediately anterior to the left common carotid artery. They demonstrate equivocal mild washout.

Question: You see the patient back in clinic to discuss her imaging findings and finalize a treatment plan. Which of the following recommendations would be appropriate

- Genetic counseling: **yes**/no. Given the patient's young age (42) at presentation, suggestion of multigland disease on imaging and history of pituitary adenoma, a diagnosis of MEN1 should be considered, and she should be referred for genetic counseling. This is best performed prior to proceeding with parathyroidectomy as the objective of surgery can be better defined preoperatively with a known diagnosis of MEN1 (Table 32.1).

In patients with multiple endocrine neoplasia type I-associated hyperparathyroidism, subtotal parathyroidectomy is recommended as the index operation whereas in patients with MEN 2a-associated hyperparathyroidism, resection of only visibly enlarged glands is recommended.

CASE 32   (continued)

(a)

(b)

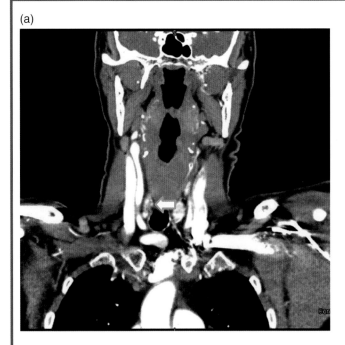
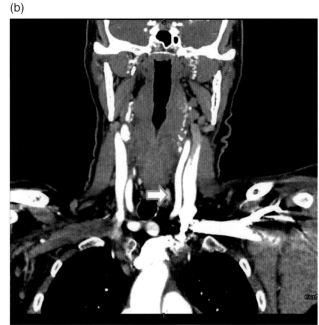

FIGURE 32.1   (a) 4D CT angio of the neck demonstrating right paratracheal enhancing nodule. (b) 4D CT angio of the neck demonstrating enhancing nodule above left thyroid lobe.

TABLE 32.1   **Multiple endocrine neoplasia: summary of associated neoplasms.**

MEN 1	Parathyroid hyperplasia, pancreatic tumors, pituitary adenoma, angiofibroma
MEN 2a	Parathyroid hyperplasia, medullary thyroid carcinoma, pheochromocytoma
MEN 2b	Medullary thyroid carcinoma, pheochromocytoma, mucosal neuroma

- Bilateral parathyroid exploration is indicated: **yes**/no. In patients with nonlocalizing preoperative imaging, hyperfunctional glands can be found in any normal anatomic location and bilateral exploration is indicated. Ectopic location is common, and intraoperative PTH monitoring should be used. The intraoperative availability of PTH assays and experienced frozen section analysis are paramount to successful surgical cure of these patients. In patients with true parathyroid hyperplasia, three and a half gland (subtotal) excision should be performed.

Question: You consent the patient for bilateral exploration and initiate exploration on the left side of the neck, the side of the larger nodule seen on CT. You identify both parathyroid glands, the superior gland being larger than the inferior. You remove this and the PTH level at 10 minutes is 159.6, pre-excision level was 168.8. How would you proceed?

Answer: Biopsy the inferior gland on the left and explore the contralateral neck.

Given the imaging findings, this is either a patient with "double adenoma" or four gland hyperplasia. It would be prudent to biopsy the ipsilateral gland to determine whether this is hypercellular or not, and to confirm parathyroid tissue. Given inconclusive preoperative scans, all parathyroid glands should be visualized prior to removing any additional glands.

Key Points

- In patients undergoing dual modality imaging, the rate of nonlocalization is approximately 8–15%.
- Intraoperative availability of PTH assays and experienced frozen section analysis are paramount to successful surgical cure for patients with parathyroid hyperplasia.
- 4D CT angiogram of the neck can be helpful in patients with negative or discordant US and sestamibi results.
- In a patient with suspected parathyroid hyperplasia, all four parathyroid glands should be visualized at the time of surgery.
- Young patients with multigland disease or concurrent/historical endocrine neoplasms should undergo genetic counseling prior to surgery.

CASE 33

Liana Puscas

History of Present Illness

A 47-year-old woman with end-stage renal disease (ESRD) is referred for possible surgical treatment of her hypercalcemia.

Question: What additional questions would you want to ask in the initial evaluation?

- Why do you have ESRD? Type 1 diabetes.
- Are you on dialysis? Yes.
- Are there any symptoms of hypercalcemia (e.g., stones: urinary, gallbladder, salivary gland; abdominal issues; etc.)? She has had several bouts of kidney stones and parotitis. She also has significant itching.
- Are there any symptoms of cardiovascular disease? Patient denies.
- What medications are you taking for your calcium levels? Calcitriol and sevelamer.

Question: What additional aspects of the history/medical record are important?

- Laboratory values:
  - Calcium: normal at 9.7 mg/dl.
  - Phosphorus: elevated at 6.4 mg/dl.
  - PTH level: elevated at 850 pg/ml.
  - Vitamin D: low normal at 20 ng/ml.
- Confirmation of patient's medication regimen.
- X-ray imaging demonstrates the presence of brown tumors and extraskeletal calcification. The presence of these lesions is another indication of the severity of disease.

Physical Examination

Well-developed female in no distress with a normal voice.
Normal head and neck examination.
No palpable neck masses. No thyroid nodules.

Management

Question: You explain to the patient that parathyroidectomy surgery is primarily considered in ESRD patients who are refractory to medical management. What medical therapies are considered "primary medical therapy" for ESRD patients?

- Phosphate binders: **yes**/no. Phosphate binders prevent the body from absorbing dietary phosphorus thereby reducing hyperphosphatemia that is secondary to ESRD.
- Active vitamin D analogs: **yes**/no. Patients with kidney disease have reduced conversion of 25-hydroxyvitamin D (25[OH]D) to its more active form, 1,25-dihydroxyvitamin D (1,25[OH]$_2$D) due to decreased enzyme levels

and are given vitamin D replacement with active, 1,25-dihydroxvitamin D.
- Calcimimetics: **yes**/no. Calcimimetics mimic the action of calcium on tissues by activation of the calcium receptors. Cinacalcet is a commonly used calcimimetic that mimics calcium at the parathyroid hormone receptor and reduces parathyroid hormone secretion.

You review the patient's medical history with her referring endocrinologist and determine that her hyperparathyroidism is refractory to all of the above listed medical interventions.

Question: Which of the following would be an indication for surgical management of hyperparathyroidism?

- Failure of medical management to control calcium and phosphorus levels: **yes**/no.
- The presence of extraskeletal calcification: **yes**/no.
- Dialysis dependence: **yes**/no.
- Debilitating bone disease: **yes**/no.
- Refractory pruritus: **yes**/no.
- Constipation: **yes**/no.
- Calciphylaxis: **yes**/no.
- Asymptomatic PTH >1000 pg/ml: **yes**.

There is no consensus on the acceptable PTH target level that defines refractory hyperparathyroidism and no formal recommendation on when to proceed with parathyroidectomy for patients with secondary or tertiary hyperparathyroidism. Many clinicians use a threshold PTH of 800 pg/ml for patients who are considered symptomatic. Symptoms of hyperparathyroidism include as listed above: extraskeletal calcification, bone disease, pruritus, calciphylaxis in addition to pain and weakness. The threshold of 800 pg/nl is important as many of these symptoms are nonspecific.

For asymptomatic patients, many consider a PTH >1000 pg/ml as a threshold for parathyroidectomy. There is some evidence to support that parathyroidectomy in these patients may reduce mortality, cardiovascular risk and risk of fracture.

Question: What are appropriate imaging modalities for a patient with ESRD and suspected secondary or tertiary hyperparathyroidism?

- 99-Tc sestamibi scan: yes.
- US: yes.
- MRI neck: maybe.
- CT neck: maybe.

Either a sestamibi scan or an US is considered adequate preoperative imaging to predict parathyroid gland location. Sestamibi scanning can indicate whether all four glands are hyperplastic in function versus one or two dominant glands. US can also measure gland size and predict location. MRI and especially 4D CT Neck Angiogram can also be of use in localizing enlarged glands.

CASE 33   (continued)

Question: Describe operative techniques that increase the chances of success in parathyroidectomy for patients with tertiary hyperparathyroidism.

- Use of rapid PTH assay (this will determine if the correct, hyperfunctioning gland[s] have been removed): **yes**/no. Just as in parathyroidectomy for primary hyperparathyroidism, intra-operative PTH evaluation can be used to confirm biochemical cure.
- Removal of the thyroid gland as well as abnormal parathyroid tissue: yes/**no**. Thyroid tissue should not routinely be removed during parathyroidectomy. This should only be considered when there is high suspicion for an intra-thyroidal parathyroid gland.
- Subtotal parathyroidectomy (3.5 gland removal) or complete gland removal with immediate auto-transplantation into the sternocleidomastoid or forearm muscle: **yes**/no. Subtotal parathyroidectomy, either leaving a half gland in-situ or with transplantation to distant muscle, is typically required

to achieve biochemical cure in patients with tertiary hyperparathyroidism. If auto-transplantation is undertaken, it will take about 6–8 months for the gland tissue to begin to function. Patients may develop hungry bone syndrome so they may require intensive calcium supplementation postoperatively.

Question: A 2.1 cm nodule is noted in the right thyroid lobe on preoperative US. An FNA is performed, which is interpreted as suspicious for papillary thyroid carcinoma. How would you proceed?

Answer: Perform right thyroid lobectomy at time of parathyroid surgery. The indications for thyroidectomy for concomitant thyroid disease during parathyroidectomy for primary hyperparathyroidism are the same as those for patients with isolated thyroid disease and should follow evidence-based guidelines. Surgery for any concomitant thyroid pathology can and should be performed at the time of parathyroidectomy.

Key Points

- Parathyroidectomy should be considered in patients with ESRD and symptomatic secondary hyperparathyroidism with PTH >800 pg/ml that is refractory to medical management.
- Medical management includes use of phosphate binders, active vitamin D analogs and calcimimetics.
- Symptoms of secondary hyperparathyroidism include extraskeletal calcification, debilitating bone disease, calciphylaxis, pruritis, pain and fatigue.
- Asymptomatic patients should be considered for surgery if they have refractory secondary hyperparathyroidism with PTH >1000 pg/ml.

Multiple Choice Questions

1. What defines successful surgical intervention for hyperparathyroidism per the original Miami criteria?
   a. Decrease in intraoperative PTH levels >50% from preincision hormone level at 5 minutes after removal of all abnormal parathyroid tissue.
   b. Decrease in intraoperative PTH levels >50% from preincision OR pre-excision hormone level at 10 minutes after removal of all abnormal parathyroid tissue.
   c. Decrease in intraoperative PTH levels >50% AND into the normal range from preincision hormone level at 5 minutes after removal of all abnormal parathyroid tissue.
   d. Decrease in intraoperative PTH levels to the normal range at 10 minutes after removal of all abnormal parathyroid tissue.

   Answer: b. Per the original Miami criteria, successful parathyroidectomy is defined by a decrease of intact intraoperative PTH levels >50% from the highest preincision or pre-excision hormone level in a peripheral blood sample obtained 10 minutes after removal of all abnormal parathyroid tissue. If these criteria are met, the neck exploration is completed and the incision is

closed. If the 10-minute sample does not meet criteria, further neck exploration is continued until all hypersecreting glands are removed and confirmed by a >50% drop from the highest subsequent pre-excision sample. The pre-excision sample is performed to account for parathyroid hormone spikes from gland manipulation. Although some surgeons require intraoperative PTH to fall into the normal range, this potentially increases the rate of false negatives and unnecessary bilateral neck exploration.

2. Which of the follow are true regarding the diagnosis of familial hypocalciuric hypercalcemia?
   a. It is an autosomal recessive disorder.
   b. It is a disorder of the renal phosphorus-sensing receptor.
   c. 24-hour urinary calcium levels should be less than 100 mg/24 hours.
   d. Calcium to creatinine clearance ratio should bee more than 0.01.

   Answer: c. Familial hypocalciuric hypercalcemia is an autosomal dominant disorder of the renal calcium-sensing receptor that can mimic primary hyperparathyroidism. This diagnosis should be considered in patients with long-standing hypercalcemia, urinary calcium levels less than 100 mg/24 hours, and a calcium to creatinine clearance ratio less than 0.01.

3. Which of the following is TRUE regarding parathyroid carcinoma?

   a. It accounts for approximately 10% of all cases of primary hyperparathyroidism.

   b. It typically presents with very high PTH and low calcium levels.

   c. Surgery should entail complete resection avoiding capsular disruption.

   d. Prophylactic central or lateral neck dissection should be performed.

   e. Diagnosis depends of histologic identification of perineural invasion.

   Answer: c. Parathyroid carcinoma accounts for approximately 1% of all cases or primary hyperparathyroidism. It typically presents with very high PTH AND very high calcium levels. Surgery should entail complete resection and typically does not require radical resection of surrounding structures. Prophylactic central and lateral neck dissection is not routinely recommended. The diagnosis depends on the histologic identification of angioinvasion.

4. Which of the following is TRUE regarding primary hyperparathyroidism?

   a. Calcium levels may fluctuate between high and normal values, therefore repeated measurements over time can be important in establishing a diagnosis.

   b. Multigland disease affects approximately 15% of patients with primary hyperparathyroidism and should be routinely considered in preoperative planning.

   c. Many pharmacologic agents are not as effective as operative management.

   d. All of the above.

   Answer: d. All of the above are true.

5. Which of the following are TRUE regarding parathyroidectomy?

   a. Surgeon volume inversely correlates with complications, cost, and length of stay.

   b. Short-term preoperative calcium and/or vitamin D supplementation should be considered.

   c. Recurrent hyperparathyroidism is defined by recurrence of hypercalcemia after a normocalcemic interval at more than 6 months after parathyroidectomy.

   d. All of the above.

Answer: d. All of the above are true. High-volume surgeons have been demonstrated to have better outcomes including lower rates of complications and lower cost of care. Prophylactic Ca and/or vitamin D supplementation has been demonstrated to reduce frequency/severity of postop hypocalcemia. Recurrent hyperparathyroidism is defined by recurrence of hypercalcemia after a normocalcemic interval at more than 6 months after parathyroidectomy.

Suggested Reading

Amin, A.L., Wang, T.S., Wade, T.J. et al. (2011). Nonlocalizing imaging studies for hyperparathyroidism: where to explore first? *J. Am. Coll. Surg.* 213 (6): 793–799.

Bilezikian, J.P., Brandi, M.L., Eastell, R. et al. (2014). Guidelines for the management of asymptomatic primary hyperparathyroidism: summary statement from the fourth international workshop. *JCEM* 99 (10): 3561–3569.

Bunch, P.M. and Kelly, H.R. (2018). Preoperative imaging techniques in primary hyperparathyroidism – a review. *JAMA Otolaryngol. Head Neck Surg.* https://doi.org/10.1001/jamaoto.2018.1671.

Cunningham, J., Locatelli, F., and Rodriguez, M. (2011). Secondary hyperparathyroidism: pathogenesis, disease progression, and therapeutic options. *CJASN* 6 (4): 913–921. https://doi.org/10.2215/CJN.06040710.

Duke, W.S., Hampton, M.V., and Terris, D.J. (2016). Reoperative parathyroidectomy: overly descended superior adenoma. *Otolaryngol. Head Neck Surg.* 154 (2): 268–271.

Lew, J.I. and Irvin, G.L. 3rd (2009). Focused parathyroidectomy guided by intra-operative parathormone monitoring does not miss multiglandular disease in patients with sporadic primary hyperparathyroidism: a 10-year outcome. *Surgery* 146 (6): 1021–1027.

Oltmann, S.C., Madkhali, T.M., Sippel, R.S. et al. (2015). KDIGO guidelines and parathyroidectomy for renal hyperparathyroidism. *J. Surg. Res.* (1): 199, 115–120. Published online 2015 Apr 18. doi:https://doi.org/10.1016/j.jss.2015.04.046.

Wetmore, J.B., Liu, J., Do, T.P. et al. (2016). Changes in secondary hyperparathyroidism-related biochemical parameters and medication use following parathyroidectomy. *Nephrol. Dial. Transplant.* 31 (1): 103.

SECTION 8

Paraganglioma

Kenneth Byrd

CASE 34

Thomas J. Ow

History of Present Illness

A 74-year-old woman is referred to your office for evaluation of a left neck mass. She was admitted for an episode of "dizziness" 1 month ago. She says she felt like the room was spinning and she became nauseous and felt weak for several minutes. The dizziness has since subsided, but she feels persistently light-headed.

Question: What additional questions would you want to ask?

- Any voice changes? Patient denies. New hoarseness in the setting of neck mass can be suggestive of vocal cord paralysis and underlying involvement of the vagus or recurrent laryngeal nerve.
- Any dysphagia? Patient denies. New dysphagia in the setting of neck mass can be suggestive of vocal cord paralysis and underlying malignancy.
- History of tobacco use? Patient denies. One should have an increased suspicion for malignancy in patient with a history of heavy tobacco use.
- Thyroid disorders? Patient denies. A hyperfunctioning thyroid nodule could present as a neck mass with associated metabolic dysfunction.
- History of neck radiation? Patient denies. Prior radiation may predispose to radiation-induced cancers and/or dysphagia and also can impact options for treatment depending on the ultimate diagnosis of this patient.

Past Medical History

Significant for hypertension, hyperlipidemia, and obesity.

Physical Examination

General: pleasant and well-appearing female in no distress.

Eyes: extraocular motions intact, vision grossly normal.

Ears: external auditory canals are clear, tympanic membranes are intact.

Anterior rhinoscopy without mass or lesion.

Oral cavity and oropharynx normal.

There is palpable 4 cm left neck mass in level II/III, mobile laterally but not vertically.

No nystagmus.

Cranial nerves II–XII are grossly intact, bilaterally.

Fiberoptic nasolaryngoscopy was performed: this shows intact vocal fold mobility and some fullness in the left hypopharynx, obscuring the left pyriform sinus. There are no mucosal lesions of pharynx or larynx.

Management

Question: What type of imaging would you consider at this point?

- Computed tomography (**CT**) neck with contrast: **yes**/no. A CT scan is a useful initial study for a neck mass of unclear etiology. CT allows for assessment of deep structures of the neck including the larynx and carotid sheath that are more difficult to evaluate on ultrasound (see Figure 34.1).
- Magnetic resonance imaging (**MRI**) neck with contrast: **yes**/no. MRI would also be a useful study to assess for carotid space involvement. A contrast-enhanced MRI is optimal for tumors at the skull base or of neural origin

(Continued)

Essential Cases in Head and Neck Oncology, First Edition. Edited by Michael G. Moore, Arnaud F. Bewley, and Babak Givi.
© 2022 American Head and Neck Society. Published 2022 by John Wiley & Sons Ltd.

CASE 34 (continued)

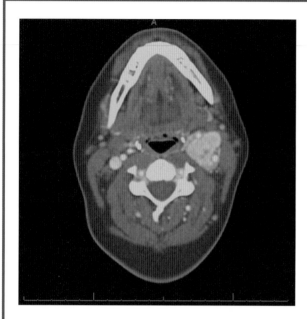

FIGURE 34.1 **This CT angiogram using contrast demonstrates a left neck mass in the parapharyngeal space splaying the carotid sheath structures.**

- Ultrasound (**US**) of the neck: **yes**/no. Though US can be useful for defining structures in the lateral neck, it is less useful for deep neck structures or vascular tumors. In this case an US would likely demonstrate the mass, but further imaging would be needed to define its extent.
- Positron emission tomography (PET)/CT scan: yes/**no**. PET/CT scans are typically ordered *after* there has been histologic confirmation of malignancy. While DOTATATE PET imaging can be used to assess for multifocal disease, it would not be appropriate at this stage of the workup.

Question: Based on the imaging results, what lesion(s) are at the top of your differential diagnosis?

- A pleomorphic adenoma: yes/**no**: The lesion appears in the post-styloid parapharyngeal space. Pleomorphic adenomas of the parapharyngeal space or deep lobe of the parotid are pre-styloid tumors. A pleomorphic adenoma is also typically a hypovascular tumor and should not enhance on the CT angiogram.
- Lymphoma: yes/**no**. Lymphoma can arise in the retropharyngeal space in the nodes of Rouviere. This would typically be medial to the internal carotid artery and cause lateral displacement of the carotid sheath. Though lymph nodes can enhance, it would also not be expected to do so as avidly on CT angiogram.

- Metastatic squamous cell carcinoma to a cervical lymph node: yes/**no**. As described above, metastatic disease would arise in the retropharyngeal space in the nodes of Rouviere or in other cervical lymph node levels more lateral in the neck.
- Paraganglioma: **yes**/no. This is a well-circumscribed lesion within the carotid sheath – the post-styloid parapharyngeal space, specifically. Tumors from neurovascular origin are highest on the differential diagnosis and include paragangliomas, schwannomas, and neurofibromas. While salivary tumors and lymph nodes can be located in the parapharyngeal space, they are typically in the prestyloid portion pushing the vessels posteriorly.

Question: Based on imaging, what type of paraganglioma is most likely?

Answer: The epicenter of the tumor appears to be between the jugular vein and the carotid artery pushing the internal carotid medially. This is most consistent with a glomus vagale or vagal paraganglioma. A carotid body tumor is less likely, as these usually are located at the carotid bifurcation and splay the internal and external carotid ("lyre" sign).

Question: What additional imaging modality would be appropriate for the next step in the diagnostic workup?

Answer: Imaging specific for neuroendocrine tumors can aid in solidifying the diagnosis and can also provide assessment for multiple concurrent lesions, as might be seen in a patient with hereditary paragangliomas. For an octreotide scan (somatostatin receptor scintigraphy), radiolabeled octreotide is given, which is preferentially taken up by tumors that have somatostatin receptors (such as carcinoid tumors, medullary thyroid carcinomas, and paragangliomas; see Figure 34.2). 68-gallium DOTATATE is a radioconjugate of the somatostatin analogue tyrosine-3-octreotate (Tyr3-octreotate or TATE) labeled with the tracer gallium Ga 68, linked by the chelating agent dodecanetetraacetic acid (DOTA). Imaging with 68-gallium DOTATATE is more expensive; however, it appears to provide superior resolution and lesion detection capabilities compared to octreotide scanning, and the study is much more convenient as it can be completed in 2–3 hours instead of over the course of 12–24 hours, which is required after octreotide injection.

Question: What management options should be discussed with this patient?

Answer:
- Observation: **yes**/no. several series have now reported that a substantial number of paragangliomas (perhaps 50–60%) will remain stable or even regress over a long follow-up period (~5 years or longer). Those that grow often do so slowly. The primary risk of observation is

CASE 34   (continued)

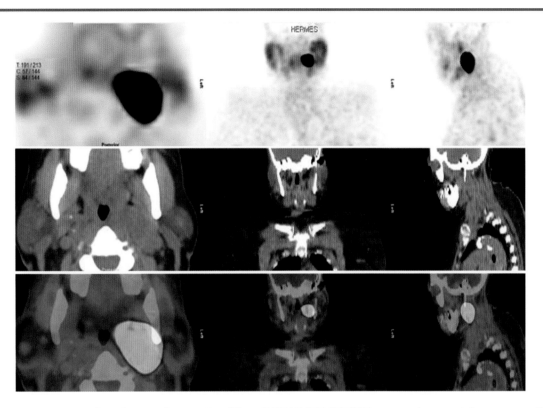

FIGURE 34.2   These images from a 68-gallium DOTATATE PET/CT are consistent with a paraganglioma.

the development of cranial nerve deficits due to tumor growth, while surgical resection often carries the same risks. In the case of vagal paragangliomas, the primary risk is that to the vagus nerve, with resulting vocal cord paralysis and dysphagia.

• Radiation: **yes**/no radiation can be delivered to a paraganglioma with the goal of tumor ablation or, more commonly, growth arrest. Radiation is typically considered for tumors <3 cm and for those where surgery would be highly morbid or where patient comorbidities preclude surgery. The preferred modality is stereotactic radiosurgery, which is given as a single fraction and has been shown to be highly effective. "Traditional" radiation treatment with intensity-modulated radiation therapy (IMRT) is also effective; however, typically 45 Gy of

radiation is delivered over 25 fractions, which requires 5 weeks of treatment.

• Surgical resection: **yes**/no details of surgical resection are described in a companion module. Briefly, surgical resection of vagal paragangliomas is typically accomplished via a lateral cervical approach and almost always requires sacrifice of the vagus nerve, which results in vocal fold immobility and dysphagia secondary to both motility and sensory deficits of the larynx/pharynx.

For this patient, all options were presented. Because of her age, the likelihood that this was a vagal paraganglioma, and because she was asymptomatic, a "wait and scan" approach was recommended. She is undergoing serial imaging with MRI, at 6 months and then annually if no progression is noted and she remains asymptomatic.

Key Points

• Imaging with MRI/magnetic resonance arteriography (MRA) is adequate for diagnosis of cervical paragangliomas. Biopsy is not required and is associated with risk of bleeding.
• The clinician should note the pattern of displacement of

the internal and external carotid arteries to determine the origin of cervical paragangliomas.
• Treatment options for paragangliomas include observation, radiation, and surgery.
• Treatment selection should take the patient's symptoms, age, and comorbidities into consideration.

CASE 35

Camilo Reyes and J. Kenneth Byrd

History of Present Illness

A 55-year-old Caucasian female presented to her primary care physician with a 6-month history of a progressively enlarging painless left neck mass. She denies any other lesions or masses of the head or neck.

Question: What additional questions would you want to ask?

- Any trouble swallowing? Patient denies. New dysphagia in the setting of neck mass can be suggestive of vocal cord paralysis and underlying malignancy.
- Any voice changes? Patient denies. New hoarseness in the setting of neck mass can be suggestive of vocal cord paralysis and underlying malignancy.
- Any difficulty opening and closing the mouth? Patient denies. Perineural invasion or direct extension to the pterygoid muscles can contribute to trismus.
- Any recent infection? Patient denies. Lymphadenitis can mimic malignancy.
- Any history of radiation exposure? Patient denies. Can predispose to thyroid cancer and other malignancies.
- Any sexually transmitted diseases? Patient denies. May increase likelihood of human papillomavirus (**HPV**) exposure.

Past Medical History

Patient is otherwise healthy.

Social History

No history of tobacco use or heavy alcohol consumption. No illicit drug use.

Physical Examination

Well-developed female in no distress. Voice strong.

Skin: no suspicious lesions.

Salivary: no fullness or masses within parotid or submandibular glands.

Oral cavity and oropharyngeal examination were without suspicious lesions.

Cervical exam revealed a large pulsatile mass that extended deep to the mandibular angle, mobile laterally but not superior/inferior.

No other lymphadenopathy.

Cranial nerves II–XII intact.

Fiberoptic nasolaryngoscopy is performed: There was fullness of the left posterolateral wall of the pharynx and full mobility of the vocal folds.

Management

Question: What type of imaging would you consider at this point?

CT neck with contrast: **yes**/no. Primary evaluation of a neck mass with contrasted CT is fast and relatively inexpensive. CT allows for assessment of deep structures of the neck including the larynx and carotid sheath that are more difficult to evaluate on ultrasound (see Figure 35.1).

- MRI neck with contrast: **yes**/no. MRI would also be a useful study if a neuroendocrine or other carotid space tumor is suspected. A contrast enhanced MRI is optimal for tumors at the skull base or of neural origin. (see Figure 35.2).
- Ultrasound of the neck: **yes**/no. Though US can be useful for defining structures in the lateral neck, it is less useful for deep neck structures or vascular tumors. In this case an US would likely demonstrate the mass, but further imaging would be needed to define its extent.

MRI/MRA with gadolinium was performed (see Figure 35.2).

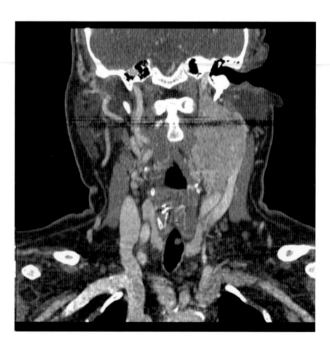

FIGURE 35.1 Coronal contrasted CT of the neck demonstrates an avidly enhancing mass of the left carotid space, displacing the internal and external carotid arteries. The mass spans from the level of the base of the styloid process down to the level of the carotid bifurcation.

CASE 35   (continued)

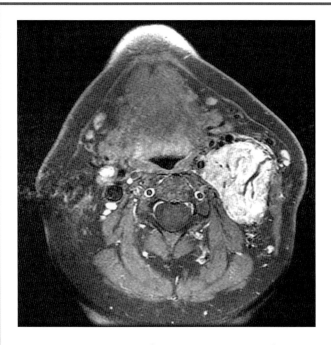

FIGURE 35.2   MRA reveals a 4.9 × 4.5 × 6.7 cm enhancing soft-tissue mass at the bifurcation the left common carotid artery (CCA) with medial splaying of the left internal and external carotid arteries and multiple flow voids.

Question: Based on history, exam, and imaging, what is the most likely diagnosis for this patient?

Answer: This is consistent with a paraganglioma based on its avid enhancement and flow voids. Because the internal and external carotid arteries are displaced anteromedially, the lesion is more consistent with a vagal paraganglioma than a carotid body tumor.

Question: What other surgical service would be important to involve in this patient's care prior to surgery?

Answer: Vascular surgery consultation is appropriate for large tumors in case of vascular injury during resection. A balloon occlusion study with a nuclear medicine brain perfusion can be considered as a means of assessing the risk of carotid sacrifice. In patients with symptomatic decreased cerebral perfusion, the vascular surgery team can plan carotid replacement with a graft in the setting or irreparable injury to the carotid bulb or internal carotid artery.

Question: What deficit will be expected from resection of this tumor?

Answer: Because the tumor most likely arises from the vagus nerve, the patient should be counseled that vocal cord paralysis is likely to occur. The patient will experience dysphonia and dysphagia postoperatively, particularly if hypoglossal nerve dissection is necessary. With rehabilitation, long-term recovery of swallowing recovery is expected for most patients. However, patients should be counseled that they may require a gastrostomy tube and/or vocal cord medialization in the short term.

Question: What step should be considered to minimize intraoperative blood loss?

Answer: Embolization of paragangliomas may be effective in decreasing intraoperative blood loss for tumors >4–5 cm. It should be performed within 1–2 days of surgery because it creates a brisk inflammatory reaction that can make removal more difficult. Control of the common, internal, and external carotid artery is an important step in surgery. However, ligation of the CCA may cause a stroke and does not control retrograde distal flow.

Treatment options were discussed with the patient, including observation, radiation, and surgery. Because of the large size of the tumor and the patient's age, she elected for treatment given the likelihood of continued growth over her expected lifespan. The patient was concerned with the appearance of her neck, and therefore radiation to arrest growth was not appropriate. Given her lack of medical comorbidities and the resectable nature of the tumor, surgery was elected.

The patient was scheduled for transcervical resection and planned medialization laryngoplasty, with preoperative embolization and vascular surgery on standby. Figure 35.3 demonstrates preoperative angiography, which identified the occipital artery as the primary feeding vessel and allowed selective embolization.

Surgery was performed via a transverse cervical incision. The internal jugular vein, CCA, and vagus nerve were identified below the mass. Vessel loops were used to control and retract the vessels (see Figures 35.4 and 35.5). The digastric muscle was retracted superiorly to reveal the upper pole of the mass, spinal accessory nerve, and hypoglossal nerve, which were noted to be stretched over the mass. The hypoglossal nerve was meticulously freed from the mass and was reflected superiorly. This allowed identification of the external carotid artery branches and partial distal control. Dissection of the tumor off the common and external carotid arteries with bipolar cautery and scissors was then performed to expose the carotid bulb. Clip ligation of the ascending pharyngeal artery further decreased the vascularity of the mass. The mass was then freed off the internal carotid artery and was pedicled on the vagus nerve, which was sacrificed. Fat injection medialization laryngoplasty was performed after layered wound closure due to anticipated true vocal fold paralysis.

(Continued)

CASE 35   (continued)

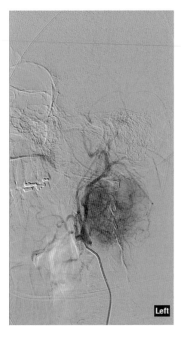

FIGURE 35.3   This image demonstrates the vascular nature of paragangliomas evident on pre-embolization angiography.

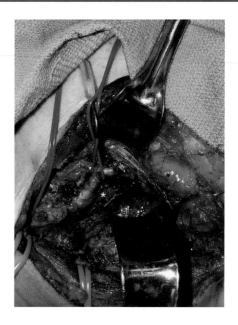

FIGURE 35.5   Careful dissection in the subadventitial plane has allowed distal control of the external carotid artery. The tumor has been dissected off the internal carotid artery (*) and is pedicled on the vagus nerve.

Speech therapy was consulted on postoperative day 1, and she was started on thickened liquids with head turn and discharged with an oral diet. She recovered uneventfully with speech therapy and advanced to normal diet without thickener. The pathology report confirmed paraganglioma as the diagnosis.

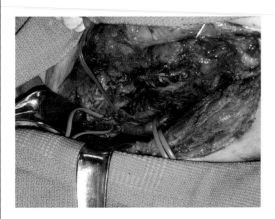

FIGURE 35.4   Proximal control of the left internal jugular vein (blue loop, right), distal vagus nerve (blue loop, left), and CCA (red loop). The tumor is present on the right side of the picture and has darkened in color due to embolization and bipolar cautery.

Key Points

- Patients should be counseled about expected postoperative vocal paralysis if surgery is planned for vagal paragangliomas.
- For large tumors that necessitate significant hypoglossal nerve dissection, postoperative swallowing therapy will be needed for dysphagia due to vagal and hypoglossal weakness.
- Preoperative embolization 1–2 days prior to surgery may decrease blood loss for tumors >4–5 cm.
- Prior to tumor dissection, the carotid branches should be isolated and controlled with vessel loops in case of major bleeding.

CASE 36

Michael G. Moore

History of Present Illness

A 46-year-old male presents to your office with a chief complaint of a left neck mass and pain. He states the mass had been present for around 10 years and has been slowly enlarging.

Question: What additional questions would you want to ask?

- Any other symptoms from it? Yes. He has had pain in the left neck that has been progressive with some radiation to the left shoulder.
- Any fevers, chills, or night sweats? Patient denies. This may signify infectious/inflammatory causes of a neck mass.
- Any other adjacent lumps that have been noticed? Yes. He has had a vague fullness in the right side of his neck over the past 6 months.
- Any change to his voice or swallowing? Patient denies.
- Any throat pain or ear pain? Patient denies. Important to ask as this may be a symptom of a tumor in the pharynx or larynx.
- Any prior skin tumors removed or history of head and neck cancer? Patient denies. Good question as this could be a regional recurrence of a head and neck skin cancer.
- Any weakness or twitching of the face? Patient denies.
- Any numbness of the face? Patient denies.
- Any change in hearing? Patient denies.
- Any tinnitus? Patient denies.
- Any difficulty opening and closing the mouth? Patient denies.

Question: What additional aspects of the history are important?

- Has he had any prior evaluation of the area? Patient denies.
- Any prior head and neck surgery or radiation? Patient denies.
- Any family history of neck masses? Yes, his father and grandfather had neck masses but the type is unknown.
- Any history of tobacco use? Patient denies.
- Any history of regular alcohol use? Patient denies.
- Any heat or cold intolerance or known thyroid disease? Patient denies.
- Any palpitations or flushing? Patient denies.

Physical Examination

He is an adult male with a normal voice, breathing comfortably and in no distress.

Ears: within normal limits, bilaterally.

Anterior rhinoscopy is normal.

Oral cavity exam shows no lesions. Normal salivary flow. No obvious stones.

Oropharynx: soft palate elevates in the midline.

Neck exam shows a firm mass in the left upper lateral neck that is mobile medial to laterally but not in the cephalocaudal direction. On the right side, there is a fullness in the upper lateral neck around level II but no discrete mass.

No other palpable neck masses.

Cranial nerves II–XII grossly within normal limits.

Question: What else would you consider as part of your initial evaluation? (Choose all that apply.)

- Fiberoptic exam: **yes**/no. There were no obvious mucosal lesions. The anatomy of the nasopharynx, oropharynx, hypopharynx, and larynx appeared normal, and the sensation and motion of the larynx were intact.
- Office ultrasound: **yes**/no. Office ultrasound demonstrates the following:
  Right side: a 2.5 × 1.9 cm hypervascular hypoechoic mass centered near the bifurcation of the carotid artery. No obvious pathologic lymph nodes.
  Left side: a 5.5 × 4.6 cm hypervascular hypoechoic mass centered near the bifurcation of the carotid artery. No obvious pathologic lymph nodes.
- Office ultrasound guided fine needle aspiration: yes/**no**. While fine needle aspirations can often be done safely, in this instance, due to the characteristic appearance of the lesions, it is not necessary.

Question: Which of the following would be the most appropriate next step in the evaluation of this patient?

- Oral HPV testing: yes/**no**. This would only signify an oral infection with HPV and would not provide meaningful information related to the neck mass. While an HPV-related oropharyngeal cancer with cervical metastases would be on the differential diagnosis, an oral HPV test is not helpful in ruling in or ruling out the diagnosis.
- Ultrasound guided core biopsy: yes/**no**. Given the highly vascular nature of these tumors, diagnosis is typically made based on radiographic findings. Core needle biopsy could result in life-threatening cervical hematoma. Core biopsies are not recommended for highly vascular lesions.
- CT/computed tomography angiography (CTA) of the head and neck: **yes**/no. In this patient with bilateral neck masses, getting a formal CT of the neck would be appropriate to further classify the lesions. Since the suspicion for paraganglioma is high, getting a CTA and including the head are important.
- Thyroid function tests: yes/**no**. Ultrasound findings are not suggestive of a thyroid mass. Thyroid function tests are helpful in the assessment of thyroid lesions or for patients with hypo- or hyperthyroid symptoms.

Figure 36.1 shows two representative CT images from the patient.

(*Continued*)

CASE 36   (continued)

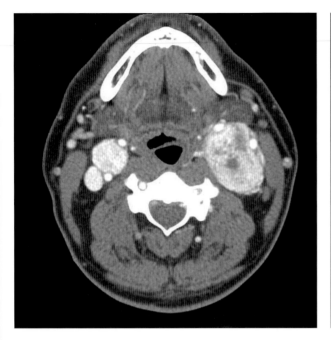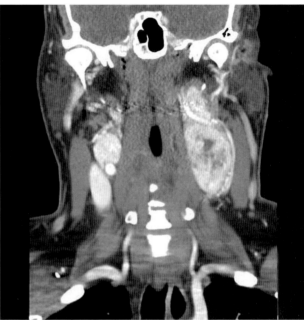

FIGURE 36.1   These are representative axial and coronal images from this patient's contrast-enhanced CT of the neck.

Due to the patient's young age and the size of the tumors, the decision was made for surgical management of the larger tumor.

Question: Which of the following should be discussed with the patient as a risk from the surgery? (Choose all that apply.)

- Tumor recurrence: **yes**/no. Given the size of the tumor, this patient would be at risk for local recurrence and the development of an additional primary tumor within the neck.
- Dry mouth: yes/**no**. Carotid body tumor resection is not likely to result in clinically significant xerostomia.
- Injury to the carotid artery with stroke: **yes**/no. Although unlikely, carotid injury can occur. Preoperative vascular surgery consultation should be considered, especially for larger tumors.
- Change in speech: **yes**/no. For tumors larger than 5 cm, the risk of postoperative cranial nerve deficit is 67%. The hypoglossal nerve is commonly affected by neuropraxia related to dissection off of the superficial aspect of the tumor, retraction to access the upper margin of the tumor, and due to devascularization.
- Change in voice or swallowing: **yes**/no. The vagus nerve proper is often preserved but commonly smaller branches making motor and sensory contributions (including

the superior laryngeal nerve branch) to the pharyngeal plexus may be compromised by the surgery leading to a change in voice and swallowing.
- Development of first bite syndrome: **yes**/no. This is a common occurrence after carotid body paraganglioma removal. It is presumably related to disruption of the sympathetic plexus that courses along the carotid artery, leading to unopposed parasympathetic stimulation of the parotid gland when eating and drinking are initiated.
- Injury to marginal mandibular nerve: **yes**/no. This can occur due to direct nerve injury or from retraction to access the superior limit of the tumor.
- Need for further treatment: **yes**/no. Residual, recurrent, or malignant tumors may need further treatment such as radiation therapy.
- Shoulder weakness: **yes**/no. This is less common for carotid body tumor surgery but should always be discussed, especially for large tumors.
- Significant lability in blood pressure: yes/**no**. This is not likely from removal of one carotid body tumor, but it can be a significant factor if surgery is performed on the contralateral side.

The patient underwent surgical resection of his left carotid body paraganglioma. All cranial nerves were able to be anatomically preserved, and he required a patch repair of his

CASE 36   (continued)

carotid bulb as well as the proximal internal carotid artery. There were no intraoperative changes in his electroencephalogram (**EEG**) signal.

Postoperatively, he was grossly neurologically intact except he was noted to have tongue protrusion to the left. He tolerated oral diet well and began therapy with speech-language pathology.

Question: What would be the appropriate course of action with regards to his right-sided tumor?

Answer: While resection of the contralateral tumor likely will be needed at some point, it would be ideal to wait at least 6 months to ensure recovery of the left hypoglossal nerve and also to allow for a steady state to be obtained after resection of the left carotid body. Continued observation would be an option as would external beam radiation therapy to the contralateral tumor. However, given the patient's young age and familial pattern of tumor development, saving radiation for disease that is truly unresectable would be ideal.

Key Points

- Genetic testing should be considered for patients with multifocal paragangliomas, family history of paraganglioma or pheochromocytoma, malignant paraganglioma, or young age at diagnosis.
- Succinyl dehydrogenase mutation is most commonly associated with hereditary paragangliomas.
- Patients should be counseled that resection of tumors >5 cm is associated with increased risk of postoperative cranial neuropathies.
- Resection of bilateral carotid body tumors carries the risk of baroflex failure syndrome, resulting in blood pressure lability.

CASE 37

Charles Yates and Michael G. Moore

History of Present Illness

A 51-year-old Caucasian female presents with a 2-month history of right-sided hearing loss and tinnitus. She denies any pain in the ear or any history of drainage from the ear.

Question: What additional questions would you want to ask?

- Any dizziness? Patient denies. Important question.
- Any history of chronic ear infections? Patient denies. Hearing loss and tinnitus can have many causes.
- Is tinnitus pulsatile? Yes. Important, as this may suggest either a vascular origin such as a tumor, dehiscent carotid or jugular bulb, or other hemodynamic cause such as anemia.
- Any history of head or ear trauma? Patient denies. Appropriate question.
- Any exposure to loud noises? Patient denies. Could be a cause of hearing loss and nonpulsatile tinnitus.
- Any weakness or twitching in the face? Patient denies.
- Any facial numbness? Patient denies.

Question: What additional aspects of the history are important?

- Tobacco or alcohol use? No regular tobacco use. She drinks one to two drinks of alcohol per week.
- Any history of head and neck cancers? Patient denies.
- Any family history of neck masses? Patient denies.

Past Medical History

She is very active with no known coronary artery disease or other major medical comorbidities.

Physical Examination

Well-developed female in no distress. Voice strong.

Skin: no suspicious lesions.

Salivary: no fullness or masses within parotid or submandibular glands.

Oral cavity examination shows moist mucosa with intact dentition. No visible or palpable mucosal lesions.

Neck exam shows no palpable neck masses or lymphadenopathy.

Cranial nerves II–XII intact.

Left ear: external ear, external auditory canal, and tympanic membrane were within normal limits.

Right ear: external ear is within normal limits. In the inferomedial aspect of the external auditory canal, there is hypervascularity and a purple bulge that appears to extend deep to the tympanic membrane. No ulcerations (see Figure 37.1).

Weber exam lateralizes to the right side.

Rinne: AD: Air<Bone; AS: Air>Bone.

(*Continued*)

CASE 37 (continued)

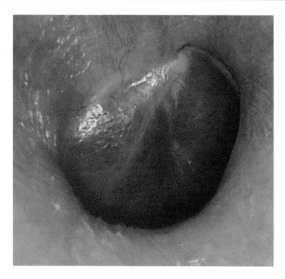

FIGURE 37.1   This otomicroscopic view of the right ear shows a vascular lesion filling the middle ear space.

Management

Question: Which of the following would be appropriate next steps in the evaluation and management of this patient? (Choose all that apply.)

- A flexible fiberoptic laryngoscopy: **yes**/no. This would be helpful to most definitively assess for any impairment in function of cranial nerve X. A mirror exam would also be an appropriate alternative to this.
- An audiogram with tympanometry: **yes**/no. In this instance, there appears to be a mass involving the right temporal bone. This, combined with the underlying hearing loss and tinnitus, would be indications for an audiogram and tympanometry (see Figure 37.2).
- A CT of the neck with IV contrast: **yes**/no. This is an excellent next step. In this instance, there is concern for a lesion in the temporal bone and/or middle ear (see Figure 37.3).
- Chest CT: yes/**no**. This would not be indicated at this point in the workup.
- A PET/CT: yes/**no**. This would be reasonable as a means to evaluate for multifocal tumor sites; however, it is typically not done as the part of the initial evaluation.

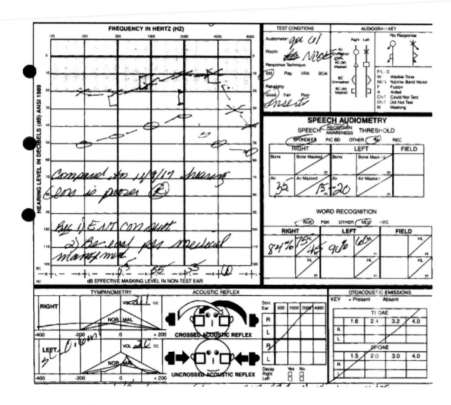

FIGURE 37.2   This is the audiogram obtained for this patient. It shows a moderate mixed hearing loss on the right side along with a mild sensorineural hearing loss bilaterally.

CASE 37   (continued)

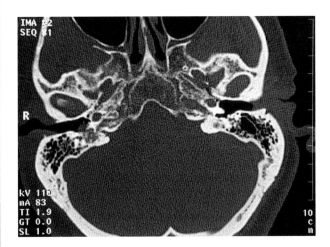

FIGURE 37.3   This is an axial cut of a temporal bone CT that demonstrates a lesion of the right middle ear and temporal bone with a smudged appearance of the bone around the jugular bulb.

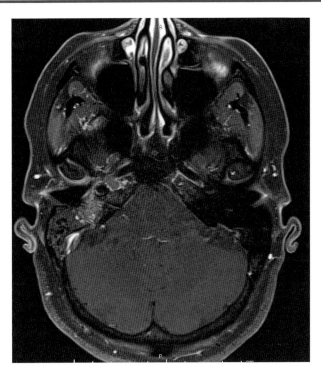

FIGURE 37.4   This is an axial cut of a T1 weighted, contrast-enhanced MRI of the temporal bone. On the right side, there is an enhancing lesion involving the right jugular foramen.

- MRI of the neck/internal auditory canal: **yes**/no. In patients where there is a concern for a neoplasm in the ear and temporal bone, an MRI can allow for improved soft-tissue resolution to best predict intracranial involvement and extension into the infratemporal fossa (see Figure 37.4).
- In-office biopsy of the right ear lesion using the otomicroscope and local anesthesia: yes/**no**. In this patient, where there is concern for a vascular neoplasm of the ear/temporal bone, an in-office biopsy is not recommended for two primary reasons. First, due to the vascular nature of the lesion, biopsy could result in life-threatening bleeding. This can occur for vascular neoplasms or in instances of anatomic variants such as a high-riding jugular bulb or aberrant internal carotid artery. The other primary reason to avoid in-office biopsy prior to obtaining imaging is to ensure that there is no communication with the intracranial space (in instances such as an encephalocele).

Question: Based on your current assessment, what would be the most likely diagnosis for this patient?

Answer: This patient most likely has a paraganglioma of the right jugular foramen with extension to the right middle ear and external auditory canal.

Question: Given the above information, what would be appropriate approaches to management of this patient?

Answer: With the presumed diagnosis of a jugular foramen paraganglioma, options for management include observation or definitive treatment with external beam or stereotactic radiation therapy or surgery. There also are descriptions of subtotal tumor resections with use of postoperative radiation therapy, if total tumor resection would lead to unacceptably high morbidity.

This patient ultimately underwent a combined transmastoid and transcervical resection of his primary tumor with preoperative embolization. In patients undergoing resection of head and neck paragangliomas, preoperative embolization around 24–48 hours before surgery can be used in an effort to reduce intraoperative blood loss. This window is believed to optimize devascularization of the tumor with reduced inflammation and by not allowing time for neovascularization. It has been shown to be particularly helpful in larger tumors where the ability to get circumferential vascular control is challenging, as in tumors with skull base extension. In all instances where embolization is considered, the benefits must be weighed with the potential risks of embolic events resulting in cerebrovascular accidents and/or isolated cranial nerve deficits.

(Continued)

CASE 37 (continued)

Question: In this patient with a right jugular foramen paraganglioma, what is the most likely indicator of the tumor being malignant?

Answer: Unlike many neoplasms, malignant and benign paragangliomas look similar in both their local behavior and on histopathology. Benign tumors may erode bone and even create cranial nerve deficits. The most reliable indicator of malignancy in a paraganglioma is evidence of spread to a site that lacks paraganglia tissue such as the cervical lymph nodes.

Key Points

- Evaluation of lesions of the temporal bone typically involves a detailed history, physical examination, and imaging with CT and MRI. In instances where a paraganglioma is considered likely, a biopsy is usually not recommended.
- Management options for jugular foramen paragangliomas include observation or treatment with external beam radiation therapy, stereotactic radiosurgery, surgical excision, or combinations of these approaches.
- Detailed counseling should be performed, weighing the risks and benefits of all approaches to management. Special considerations include the patient's age and comorbidity status, current symptoms including hearing loss and any pre-existing swallowing or cranial nerve deficits, and concern for malignancy.
- Surgical resection, when pursued, is usually accomplished through a joint effort with a neurotologist as well as a head and neck surgeon. The approach used is dictated by the tumor extent and, in some instances, collaboration with neurosurgery is needed for intracranial extension.
- Preoperative embolization may be implemented in an effort to reduce intraoperative blood loss. However, patients should be counseled on risks such as cerebrovascular accidents as well as iatrogenic cranial nerve injury using this approach.

Multiple Choice Questions

1. Which of the following is true regarding resection of a 4 cm left vagal paraganglioma?

   a. It is likely to result in mild dysphagia with solids.

   b. A perioperative tracheostomy is often needed for airway management.

   c. There is approximately a 40% risk of loss of vocal fold mobility after surgical resection.

   d. Preoperative embolization runs the risk of vocal fold paralysis.

   Answer: d. Resection of vagal paragangliomas runs a very high risk of permanent loss of vagal nerve function resulting in severe dysphagia related to loss of vocal fold mobility (dysphagia often worse with liquids), reduced pharyngeal muscle strength due to loss of vagal contribution to the pharyngeal plexus, and numbness in the ipsilateral larynx and hypopharynx. One series showed that in 40 tumors resected, 37 required vagal nerve resection, and the remaining 3 patients suffered permanent vocal fold paralysis. While a loss of vagal nerve function impacts voice and swallowing function, a tracheostomy is not needed as long as contralateral function is adequate.

2. A 53-year-old female presents with imaging suggestive of a 5 cm right vagal paraganglioma. What would be an expected finding on this patient's imaging?

   a. Displacement of the right internal carotid artery medially.

   b. Displacement of the parapharyngeal fat posterolaterally.

   c. It would be expected to grow at a rate of 8 mm per year.

   d. The mass would show homogeneous enhancement with contrast on MRI.

   Answer: a. Vagal tumors lie in the post-styloid parapharyngeal space/carotid space and will originate between the internal carotid artery and internal jugular vein. The artery will typically be displaced medially or anteromedially. The parapharyngeal fat will be pushed anteriorly. Rate of growth of these tumors is typically slow, with a series of observed jugular foramen paragangliomas growing at a rate of 0.8 mm/year. When enhancement is typical for these tumors, flow voids result in a "salt and pepper" appearance.

3. A 43-year-old male patient is 1 day s/p transcervical resection of a left vagal paraganglioma. He complains of dysphagia with liquids. What would be helpful to allow this patient to swallow more safely?

   a. Initiate a course of decadron 10 mg IV every 8 hours.

   b. Perform a tracheostomy to assist with pulmonary toilet.

   c. Recommend a chin tuck to the right side when swallowing.

   d. Recommend a chin tuck to the left side when swallowing.

   Answer: d. A chin tuck to the affected side can aid in swallowing in patients with loss of vocal fold mobility. This helps obliterate the nonfunctional and insensate pharynx. Thickening of liquids and ongoing swallowing therapy are also helpful. Use of decadron and placement of a tracheostomy would not aid in swallowing function.

4. You are evaluating an 82-year-old male patient for an incidentally found 4 cm left upper neck mass that is consistent with a vagal paraganglioma on imaging. The patient is currently

asymptomatic. What would be the most appropriate next step in management of this patient?

a. Repeat imaging in 6 months.

b. Arrangement of a neck angiogram with embolization of the mass.

c. Transcervical resection of the tumor.

d. Stereotactic radiosurgery for the mass.

Answer: a. In this asymptomatic elderly patient, surgical resection is typically contraindicated. While radiation can be considered, stereotactic radiosurgery is typically reserved for masses 3 cm or smaller. The most appropriate management here would be a period of observation with repeat imaging.

5. In preparation for surgery, a patient undergoes a left-sided carotid artery balloon occlusion test and selective embolization preoperatively. Which of the following is true regarding this procedure?

a. The risk of stroke for carotid resection in a patient with a balloon occlusion test showing normal collateral circulation is 1%.

b. Embolization of carotid body paragangliomas is very safe and should be performed on all patients undergoing resection of these tumors.

c. The ideal timing of embolization is 7–10 days before surgical resection.

d. Isolated cranial neuropathies can occur following paraganglioma embolization.

Answer: d. Isolated cranial neuropathies have been reported after embolization of head and neck paragangliomas. They are less common in carotid body tumors but have been described. In patients where there is a risk of need for carotid resection, a preoperative carotid artery balloon occlusion test with postocclusion single-photon emission computerized tomography (**SPECT**) scan is recommended. However, even with a normal result, false-negative rates up to 10% have been observed, and patients should be counseled appropriately. In addition to the risks of isolated cranial neuropathies from embolization, there is around a 0.5–1% risk of stroke from the embolization itself. As a result, it should be reserved for larger tumors (some studies use 5 cm as a cutoff) or when there is concern for challenging access to control the proximal and distal vessels (as in jugular foramen and vagal paragangliomas). When performed, it is ideally done 24–48 hours before the surgery to minimize inflammation and collateral vessel formation.

6. With the leading candidate diagnosis being multifocal neck paragangliomas in a patient with a family history of neck masses, a genetics consult is obtained. Mutations in which of the following gene families is most likely to be associated with such multifocal disease?

a. NF1.

b. Succinate dehydrogenase.

c. MEN1.

d. p53.

Answer: b. In approximately 10% of individuals affected by paragangliomas, multifocal disease is identified, with the most common being bilateral carotid body tumors. In recent years, the succinate dehydrogenase gene family has been found to be altered in up to one-third of head and neck paragangliomas with strong predictors of germline mutations including a positive family history, multifocal disease, a prior pheochromocytoma, malignant paragangliomas, male sex, and disease diagnosis before age 50. Paragangliomas can be associated with MENIIA and IIB, as well as in neurofibromatosis and von Hippel–Lindau disease, but they are significantly less common.

7. The patient undergoes a successful transcervical resection of his left-sided carotid body paraganglioma. He has transient dysarthria related to left hypoglossal nerve paresis and mild dysphagia, both of which resolve with time and speech therapy. Approximately 6 months following the surgery, repeat imaging is performed showing continued growth of the right-sided tumor. What special consideration must be made for surgery on the right-sided tumor?

a. He is at high risk for hemodynamic instability if the other tumor is removed.

b. Surgery on the right-sided tumor likely will result in the need for a tracheostomy.

c. Surgery is not an option for the right-sided tumor.

d. He should have a preoperative gastrostomy tube placed.

Answer: a. When surgery is performed on the second side in patients with bilateral carotid body paragangliomas, they are at risk for baroreflex failure syndrome that is characterized by blood pressure lability with severe hypertension as well as profound hypotension, which can be triggered by sedation or induction of anesthesia. Patients requiring surgery should be followed closely by a medical consultant and often require sodium nitroprusside to avoid hypertension. Clonidine (a peripheral and central alpha-2 receptor agonist) or phenoxybenzamine (an alpha-1 and alpha-2 antagonist) have a longer half-life and may be used for more chronic management. Given that the patient did not have any vagal nerve injury during the first surgery, it is not likely that a tracheostomy would be needed following removal of the right-sided tumor. While dysphagia is possible following this surgery, prophylactic gastrostomy tube placement would not be appropriate.

8. A 63-year-old male patient presents for evaluation of left-sided hearing loss. Workup demonstrates a 3 cm mass arising in the left jugular foramen with surrounding bone destruction. Which of the following is true for this patient?

a. Surgical resection is recommended as it is unlikely to result in significant morbidity.

b. External beam radiation therapy will offer a high rate of local control.

c. Bone erosion suggests a malignant process, and therefore a systemic workup is recommended.

d. Observation of the tumor would likely result in a rate of growth of 5 mm per year.

Answer: b. Jugular foramen paragangliomas present a challenge to patients and managing providers. The use of external beam radiation therapy has been shown to result in an excellent rate of local control and is often preferred over resection due to the high rate of cranial neuropathies that may result from surgery. The local clinical behavior of paragangliomas has not been shown to be different between benign and malignant lesions. Diagnosis of malignancy requires confirmation of disease spread to other sites lacking neuroendocrine tissue. Growth rates of these tumors is typically less than 1 mm per year, when observation is employed.

9. A 42-year-old female presents for evaluation of 1 year of progressive left facial paralysis, hearing loss, and bleeding from the left ear canal. Workup identifies a vascular tumor at the left lateral skull base with extension into the left middle ear and mastoid, consistent with a jugular foramen paraganglioma. Which of the following is true for this patient?

   a. External beam radiation therapy is likely to result in complete resolution of the tumor.

   b. Surgical debulking provides a high likelihood of return of facial movement.

   c. A biopsy of tissue in the external auditory canal is important to determine a pathologic diagnosis.

   d. Surgical debulking with postoperative external beam radiation would be an appropriate option for management.

   Answer: d. While surgery for jugular foramen paragangliomas may result in significant morbidity due to potential involvement of the facial nerve and lower cranial nerves, it may still be appropriate in young patients, especially those with pre-existing cranial neuropathies, hearing loss, and/or significant ear canal bleeding. While external beam radiation therapy alone may provide good local tumor control, it halts progression but does not result in resolution. As a result, due to the issue of bleeding, it may be inadvisable here. Due to the progressive onset of facial paralysis, functional improvement with either surgery or radiation therapy is unlikely. Due to the highly vascular nature of these tumors, biopsies should be avoided.

Suggested Reading

Baysal, B.E., Ferrell, R.E., Willett-Brozick, J.E. et al. (2000). Mutations in SDHD, a mitochondrial complex II gene, in hereditary paraganglioma. *Science* 287 (5454): 848–851. https://doi.org/10.1126/science.287.5454.848.

Chun, S.G., Nedzi, L.A., Choe, K.S. et al. (2014). A retrospective analysis of tumor volumetric responses to five-fraction stereotactic radiotherapy for paragangliomas of the head and neck (glomus tumors). *Stereotact. Funct. Neurosurg.* 92: 153–159.

Gimenez-Roqueplo, A.P., Dahia, P.L., and Robledo, M. (2012). An update on the genetics of paraganglioma, pheochromocytoma, and associated hereditary syndromes. *Horm. Metab. Res.* 44: 328–333.

Gur, I. and Katz, S. (2010). Baroreceptor failure syndrome after bilateral carotid body tumor surgery. *Ann. Vasc. Surg.* 24: 1138.

Hinerman, R.W., Amdur, R.J., Morris, C.G. et al. (2008). Definitive radiotherapy in the management of paragangliomas arising in the head and neck: a 35-year experience. *Head Neck* 30: 1431–1438.

Hirsch, B.E., Johnson, J.T., Black, F.O., and Myers, E.N. (1982). Paraganglioma of vagal origin. *Otolaryngol. Head Neck Surg.* 90 (6): 708–714. https://doi.org/10.1177/019459988209000607.

Ivan, M.E., Sughrue, M.E., Clark, A.J. et al. (2011). A meta-analysis of tumor control rates and treatment-related morbidity for patients with glomus jugulare tumors. *J. Neurosurg.* 114: 1299–1305.

Langerman, A., Athavale, S.M., Rangarajan, S.V. et al. (2012). Natural history of cervical paragangliomas: outcomes of observation of 43 patients. *Arch. Otolaryngol. Head Neck Surg.* 138: 341–345.

Lim, J.Y., Kim, J., Kim, S.H. et al. (2010). Surgical treatment of carotid body paragangliomas: outcomes and complications according to the Shamblin classification. *Clin. Exp. Otorhinolaryngol.* 3: 91–95.

Mojtahedi, A., Thamake, S., Tworowska, I. et al. (2014). The value of (68)Ga-DOTATATE PET/CT in diagnosis and management of neuroendocrine tumors compared to current FDA approved imaging modalities: a review of literature. *Am. J. Nucl. Med. Mol. Imaging* 4 (5): 426–434.

Moore, M.G., Netterville, J.L., Mendenhall, W.M. et al. (2016). Head and neck paragangliomas: an update on evaluation and management. *Otolaryngol. Head Neck Surg.* 154 (4): 597–605.

Netterville, J.L., Jackson, C.G., Miller, F.R. et al. (1998). Vagal paraganglioma: a review of 46 patients treated during a 20-year period. *Arch. Otolaryngol. Head Neck Surg.* 124 (10): 1133–1140.

Power, A.H., Bower, T.C., Kasperbauer, J. et al. (2012). Impact of preoperative embolization on outcomes of carotid body tumor resections. *J. Vasc. Surg.* 56: 979–989.

Sniezek, J.C., Netterville, J.L., and Sabri, A.N. (2001). Vagal paragangliomas. *Otolaryngol. Clin. North Am.* 34 (5): 925–939. vi.

Suárez, C., Rodrigo, J.P., Bödeker, C.C. et al. (2013). Jugular and vagal paragangliomas: systematic study of management with surgery and radiotherapy. *Head Neck* 35 (8): 1195–1204. https://doi.org/10.1002/hed.22976.

Sugawara, Y., Kikuchi, T., Ueda, T. et al. (2002). Usefulness of brain SPECT to evaluate brain tolerance and hemodynamic changes during temporary balloon occlusion test and after permanent carotid occlusion. *J. Nucl. Med.* 43: 1616–1623.

Wasserman, P.G. and Savargaonkar, P. (2001). Paragangliomas: classification, pathology, and differential diagnosis. *Otolaryngol. Clin. North Am.* 34 (5): 845–862, v-vi.

SECTION 9

Neck

Jason Kass

CASE 38

Chase Heaton

History of Present Illness

A 42-year-old woman who has never smoked is referred by her dentist for a painful right lateral tongue lesion. This has been present for 4 months. It was initially thought to be due to rubbing against her molar caps but has persisted after having the caps smoothed. An oral surgeon performed an incisional biopsy that showed invasive squamous cell carcinoma (SCC).

Question: What additional questions would you want to ask?

- Any trouble swallowing or weight loss? Patient denies. Important to ask as the degree of pain and dysfunction is typically correlated to the extent of invasion into the tongue muscle.
- Any other lumps or bumps in the head or neck? Patient denies. Regionally metastatic disease should always be screened for in patients presenting with oral cavity tumors.
- Any difficulty with opening the mouth? Patient denies. Important to ask because either perineural invasion (PNI) or direct extension to the pterygoid muscles can contribute to trismus.

Past Medical History

She is otherwise healthy. Nonsmoker.

Physical Examination

General: pleasant and well-appearing female in no acute distress.

Ears: external auditory canals are clear, tympanic membranes are intact, no evidence of fluid.

Nose: external nose normal. Anterior rhinoscopy shows straight septum, no lesions.

Oral cavity: 1.2 cm right lateral tongue lesion, slightly exophytic, with leukoplakic changes on the periphery. It is painful to the touch due to the recent biopsy, so you are unable to feel an underlying mass (see Figure 38.1).

Oropharynx: no lesions or masses visible, soft to palpation throughout, tonsils are 2+ and symmetric.

Face: symmetric, no lesions or masses.

Neck/lymph: normal landmarks, no palpable masses.

Neuro: cranial nerves are grossly intact including facial sensation, facial motion, tongue motion, and shoulder shrug.

Respiratory: no abnormal effort of breathing, mild dysphonia.

Management

Question: Which of the following would be appropriate next steps in this patient's care? (Choose all that apply.)

- Narrow excision of the right lateral tongue cancer with 3 mm margins: yes/**no**. Excisional biopsies should be avoided as it may impact the ability to formally resect the tumor with clear margins. Surgical excision should follow completion of workup including imaging.
- Computed tomography (CT) scan of the neck with IV contrast: **yes**/no. In this patient, the next part of the evaluation is to obtain imaging to evaluate for subclinical lymphadenopathy. A CT of the neck with IV contrast is ideal for this but an ultrasound may also be performed as long as there is no concern for bone involvement by the primary lesion.

(Continued)

Essential Cases in Head and Neck Oncology, First Edition. Edited by Michael G. Moore, Arnaud F. Bewley, and Babak Givi.
© 2022 American Head and Neck Society. Published 2022 by John Wiley & Sons Ltd.

CASE 38   (continued)

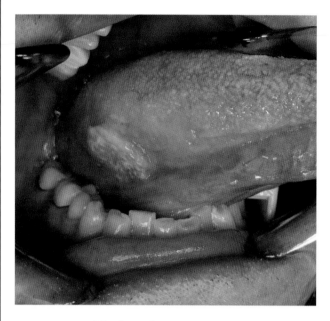

FIGURE 38.1   This photo demonstrates the exophytic lesion of the patient's right lateral tongue. It measures approximately 1.2 cm in maximal dimension.

- CT scan of the chest with IV contrast: **yes**/no. With a diagnosis of early stage tongue cancer, a CT of the chest is typically adequate to rule out distant metastatic disease rather than a positron emission tomography (PET)/CT.
- Referral to radiation oncology: yes/**no**. Though this patient may require adjuvant radiation or may be interested in discussing nonsurgical treatment, referral to radiation oncology and medical oncology can be reserved for after completion of workup. Also, oral cavity cancers are treated most effectively with upfront surgery so referral to radiation oncology for this patient with an early stage lesion is not appropriate.
- Discussion at a multidisciplinary tumor board: **yes**/no. After completion of imaging, the patient's case should be discussed at a multidisciplinary tumor board.

A same-day CT scan is performed. Due to dental artifact, the tongue lesion is not visualized. There is no suspicious neck lymphadenopathy. A chest CT is negative for distant metastatic spread.

Question: You review the case at the upcoming multidisciplinary head and neck tumor board. Review of outside biopsy pathology demonstrates a moderately differentiated SCC without obvious lymphovascular invasion (LVI) or perineural invasion (PNI). Depth of invasion

(DOI) cannot be determined as tumor extends to the deep margin of the biopsy. You recommend a wide local resection of the tongue cancer. What would be an appropriate way to manage this patient's neck? (Choose all that apply.)

- Concurrent neck dissection: **yes**/no.
- Staged neck dissection: **yes**/no.
- Sentinel lymph node dissection: **yes**/no.
- Observation of the neck: **yes**/no.

The greatest predictor of occult nodal spread to the neck from oral cavity cancer is DOI, a finding that has been corroborated across many studies. The threshold of when to perform an elective neck dissection has been a subject of broader debate. A prospective randomized controlled trial published by D'Cruz et al. (2015) found that in patients with DOI>3 mm, upfront elective neck dissection yielded better survival than observation. The challenge in clinical management is that the DOI is typically not known prior to surgery. Performing a staged neck dissection is therefore an appealing option that allows for final pathologic analysis prior proceeding with elective neck dissection. Alternatively, if other risk factors are present it would also be appropriate to proceed with upfront concurrent neck dissection. A growing body of literature also supports the use of sentinel lymph node dissection in early tongue cancer.

Question: The patient undergoes a wide local resection of his tongue cancer. The pathologist reports that there is no PNI or LVI. The DOI is estimated at 6 mm. Based on these histologic findings, what is the stage of the tumor?

Answer: cT2N0.

Per the AJCC 8th Edition, a tumor less than or equal to 2 cm can be upstaged depending on DOI. A tumor that has greater than 5 mm depth of invasion and is less than or equal to 4 cm in diameter is staged as T2. A tumor that has greater than 1 cm depth of invasion or is greater than 4 cm in diameter is staged as T3.

Question: Based on the above pathologic findings, you recommend an elective ipsilateral neck dissection. What lymph node levels will you dissect?

Answer: Ipsilateral, right, levels I–III.

In large retrospective studies, oral cavity SCC elective neck dissection specimens show rare occult nodal metastases to level IV (~3%), and no metastases to level V. An elective, selective supraomohyoid neck dissection level I–III is sufficient for management of cN0 oral cavity SCC, when elective neck dissection is deemed appropriate. There is some debate to whether or not level IV should be dissected for patients with lateral oral tongue cancers. A publication by Byers demonstrated a 16% of skip lesions in these individuals.

Neck level anatomy for supraomohyoid neck dissection (levels I–III):

CASE 38   (continued)

- Level I:
  - Level Ia (submental): midline, triangular boundary between the anterior belly of the digastric muscles, from the mandible superiorly down to the hyoid inferiorly. Deep aspect is the mylohyoid muscle.
  - Level Ib (submandibular): within the boundaries of the anterior belly of the digastric, the stylohyoid muscle, and the mandible. Deep aspect is floor of neck/mouth. The submandibular gland (SMG) is part of this nodal group.
- Level II (upper jugular):
  - Level IIa: posterior (lateral) border is CN XI, anterior (medial) border is the stylohyoid muscle (radiographic correlate is the posterior border of SMG). Skull base down to inferior border of the hyoid bone. Deep aspect is floor of neck.
  - Level IIb: posterior (lateral) border is the posterior border of sternocleidomastoid muscle (SCM), CN XI anteriorly (medially). Skull base down to inferior border of the hyoid bone. Deep aspect is levator scapuli muscle, and floor of neck.
- Level III (middle jugular): posterior (lateral) border is the posterior border of the SCM, and anterior (medial) border is the sternohyoid muscle. Superiorly from inferior border of the hyoid bone to the inferior border of the cricoid cartilage. Deep aspect is the floor of the neck.

Key Points

- Patients with a tongue cancer with DOI >3 mm should undergo upfront elective nodal dissection as this has been shown to reduce recurrence and increase survival.
- DOI is an important staging criteria with DOI >5 mm upstaging to at least a T2 and DOI >10 mm upstaging to at least a T3.
- A selective supraomohyoid, level I–III neck dissection is sufficient for elective nodal dissection in most oral cavity SCCs.

CASE 39

Tanya Fancy

History of Present Illness

A 55-year-old gentleman presents with a right forehead lesion that has progressively enlarged over the past several months. He has undergone excision of two prior lesions on his scalp that per patient report were completely excised. Pathology unknown.

Question: What additional questions would you want to ask?

- Any numbness or shooting pains around the tumor site? Patient denies. Important to ask as PNI from cutaneous malignancies can manifest neuropathic symptoms.
- Any limitation in brow motion or eyelid contraction? Patient denies. Important as retrograde PNI along the frontal branch of the facial nerve could cause facial nerve weakness.
- Any other lumps or bumps in the neck parotid? Patient denies. Important as large, recurrent tumors have a higher risk of regional metastatic spread.

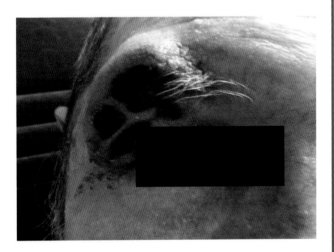

FIGURE 39.1   This photo demonstrates the 3.5 cm ulcerative lesion of the patient's right periorbital skin. It is mobile from the adjacent bone, and his extraocular motions are intact.

(Continued)

CASE 39   (continued)

Past Medical History

He is diabetic and has a history of Chronic Lymphocytic Leukemia (CLL), currently maintained on ibrutinib.

He has a 50 pack-year history of smoking cigarettes.

Physical Examination

General: pleasant and well-appearing male in no distress.
Ears: external auditory canals are clear, tympanic membranes are intact, no evidence of fluid.
Nose: external nose normal. Anterior rhinoscopy shows straight septum, no lesions.
Oral cavity: no lesions or masses. Healthy dentition.
Oropharynx: no lesions or masses visible, soft to palpation throughout, tonsils are 2+ and symmetric.
Face: see Figure 39.1.
Neck/lymph: normal landmarks, no palpable masses.
Neuro: there is some reduction of his visual field in the right upper outer quadrant but extraocular movements are otherwise intact. All other cranial nerves are grossly intact including facial sensation, facial motion, tongue motion, and shoulder shrug.

A biopsy is performed and is consistent with cutaneous SCC (CSCC).

Management

Question: Which of the following is/are risk factors for the development of metastatic disease in this patient? (Choose all that apply.)

- Immunosuppression: **yes**/no.   Immunosuppressed patients are both much more likely to develop CSCC and their tumors are more aggressive with greater risk of recurrence and metastatic spread.
- Size >2 cm: **yes**/no. Increased diameter is a well-established risk-factor for recurrence and metastasis and the primary basis for T stage determination.
- PNI: **yes**/no. PNI is one of the strongest predictors of recurrence, and metastatic disease and including in the staging criteria.
- Recurrent tumor: **yes**/no. Recurrent tumors are more likely to behave aggressively with higher rates of subsequent local and regional recurrence.

In addition, DOI and poor histologic differentiation have been identified as high-risk features associated with recurrence and metastasis.

Question: You order a contrasted CT scan that demonstrates no evidence of erosion of the underlying bone and no pathologically enlarged lymph nodes. What would be the next best step in managing this patient?

- Excision and SLNB: **yes**/no. The role of sentinel lymph node biopsy has been expanded to nonmelanoma skin cancers though not yet widely performed.

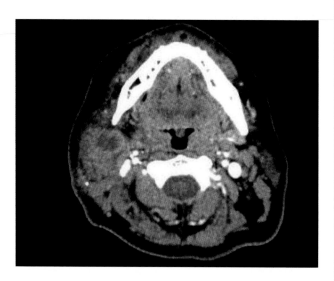

FIGURE 39.2   This cut of the patient's axial CT of the neck with IV contrast shows a mass in the right parotid gland with ill-defined margins and central hypodensity, concerning for a regional recurrence of cutaneous cancer. An ultrasound-guided fine needle aspiration (FNA) confirms SCC.

- Excision and parotidectomy: **yes**/no. It is common practice to perform neck dissection in mucosal head and neck SCC when the risk of occult disease is higher than 20–30%. However, the risk of nodal spread for a particular skin tumor hasn't been yet well established to identify which patients meet this threshold. In a patient with a high-risk tumor, however, it is reasonable to offer a elective nodal basin dissection.
- Excision with adjuvant radiation therapy: **yes**/no. Adjuvant therapy should be considered in patients with significant PNI, positive margins following resection or regional metastatic spread. If any of these criteria are identified during definitive surgical management, the patient should be referred for consideration of adjuvant radiation therapy.
- Excision with parotidectomy and ipsilateral selective neck dissection: yes/**no**. In the absence of nodal spread to the parotid, the chance of occult disease in the neck would be low and a neck dissection is unlikely to benefit the patient.

Note that in the setting of palpable cervical nodal or parotid disease, the patient should undergo upfront therapeutic neck dissection and parotidectomy. There is some debate on the appropriate extent of parotidectomy to perform in these patients. Hirshoren et al argued that a superficial parotidectomy is adequate, especially when adjuvant therapy is being used (Hirshoren et al. 2018). However, Thom et al demonstrated that 22% of patients with metastatic cutaneous lesions to the parotid had deep lobe involvement and advocated for a total/subtotal parotidectomy (Thom et al. 2014).

CASE 39 (continued)

The patient undergoes wide local excision of his tumor with sentinel lymph node biopsy. Final pathology demonstrates negative margins and no PNI or LVI. The sentinel lymph biopsy demonstrates no nodal involvement.

Three months later the patient presents for routine cancer surveillance after resection and negative sentinel node biopsies, and you palpate a nodule in his ipsilateral parotid gland. There is no palpable cervical lymphadenopathy. The remainder of the physical examination is unremarkable, forehead healing well. Figure 39.2 shows a representative axial cut from this patient's CT of the neck with IV contrast.

Question: What would be the next best step in the management of this patient's disease?

- Radiation therapy: yes/**no**. Radiation alone would offer a lower chance of achieving locoregional control.
- Chemo-radiation therapy: yes/**no**. Radiosensitizing chemotherapy would enhance locoregional control, however would likely still be inferior to surgical resec-

tion with adjuvant therapy. That said, definitive chemo-radiation should be discussed as a treatment alternative in patient where facial nerve sacrifice is anticipated during surgery.

- Parotidectomy: yes/**no**. Parotidectomy alone would be inadequate surgical therapy to address this tumor given the high likelihood of occult cervical nodal disease.
- Parotidectomy and neck dissection: **yes**/no. In the majority of patients with parotid metastases and a clinically negative neck, a combination of parotidectomy and a level II and III neck dissection is adequate for staging the patient's disease. Patients with parotid disease have an approximately 20–30% chance of harboring cervical metastases and so the neck should be addressed either surgically or with adjuvant radiation therapy. It is critical to always dissect the external jugular chain of nodes since they are at high risk for harboring disease. Following successful surgery, the patient should be considered for adjuvant therapy based on the pathologic findings.

Key Points

- Sentinel node biopsy is emerging as an effective means of managing occult disease in CSCC given the wide variability of lymphatic drainage across the head and neck.
- Patient with extensive PNI, positive margins, or regional metastatic disease should be considered for adjuvant radiation after surgery.
- Patients with parotid metastasis have a high rate of occult nodal disease in the neck and should undergo concurrent neck dissection.

CASE 40

Michael G. Moore

History of Present Illness

A 31-year-old Caucasian female presents with a 6-month history of a progressively enlarging right neck mass.

Question: What additional questions would you want to ask? (Choose all that apply.)

- Any inciting events? Patient denies. She just noted it looking in the mirror and since then it has been getting bigger.
- Any prior evaluation and treatment? Yes. She was seen by her primary doctor and thought to have cervical lymphadenitis. A course of oral antibiotics did not improve the swelling.
- Any pain in the mass? It is starting to get more uncomfortable.

- Any trouble swallowing? Patient denies. Important to ask as it could reflect involvement of the vagus or recurrent laryngeal nerve or dysfunction related to a mucosal head and neck primary tumor.
- Any voice changes? Patient denies. Important to ask.
- Any other adjacent lumps that have been noticed? Patient denies. Important to ask.

Question: What additional aspects of the history are important?

- Tobacco or alcohol use? She has never smoked. Occasionally drinks alcohol but not in excess.
- Any history of head and neck cancers? Patient denies.
- Past medical history: none.
- Family history: no known family history of neck masses or thyroid disease.

(Continued)

CASE 40 (continued)

Physical Examination

Well-developed female in no distress. Voice strong.
Skin: no suspicious lesions.
Salivary: no fullness or masses within parotid or SMGs.
Oral cavity and oropharynx examination shows normal anatomy. No obvious mucosal lesions to inspection or palpation.
Cervical exam revealed a firm mobile 4 cm neck mass just lateral to the upper aspect of the right thyroid cartilage.
No other neck masses.
Cranial nerves II–XII intact.

Management

Question: Which of the following steps would be appropriate in the continued evaluation of this patient?

- Flexible fiberoptic laryngoscopy: **yes**/no. In an adult patient with an enlarging neck mass, the potential for a malignancy of the upper aerodigestive tract with nodal metastasis needs to be considered. In a young nonsmoker, a human papillomavirus (**HPV**)-related oropharyngeal cancer, thyroid cancer, or nasopharyngeal cancer are potential sources. While oral tongue cancer may also produce nodal disease, even in a young nonsmoker, you would expect to see a primary lesion on oral exam.
- Flexible fiberoptic laryngoscopy shows normal anatomy in the nasopharynx, oropharynx, hypopharynx, and larynx, with no evidence of mucosal lesions. Sensation and movement functions also appear grossly intact.
- Oral HPV testing: yes/**no**. While a regional metastasis of an HPV-related oropharyngeal cancer is in the differential diagnosis, oral HPV screening tests only for the presence of the virus and does not provide useful information on the presence or absence of cancer.
- Office ultrasound: **yes**/no. This is a great option to assess this lesion and to evaluate for adjacent lymphadenopathy.

Office ultrasound shows a well-circumscribed 4.0 × 3.4 × 2.5 cm lesion in the right neck that appears to be posteromedial to the right carotid artery. There is no significant internal vascularity to the lesion. The lesion is relatively homogeneous.

- Office ultrasound-guided FNA: **yes**/no. This is a very appropriate next step. Since this was not seen to be particularly vascular, such a procedure should be safe and very informative.

An ultrasound-guided FNA shows spindle cells with mild atypia.

- Thyroid function tests: yes/**no**. This would be appropriate for evaluation of a thyroid nodule but not part of the initial workup of a lateral neck mass.

- Magnetic resonance imaging (MRI) of the neck with and without gadolinium: **yes**/no. Given the findings on ultrasound and FNA, it would be appropriate to obtain two-dimensional imaging at this point. While a CT would be helpful, an MRI will likely provide a little better soft-tissue detail and may allow for assessment of a neural tail that could be seen in a nerve sheath tumor (see Figure 40.1). It also allows this young patient to avoid radiation exposure.

Question: Based on the clinical history described and the MRI images depicted in Figure 40.1, which of the following is the most likely diagnosis of this patient?

- Right neck cancer, unknown primary, presumably from an oropharyngeal primary source: yes/**no**.
- An external/mixed laryngocele: yes/**no**. This lesion is not in direct continuity with the larynx.
- Metastatic thyroid cancer: yes/**no**. The location would be atypical for a metastatic lymph node, particularly for thyroid cancer, which typically metastasizes first to the central neck and then to level IV of the ipsilateral neck.
- Peripheral nerve sheath tumor: **yes**/no. This lesion is most likely a peripheral nerve sheath tumor due to the location, scant vascularity, and findings on ultrasound-guided FNA and MRI. The lesion appears to be in the post-styloid parapharyngeal space as it pushes the carotid sheath contents anteriorly.
- Paraganglioma: yes/**no**. A paragangliomas can typically present in a similar location and should be considered, however would typically present with flow voids on MRI due to the hypervascular nature of these tumors.

Question: Which of the following would be appropriate next steps in the evaluation and management of this patient? (Choose all that apply.)

- Observation with repeat scan in 6 months: **yes**/no.
  Given the presumptive diagnosis of a benign nerve sheath tumor, observation should be offered.
- Panendoscopy with guided biopsies and possible tonsillectomy: yes/**no**.
  Panendoscopy with tonsillectomies would be indicated in a patient with documented metastatic SCC to a cervical lymph node.
- Excision of the right neck mass: **yes**/no.

In this patient, the presumptive diagnosis is a peripheral nerve sheath tumor, a very reasonable option would be to observe. Because of the development of mild discomfort around the lesion there is some suspicion raised about a malignancy. Moreover, due to the lesion's size and the patient's young age, it is likely that it will

CASE 40   (continued)

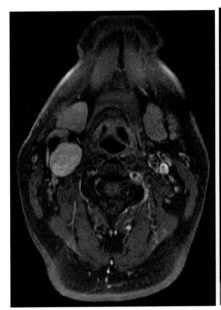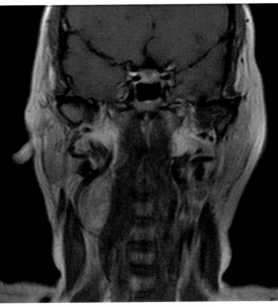

FIGURE 40.1   **These representative axial and coronal T1-weighted images after administration of gadolinium contrast demonstrate a well-circumscribed enhancing mass in the right parapharyngeal space.**

require removal at some point and delay may result in continued growth making future resection more challenging and morbid. As a result, excision of the lesion should be considered.

- External beam radiation therapy: yes/**no**.
  The use of external beam radiation therapy has been shown to be very effective in halting growth in nerve sheath tumors. However, in a young patient, the risk of long-term side effects as well as the low rate of radiation induced malignancy would argue against this approach.

Question: The patient opted initially for observation, but a repeat MRI 6 months later shows slight growth of the lesion, and she had developed worsening pain in the area. As a result, she elected to pursue transcervical excision. Which of the following would be important risks to describe to the patient? (Choose all that apply.)

- Injury to the carotid artery with stroke: **yes**/no.
- Change in speech: **yes**/no.
- Change in swallowing function: **yes**/no.
- Development of first-bite syndrome: **yes**/no.
- Change in eyelid position: **yes**/no.

The superior laryngeal nerve or the vagus nerve proper (much less likely due to the location) are possible nerves of origin of this mass. Since it is behind/medial to the vessel, it is not likely to be related to the hypoglossal nerve. Though carotid injury is very unlikely for a peripheral nerve sheath tumor, due to the proximity to the vessel, this risk should be discussed. Also, if this turned out to be an atypical presentation of a paraganglioma, the risk to the adjacent artery is more significant. In excising this tumor, the vagus nerve proper is likely to be preserved but smaller branches contributing motor and sensory contributions (including the superior laryngeal nerve branch) to the pharyngeal plexus may be compromised by the surgery leading to a change in voice and swallowing. First-bite syndrome is possible, especially if this tumor is found to arise from the sympathetic chain. It is presumably related to disruption of the sympathetic input that courses toward and along the carotid artery, leading to unopposed parasympathetic stimulation of the parotid gland when eating and drinking are initiated. Disruption of the sympathetic chain can also result in an ipsilateral Horner's syndrome (ptosis, miosis, and anhydrosis).

Figure 40.2a and b depict the intraoperative findings. The vagus and superior laryngeal nerve branch appeared to be spared and the mass appeared to arise from a nerve medial and posterior to the carotid artery.

(*Continued*)

CASE 40 (continued)

(a)   (b)

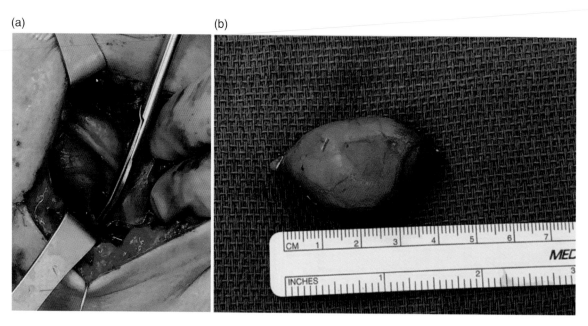

FIGURE 40.2 (a) and (b) These intraoperative photos show the right neck mass adjacent to the patient's carotid artery and vagus nerve. This tumor arose from the patient's right sympathetic chain. Final pathology demonstrated a benign ganglioneuroma. The patient postoperatively had normal speech and swallowing but did complain of right eye ptosis and mild first-bite syndrome.

Key Points

- In an adult patient with an enlarging neck mass, the potential for a malignancy of the upper aerodigestive tract with nodal metastasis needs to be considered.
- MRI is best suited to evaluating neurogenic tumors of the neck.
- Surgical resection, radiation therapy, and observation are all reasonable options for managing a benign nerve sheath tumor of the neck.
- First-bite and Horner's syndrome can result from sympathetic chain ganglioneuroma excision.

CASE 41

Chase Heaton

History of Present Illness

A 66-year-old male with a history of a reportedly benign skin lesion removed from his right forehead presented with a 7-month history of double vision and pain on the right side of his forehead.

Question: What additional questions would you want to ask?

- Any numbness or shooting pains around scar? Patient denies. Important to ask as PNI from cutaneous malignancies can manifest neuropathic symptoms.
- Any limitation in brow motion or eyelid contraction? Patient denies. Also important as retrograde PNI of a tumor along the frontal branch of the facial nerve could cause facial nerve weakness.
- Any other lumps or bumps in the neck parotid? Patient describes some slight fullness of his right upper neck. Important as large, recurrent cutaneous tumors have a higher risk of regional metastatic spread.

CASE 41   (continued)

Past Medical History

He is a type II diabetic.

Social History

He has a 10 pack-year history of smoking cigarettes.

Physical Examination

General: pleasant and well-appearing male in no distress.
Ears: external auditory canals are clear, tympanic membranes are intact, no evidence of fluid.
Nose: external nose is normal. Anterior rhinoscopy shows straight septum, no lesions.
Oral cavity: no lesions or masses. Healthy dentition.
Oropharynx: no lesions or masses visible, soft to palpation throughout, tonsils are 2+ and symmetric.
Face: well-healed incision on his right forehead.
Neck/lymph: subtle right level II enlarged lymph node. Mobile, nontender.
Neuro: right-sided lagophthalmos, diplopia on upward gaze, and CN V1 (ophthalmic) neuropathy. All other cranial nerves are grossly intact including facial sensation, facial motion, tongue motion, and shoulder shrug.

Management

Question: You decide to proceed with cross-sectional imaging. Which of the following would be appropriate next steps in the workup of this patient? (Choose all that apply.)

- CT neck with contrast: **yes**/no. CT scan is a good low-cost method for assessing any head and neck tumor. It allows for evaluation of the soft-tissue extent of a tumor, delineates underlying bone involvement, and assesses for the presence of lymphadenopathy.
- MRI neck with contrast: **yes**/no. In the setting of an advanced cutaneous malignancy with symptoms concerning for PNI, an MRI is essential for delineating any involvement of the supraorbital branch of the of the trigeminal nerve and evaluate for extent into the orbit or trigeminal ganglion.
- Ultrasound of the neck: yes/**no**. Though ultrasound can be useful in looking for evidence of lateral neck disease it will have limited ability to delineate the extent of a primary tumor.
- PET/CT: **yes**/no. Given the presence of an enlarged regional lymph node, a PET/CT would be an appropriate method of assessing for regional and distant metastatic spread.

MR imaging with gadolinium revealed right-sided cavernous sinus, superior orbital fissure, and intraorbital ophthalmic nerve enlargement and enhancement. Incidentally, an enhancing ipsilateral level IIA neck mass measuring 2.0×1.6×1.7 cm was noted (see Figure 41.1).

Question: The right neck mass and a supraorbital nerve biopsy both demonstrate p16+ SCC. What further testing on the biopsy specimens would you recommend to help identify a primary lesion?

Answer: Polymerase chain reaction (PCR) amplification and genotyping for high-risk HPV virus (HPV-16 and HPV-18).

HPV can be tested for using PCR amplification and genotyping for high-risk HPV virus (HPV-16 and HPV-18). S-100 immunohistochemistry (IHC) is a biomarker for melanoma, schwannoma, and neurofibroma. p53 mutations are common in head and neck SCC (HNSCC) but not routinely tested.

HPV DNA in situ hybridization testing was performed on both biopsy samples. The right neck mass was HPV+ and the supraorbital nerve tumor was HPV-.

Oculoplastic surgery performed a right anterior orbitotomy and excision of the frontal nerve for a presumed delayed perineural recurrent cutaneous skin cancer.

For the HPV-associated oropharyngeal disease, you recommend further workup to find the primary. After performing bilateral palatine tonsillectomy and a transoral robot-assisted surgical (TORS) resection of the right and 1/3 left lingual tonsils, pathology reveals a 0.3 cm focus of SCC within the right palatine tonsil, excised with negative margins and no LVI or PNI. For potential single-modality treatment of his HPV-associated oropharyngeal SCC (OPSCC), you recommend an ipsilateral neck dissection.

Question: What lymph node levels will you address in your right (ipsilateral) neck dissection?

Answer: levels II–IV.

The draining nodal basins for oropharyngeal primary tumors are levels II–IV. Level I is dissected in the case of oral cavity primary tumors. Rarely are level V lymph nodes involved, and therefore are often excluded from neck dissection specimens in OPSCC.

Two of 29 lymph nodes were positive for metastatic disease, and extracapsular extension was present. The patient then received concurrent chemoradiation (seven cycles of cisplatin and concurrent intensity modulated radiation therapy – 6996 cGy to the oropharynx, and 7200 cGy via Cyberknife to the right V1 nerve). There was no evidence of disease at 6-month follow-up.

(Continued)

CASE 41   (continued)

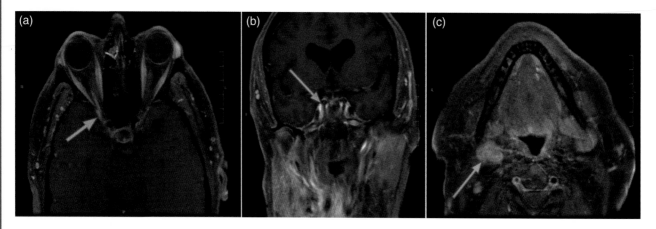

FIGURE 41.1   (a) and (b) Axial and coronal views showing enhancement and enlargement of ophthalmic (CN V1) nerve. (c) Axial view demonstrating a 2.0 cm right level IIA neck mass.

Key Points

- Synchronous head and neck primaries, while uncommon, do occur (estimates published between 2 and 3%).
- The cutoff point for p16 overexpression is diffuse (≥70%) tumor expression, with at least moderate (+2/3) staining intensity.
- Overexpression of p16 is an independent positive prognosticator and is a robust surrogate biomarker for HPV-mediated carcinogenesis.
- The primary draining nodal basins for oropharyngeal primary tumors are levels II–IV.

CASE 42

Avinash Mantravadi

History of Present Illness

A 35-year-old male presents for evaluation of a left neck mass. He states that approximately 8 months ago, he fell at work and after this noted tenderness in his left lower neck that persisted over several months. He was seen in an urgent care and was found to have a left level VB neck mass. Needle biopsies were initially inconclusive, and no further workup was pursued.

Over the next 4 months, the patient describes considerable growth in the left neck mass, with further left shoulder pain and expansion of the mass to the point that it limited his range of motion. He was referred to an outside otolaryngologist who ordered an FNA that was nondiagnostic and subsequently a core biopsy, which was suspicious for malignancy but remained inconclusive, and the patient was then referred to you.

Question: What additional questions would you want to ask?

- Is the mass enlarging? Yes, it has been slowly enlarging over the past few months.
- Any change in energy? Yes, mild decrease in energy.
- Any nasal congestion? Patient denies.
- Any oral bleeding/hemoptysis? Patient denies.
- Any voice changes? Patient denies.
- Any dysphagia/odynophagia? Patient denies.
- Any respiratory difficulty? Patient denies.
- Any unintentional weight loss? Patient denies.

Past Medical/Surgical/Social History

His review of systems is otherwise negative. He is healthy with no medical problems and no prior surgeries. He is a one-pack-per-day smoker for the past 17 years and drinks one to two beers daily. He works in a factory.

CASE 42   (continued)

Physical Examination

On physical examination, there is a 6 × 6 cm left supraclavicular mass that is firm and fixed. There is possible fixation to the skin posterolaterally, and the tumor extends to just behind the clavicle at its midpoint. It is tender to palpation. The remainder of the examination, including flexible fiberoptic nasal endoscopy and laryngoscopy, is unremarkable.

Management

The pathology report from his core biopsy sample demonstrates findings suggestive of poorly differentiated malignant cells without further characterization due to limitation on specimen size.

Representative CT imaging is demonstrated in Figure 42.1. The patient cannot undergo PET imaging due to limitations placed by his insurance carrier.

As of now, the pathology has been suggestive of malignancy, however, no further characterization has been made due to limitation of sample size. Imaging demonstrates a large enhancing mass spanning levels IV and VB in close proximity to the subclavian artery.

Question: What is the next best step in management?

- Surgical resection: yes/**no**. Surgery and its associated morbidity cannot be considered without more definitive pathology first.
- Repeat FNA: yes/**no**. The patient has already had multiple aspiration biopsies including fine needle and core samples without success in determining the diagnosis.
- Panendoscopy and biopsy with possible tonsillectomy: yes/**no**. While assessment of the mucosal access and tonsil is reasonable, on its own it neglects definitive diagnosis of the etiology of the patient's neck disease.
- Panendoscopy and biopsy with open biopsy of the left neck mass: **yes**/no. In this situation an open biopsy to obtain definitive pathology to better guide and expedite the initiation of therapy should be considered. It should be noted, however, that open biopsy may place the patient at greater risk for local recurrence or tumor seeding of the tract, and this must be balanced against the clinical suspicion for a true head and neck primary lesion. Level V and supraclavicular adenopathy alone would be unusual for an upper aerodigestive tract primary malignancy, however diagnostic upper airway endoscopy should be performed as well while the patient is under anesthesia to provide the most useful information.

It is important to note that the approach for open biopsy should take into consideration the possibility of surgery in the future, such that incisions should be designed for reuse and the assumption of tumor spillage or seeding along the tract should be considered should the patient require skin or soft-tissue resection at a later time.

Upper airway endoscopy is unremarkable and no mucosal biopsies are taken. Open biopsy is performed through a small supraclavicular incision. The tumor is found to be vascular, firm, and fixed with high-grade features noted intraoperatively. Final pathology demonstrates sheets of poorly differentiated cells with vesicular nuclei, prominent nucleoli, and grainy cytoplasm. IHC stains are positive for AE1/AE3. They are negative for p16, CK5/6, P63, Melan A, S100, TG, Napsin A, TTF-1, ALK, and CK7. The cells are also negative for EBV and HPV high-risk 16/18 via in situ hybridization. Flow cytometry shows immunophenotypically unremarkable T-cell population and polyclonal B cells with no evidence of non-Hodgkin's lymphoma.

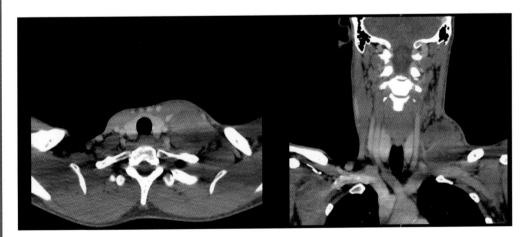

FIGURE 42.1   These axial and coronal cuts of a contrasted CT neck demonstrate a left supraclavicular mass.

(Continued)

CASE 42 (continued)

Question: Based on the pathologic description and immunohistochemical profile, which of the following best describes this patient's tumor?

- Primary lung carcinoma: yes/**no**. The immunohistochemical profile described above is negative for lung markers (Napsin A, TTF-1, CK7, and ALK)
- Poorly differentiated carcinoma: **yes**/no. This appears to represent a poorly-differentiated carcinoma without further characterization. Additional testing for specific primary sites may be performed for better delineation of the site of origin.
- High-grade lymphoma: yes/**no**. Flow cytometry is used to evaluate for lymphoma, which is negative.
- Primary head and neck SCC: yes/**no**. The immunohistochemical profile described above is negative squamous markers (p63, CK5/6, p16).
- Thyroid malignancy: yes/**no.** Thyroid malignancy is unlikely given negativity for TG and TTF-1.

PET/CT imaging is obtained, which demonstrates intense uptake in the left neck mass as well as several intrapulmonary masses, and retroperitoneal lymph nodes suspicious for metastases. The patient is admitted to an outside facility with rapidly worsening and intractable pain related to significant interval growth of his neck mass.

Without further characterization of the tumor origin, he is started on cisplatin and paclitaxel in an effort to slow tumor growth.

Over the next several days, the patient's pain improves dramatically and the tumor is decreased in size clinically. Additional immunohistochemical stains are ordered and are positive for OCT4, podoplanin, PLAP, and SALL4.

Question: What is the next best test to order to confirm the patient's primary tumor site of origin?

Answer: Testicular ultrasound.

The patient's dramatic clinical response to platinum-based chemotherapy is typical of germ cell tumors of urogenital tract origin. In addition, immunohistochemical stains including OCT4, PLAP, and SALL4 are highly specific for germ cell tumors including seminoma. The patient has undergone prior PET/CT imaging that demonstrated retroperitoneal adenopathy characteristic of metastatic testicular cancer (or other urogenital malignancies) along with a lack of FDG uptake in the primary site often seen in these tumors. There are no clinical symptoms or histopathologic indications of esophageal carcinoma thus far in this patient's workup, nor is the patient in the typical age range for patients presenting with esophageal malignancies. Germ cell tumors commonly metastasize to the liver and brain, however, dedicated imaging of these sites as a next step does not provide further characterization of the primary site. Tumor markers including AFP and HCG are used in the initial diagnosis and ongoing surveillance of these patients as well.

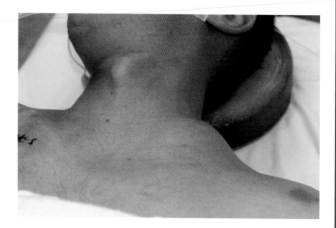

FIGURE 42.2 **This clinical photo demonstrates a left supraclavicular mass, now soft, nontender, and mobile.**

The patient receives four cycles of BEP chemotherapy (bleomycin, etoposide, and platinum) with normalization of tumor markers and significant decrease in the overall size of his left supraclavicular mass. Repeat imaging demonstrates resolution of all pulmonary and retroperitoneal lesions. However, the patient has a persistent large left supraclavicular mass that is now nontender, mobile and soft to palpation (see Figure 42.2). Representative CT imaging is noted in Figure 42.3.

Question: A needle biopsy is obtained. What is the most likely pathology?

Answer: Teratoma.

With normalization of tumor markers and resolution of symptoms and all other sites of metastatic disease, persistent active carcinoma is unlikely. Cystic fluid with necrosis is possible on FNA, however this would not explain the solid components of this tumor noted on imaging. Nonseminomatous germ cell tumors typically harbor components of teratoma and other germ cell tumor types. Although the pathogenesis is not clearly defined, it is theorized that current chemotherapy regimens for testicular cancer selectively induces transformation of malignant cells to benign cells while selecting out and preserving teratoma. The presence of teratoma after treatment is well-established phenomenon and is characterized by the presence of persistent or enlarging masses after chemotherapy, normalization of tumor markers, and histologic confirmation of teratoma on pathologic analysis. There is no defined association between lymphoma and germ cell tumors.

Question: The patient has no other sites of persistent disease radiographically. What is the next best step in management?

Answer: Left selective neck dissection levels III–VB.

Persistent teratoma in distant sites of metastases including the neck has been well documented after primary treatment of

CASE 42 (continued)

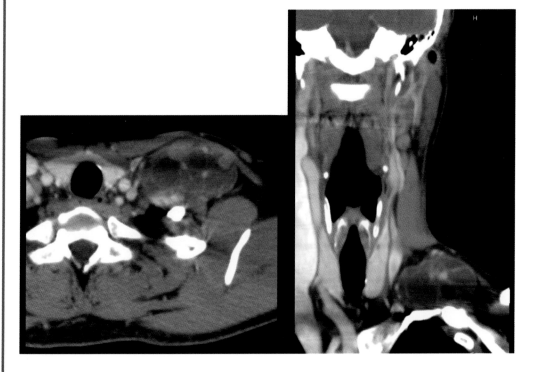

FIGURE 42.3 These respective axial and coronal cuts of a CT neck with IV contrast demonstrate a partially cystic and solid mass of left supraclavicular fossa.

metastatic testicular carcinoma. Treatment involves surgical resection of these sites of disease, which has resulted in excellent overall prognosis for these patients. Observation alone may place the patient at risk for malignant conversion in the future or possibly leaving active tumor behind which can only be proven on final pathologic assessment of the surgical specimen. The primary mechanism of spread of many non–head and neck primary malignancies to the neck is through the lymphatic route with spread through the thoracic duct and manifestation in the supraclavicular fossa. This is particularly true for urogenital malignancies, which often spread through the paraaortic route to the neck. Because of this route of spread, management of the neck involves selective neck dissection of the involved levels typically starting one level above the site of disease. Because the disease arises from inferior, addressing levels I and II in this case is not required and allows for adequate disease control without the additional morbidity and potential for cranial nerve injury with dissection of these sites. The patient's tumor has become soft, mobile, and nontender, which is characteristic of teratoma. Review of the imaging demonstrates no involvement of the jugular vein and preservation of a plane of dissection between the tumor and the SCM. In addition, given the low nature of this disease, it is likely that the branch of the spinal accessory nerve to the trapezius in level V can be dissected and preserved, such

that a radical neck dissection is not required (see Figure 42.4). Due to the intimate association between these tumors and the thoracic duct, caution must be taken during dissection to avoid chyle leak postoperatively.

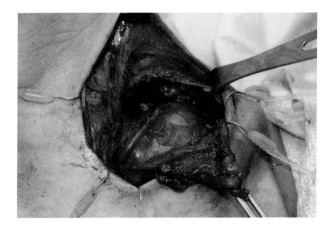

FIGURE 42.4 This intraoperative photo shows the left supraclavicular teratoma with clear plane of dissection between transverse cervical artery, SCM, and posterior branch of spinal accessory nerve to trapezius.

(Continued)

Key Points

- Metastatic urogenital malignancies are a rare cause of cervical adenopathy.
- Immunohistochemical stains for OCT4, PLAP, and SALL4 are highly specific for germ cell tumors including seminoma.
- The presence of teratoma after treatment is a well-established phenomenon and is characterized by the presence of persistent or enlarging masses after chemotherapy, normalization of tumor markers, and histologic confirmation of teratoma on pathologic analysis.
- Treatment involves surgical resection of these sites of disease, which has resulted in excellent overall prognosis for these patients.
- Because of the inferior route of spread, management of these tumors in the neck typically involves starting one level above the site of disease.

Multiple Choice Questions

1. In a patient with early stage oral cavity cancer, what pathologic finding, if present, would raise your suspicion about occult nodal metastases and prompt you to perform an elective neck dissection?

   a. PNI.

   b. DOI>3 mm.

   c. LVI.

   d. Well-differentiated tumor.

   Answer: b. A study by D'Cruz et al. (2015) concluded that among patients with early stage oral SCC, elective neck dissection resulted in higher rates of overall and disease-free survival. Waiting for disease to recur, in the subset with occult disease, had inferior survival. A subset analysis demonstrated that this benefit was only observed in patients with DOI>3 mm. While PNI and LVI both can lead to worse prognosis, they, in and of themselves have not been shown to predict occult nodal metastatic disease.

2. The most common site of regional metastatic disease from head and neck cutaneous SCC is

   a. Ipsilateral upper jugular nodes.

   b. Ipsilateral parotid gland.

   c. Occipital nodes.

   d. Retroauricular nodes.

   e. Ipsilateral lower jugular nodes.

   Answer: b. Although metastatic disease from cutaneous SCC is uncommon, high risk lesions have been reported to have metastatic rates exceeding 30%. Involvement of the regional nodes increases the risk of recurrence and lowers the survival rate. The parotid is the most commonly involved site. Among pathologically positive necks, level II is the most commonly involved.

3. Which of the following would prompt you to consider performing sentinel lymph node biopsy in a patient with skin cancer? (Choose all that apply.)

   a. 2 cm Merkel cell carcinoma.

   b. Single palpable occipital node in a patient with T1 right temple SCC.

   c. 2.0 mm deep, ulcerated melanoma with 3 mitoses/hpf.

   d. 3 cm desmoplastic SCC.

   Answer: a, c, d. There is no role for SLNB in a patient with clinically evident lymphadenopathy. In such cases therapeutic neck dissection is indicated.

4. In a patient with vagal schwannoma of the neck, which of the following would be an appropriate way to counsel a patient about expected postoperative vocal cord function following an enucleation/intracaspular dissection?

   a. TVF rarely recovers after enucleation and patient is likely to benefit from long-term medialization laryngoplasty.

   b. Immediate TVF paresis is expected but often recovers, and most patients do not need to undergo medialization laryngoplasty.

   c. TVF function is expected to be preserved immediately following the surgery.

   d. Given the high rate of recurrence associated with enucleation procedures, this method of resection should not be attempted.

   Answer: b. Netterville and Groom (2015) published clinical outcomes on a series of patients with cervical schwannoma resected with an enucleation/intracapsular dissection technique. Though most patient experience some degree of acute paresis after surgery, the majority went on to have near normal vocal cord function and 8/16 had symmetric TVF function at 1 year.

5. A PET/CT scan shows FDG avidity of the right neck mass and orbital lesion, but no other sites of hypermetabolic disease. FNA of the mass revealed metastatic SCC. You ask the pathologist to test for p16 from the FNA sample. Which of the following statements regarding p16 is false?

   a. Overexpression of p16 is an independent positive prognosticator in oropharyngeal cancer.

   b. p16 IHC staining is a robust surrogate biomarker for HPV-mediated carcinogenesis.

   c. The cutoff point for p16 overexpression is >25% tumor expression, with at least 1/3 staining intensity.

   d. Up to 32% of CSCC nodal metastases may overexpress p16, but it does not confer a survival advantage.

Answer: c. Specifically, the cutoff point for p16 overexpression is diffuse (≥70%) tumor expression, with at least moderate (+2/3) staining intensity. Per the AJCC 8th Edition, overexpression of p16 is an independent positive prognosticator and is a robust surrogate biomarker for HPV-mediated carcinogenesis. Satgunaseelan et al. (2017) found that up to 32% of CSCC nodal metastases may overexpress p16, but it does not confer a survival advantage.

6. When imaging and examination shows no evidence of enlarged cervical lymph nodes, what is the rate of occult nodal metastasis in a patient with recurrent laryngeal cancer after prior definitive nonsurgical therapy?

   a. 3%.

   b. 17%.

   c. 35%.

   d. 45%.

   Answer: b. Rates of occult nodal metastasis range from 0–30% in the literature. A review of the literature reports a comprehensive occult metastasis rate of 17%.

7. What tumor factors are the strongest predictors of pathologically positive occult nodal metastasis during salvage laryngectomy?

   a. Increasing T stage.

   b. Glottic subsite.

   c. Supraglottic subsite.

   d. a and c.

   Answer: d. Increasing T stage, especially T3 and T4 cancers, and supraglottic subsite.

8. What is the occult metastatic rate for supraglottic tumors?

   a. 10%.

   b. 18%.

   c. 28%.

   d. 38%.

   Answer: c. The largest series reports an occult nodal metastatic rate of 28% for supraglottic tumors. The rate of occult metastases for glottic tumors is 10%.

9. If a neck dissection is performed for a cN0 patient with supraglottic cancer, what levels should be included?

   a. Levels II–IV.

   b. Levels I–IV.

   c. Levels I–V.

   d. Levels II–VI.

   Answer: a. Most authors would agree on dissection of levels II-IV for supraglottic tumors and glottic tumors. For glottic and subglottic tumors, strong consideration of the paratracheal nodal basin is also recommended. In most supraglottic tumors, regardless of T stage, elective nodal dissection should be performed. Moreover, in all T3/T4 glottic tumors, elective nodal dissection should be performed, including paratracheal nodal dissection, if surgery is pursued.

References

D'Cruz, A.K., Vaish, R., Kapre, N. et al. (2015). Elective vs therapeutic neck dissection in node-negative oral cancer. *N. Engl. J. Med.* 373 (6): 521–529.

Hirshoren, N., Ruskin, O., McDowell, L.J. et al. (2018). Management of parotid metastatic cutaneous squamous cell carcinoma: regional recurrence rates and survival. *Otolaryngol. Head Neck Surg.* 159 (2): 293–299.

Netterville, J.L. and Groom, K. (2015). Function-sparing intracapsular enucleation of cervical schwannomas. *Curr. Opin. Otolaryngol. Head Neck Surg.* 23 (2): 176–179.

Satgunaseelan, L., Chia, N., Suh, H. et al. (2017). p16 expression in cutaneous squamous cell carcinoma of the head and neck is not associated with integration of high risk HPV DNA or prognosis. *Pathology* 49 (5): 494–498.

Thom, J.L., Moore, E.J., Price, D.L. et al. (2014). The role of total parotidectomy for metastatic cutaneous squamous cell carcinoma and malignant melanoma. *JAMA Otolaryngol. Head Neck Surg.* 140 (6): 548–554.

Suggested Reading

Albany, C., Kesler, K., and Cary, C. (2019). Management of residual mass in germ cell tumors after chemotherapy. *Curr. Oncol. Rep.* 21 (1): 5.

Chernock, R.D. and Lewis, J.S. (2015). Approach to metastatic carcinoma of unknown primary in the head and neck: squamous cell carcinoma and beyond. *Head Neck Pathol.* 9 (1): 6–15.

Civantos, F.J., Zitsch, R.P., Schuller, D.E. et al. (2010). Sentinel lymph node biopsy accurately stages the regional lymph nodes for T1-T2 oral squamous cell carcinomas: results of a prospective multi-institutional trial. *J. Clin. Oncol.* 28 (8): 1395–1400.

D'Souza, J. and Clark, J. (2011). Management of the neck in metastatic cutaneous squamous cell carcinoma of the head and neck. *Curr. Opin. Otolaryngol. Head Neck Surg.* 19 (2): 99–105.

Durham, A.B., Lowe, L., and Malloy, K.M. (2016). Sentinel lymph node biopsy for cutaneous squamous cell carcinoma on the head and neck. *JAMA Otolaryngol. Head Neck Surg.* 142 (12): 1171–1176.

El-Naggar, A.K. and Westra, W.H. (2012). p16 expression as a surrogate marker for HPV-related oropharyngeal carcinoma: a guide for interpretive relevance and consistency. *Head Neck* 34: 459–461.

Jordan, R.C., Lingen, M.W., Perez-Ordonez, B. et al. (2012). Validation of methods for oropharyngeal cancer HPV status determination in US cooperative group trials. *Am. J. Surg. Pathol.* 36: 945–954.

Kharod, S.M., Herman, M.P., Amdur, R.J., and Mendenhall, W.M. (2018). Fractionated radiation therapy for benign nonacoustic schwannomas. *Am. J. Clin. Oncol.* 41 (1): 13–17.

Langerman, A., Rangarajan, S.V., Athavale, S.M. et al. Tumors of the cervical sympathetic chain-diagnosis and management. *Head Neck* 35: 930–937, 3.

Robbins, K.T., Clayman, G., Levine, P.A. et al. (2002). Neck dissection classification update: revisions proposed by the American Head and Neck Society and American Academy of Otolaryngology Head and Neck Surgery. *Arch. Otolaryngol. Head Neck Surg.* 128 (7): 751–758.

Shah, J.P., Candela, F.C., Poddar, A.K. et al. (1990). The patterns of cervical lymph node metastases from squamous carcinoma of the oral cavity. *Cancer* 66 (1): 109–113.

Vauterin, T.J., Veness, M.J., Morgan, G.J. et al. (2006). Patterns of lymph node spread of cutaneous squamous cell carcinoma of the head and neck. *Head Neck* 28 (9): 785–791.

van Vledder, M.G., van der Hage, J.A., Kirkels, W.J. et al. (2010). Cervical lymph node dissection for metastatic testicular cancer. *Ann. Surg. Oncol.* 17 (6): 1682–1687.

SECTION 10

Trachea

Stephen Kang

CASE 43

David Neskey

History

A 45-year-old male presents with progressive shortness of breath and difficulty breathing. He states this initially started a few weeks ago, and he presented to an urgent care facility for persistent cough and shortness of breath. He was subsequently diagnosed with bronchitis and prescribed steroids and albuterol with minimal improvement in his symptoms. Over the past 2 weeks, his symptoms have continued to progress, and he recently presented to the ER for difficulty breathing.

Past Medical History

None.

Past Surgical History

None.

Physical Examination

Well-developed male with stable vital signs with the exception of tachycardia to the 110s. He is in mild respiratory distress, saturating 98% on room air. Inspiratory stridor is appreciated along with diffuse expiratory wheezing and increased work of breathing at rest. The remainder of the head and neck exam is normal.

Question: What would be appropriate next steps in this patient's evaluation?

Answer: In this patient with subacute dyspnea, assessment of his lungs and upper airway is needed. Here, a computed tomography (CT) scan was ordered that revealed a 3 cm mass localized

to the trachea without apparent involvement of the esophagus. The mass appeared entirely intraluminal without extension into anterior neck soft tissues. There was no cervical adenopathy appreciated (see Figure 43.1). Flexible endoscopy was subsequently performed and revealed a tracheal mass about 2 cm below the level of the vocal folds. It was soft and appears to be pedunculated off the posterior tracheal wall but obstructing >80% of the airway.

The patient was admitted to the ICU. Overnight he developed progressive shortness of breath and work of breathing. An awake fiberoptic intubation was subsequently performed without complication.

Question: What would be the next appropriate step in this patient's management?

Answer: Bronchoscopy with biopsy of the lesion. The patient was subsequently taken to the operating room for bronchoscopy. In this instance, it is important to obtain a tissue diagnosis prior to formal management of the lesion. If possible, tracheostomy should be avoided, even if it could be accomplished distal to the tumor since this may impact the ability to offer a formal resection later.

Intraoperatively, the tumor was biopsied, and at the time of endotracheal tube exchange, the patient acutely decompensated and went into ventricular fibrillation arrest. ACLS protocol was initiated, and decreased breath sounds were appreciated. Bilateral chest tubes were placed and return of spontaneous cardiac function was achieved. Over the next 2 days, he recovered, and he was neurologically intact.

Question: What would be the differential diagnosis for this patient?

Answer: Primary tracheal neoplasms can be classified as either epithelial or mesenchymal and can originate from any layer of the tracheal wall (see Table 43.1). The proximal and distal thirds

(Continued)

Essential Cases in Head and Neck Oncology, First Edition. Edited by Michael G. Moore, Arnaud F. Bewley, and Babak Givi.
© 2022 American Head and Neck Society. Published 2022 by John Wiley & Sons Ltd.

CASE 43   (continued)

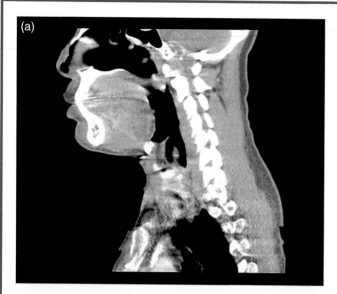

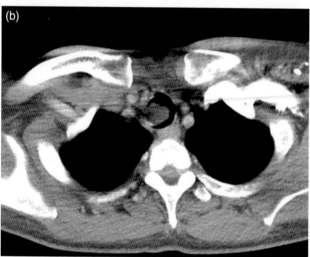

FIGURE 43.1   CT images of tracheal tumor: (a) Sagittal image demonstrating mass within the proximal trachea. (b) Axial image demonstrating a mass obstructing approximately 80% of the tracheal lumen.

TABLE 43.1   Tracheal neoplasms.

Benign	Malignant
Epithelial	Epithelial
Papilloma	Squamous cell carcinoma
Adenoma	Adenoid cystic carcinoma
Mesenchymal	Mucoepidermoid carcinoma
Granular cell tumor	Acinic cell carcinoma
Chondroma	Mesenchymal
Lipoma	Leiomyosarcoma
Schwannoma	Rhabdomyosarcoma
	Chondrosarcoma
	Lymphoma
	Melanoma

75% (bracketing Squamous cell carcinoma and Adenoid cystic carcinoma)

of the trachea along with the party wall are the most frequently affected subsites. Approximately 90% of adult tracheal neoplasms are malignant, whereas 80% of pediatric lesions are benign.

The biopsy fragments show a spindle cell neoplasm with some nuclear pleomorphism and scattered mitoses with a prominent myxoid stroma. The Ki-67 shows a relative high proliferation index. Additional testing showed the tumor was negative for AE1/AE2 and CAM5.2 (suggesting against sarcomatoid carcinoma) as well as MART-1, HMB45 and S-100, pointing against it being melanoma or a peripheral nerve sheath tumor. Given these findings and the immunoprofile (positive SMA), a low-grade leiomyosarcoma is favored.

Question: What would be the recommended management for this patient?

Answer: The patient underwent definitive surgical tracheal resection of rings 1–6 with a hilar release followed by primary anastomosis. The lesion was well circumscribed and pedicled off the party wall without extension into the esophagus. Based on the preoperative CT scan, it did not appear the lesion extended into the subglottis, which would have required a cricotracheal resection. Following the resection, the distal trachea was easily reapproximated to the proximal end. Using intermittent ventilation, the posterior wall of the anastomosis was closed with interrupted 2.0 PDS suture. With the posterior half of the anastomosis complete, the endotracheal tube was transitioned from the previous tracheotomy site to an oral intubation. With the oral endotracheal tube the anterior aspect of the anastomosis was closed again with interrupted 2.0 PDS suture. Once the re-anastomosis was complete, the infrahyoid strap muscles were reapproximated and a Penrose drain was placed. The platysma and skin was loosely closed with interrupted 3.0 vicryl and 4.0 monocryl. The patient was extubated in the operating room at the end of the case and transferred to the ICU.

Question: What adjunctive measures may need to be taken in patients undergoing segmental tracheal resection and re-anastomosis?

Answer: It is critical to minimize tension across the repair to avoid perioperative dehiscence and/or stenosis. In this case, a hilar release was performed. Other options include mobilization of the trachea by anterior and posterior blunt dissection minimizing violation of the lateral vasculature, and division of the infrahyoid or suprahyoid musculature. Additionally, a Grillo stitch (suture of the mandible periosteum toward the clavicle periosteum) is typically placed for 4–5 days to ensure the anastomosis heals. It also is recommended that the patient perform voice rest to minimize intratracheal pressure to lessen pressure on the repair. A nasogastric tube may also be

CASE 43   (continued)

beneficial to reduce hyolaryngeal elevation with swallowing that will increase tension across the repair.

This patient recovered well and was discharged home on postoperative day 5. On outpatient follow-up, the anastomotic site was noted to be healed without stenosis (see Figure 43.2). Review of the final pathology revealed a low-grade leiomyosarcoma pT2aNxM0 excised with negative margins. Postoperative radiation was not recommended given negative margins and low-grade features. He is seen in follow up every 3 months, and flexible endoscopy or bronchoscopy is performed to ensure there is no evidence of recurrent disease or stenosis at the anastomotic site.

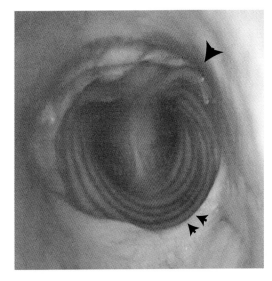

FIGURE 43.2   Flexible bronchoscopy image of anastomotic site. Single arrowhead delineates anastomosis suture line. Double arrowhead demonstrates an anterior area of mild stenosis.

Key Points

- Patients with primary tumors of the trachea tend to present with slow onset of respiratory difficulty and hemoptysis and cough occurring with more advanced disease.

- Airway management strategies should always be a primary consideration when assessing patients with tracheal pathologies.
- When segmental surgical resection is performed for tracheal neoplasms, care must be made to minimize tension across the anastomosis, postoperatively.

CASE 44

Basit Jawad and Rizwan Aslam

History of Present Illness

A 70-year-old male presents with a 3-month history of progressively worsening inspiratory stridor, exercise intolerance, and decreased PO intolerance. The symptoms began following a prolonged hospitalization in Puerto Rico 4 months prior, where he was intubated for nearly 3 weeks for a hypoglycemic coma. The patient has subsequently been hospitalized twice for aspiration pneumonitis. On presentation to your institution, Interventional Pulmonology first evaluated the patient and performed a bronchoscopy. This was notable for high tracheal stenosis with associated granulation tissue. The tracheal stenosis was unsuccessfully balloon dilated on two separate occasions, each time failing to resolve his symptomatology. The patient was ultimately referred to Otolaryngology for definite surgical management.

Past Medical History: diabetes mellitus, hypertension, prolonged intubation for hypoglycemic coma.

Past Surgical History: hernia repair, right upper extremity lipoma excision.

Medications: hydrochlorothiazide, aspirin, Claritin.

Social History: no alcohol/tobacco history.

Family History: coronary artery disease and hypertension in maternal family.

Allergies: none.

Physical Examination

Constitutional: in no acute distress, friendly 70-year-old male.

Skin/scalp: Fitzpatrick IV, no gross mass/ulcerated lesions.

Ear: bilateral auricles WNL. EAC patent. TMs intact.

Anterior rhinoscopy: septum midline, no mass lesion.

Oral cavity/OP: no oral lesions. FOM soft.

Neck: soft, no LAD. Landmarks palpable. No external scars/fibrosis.

Neuro: alert and oriented x 3. Cranial nerves II–XII grossly intact on external exam (review laryngeal exam below).

Respiratory: NAD, mild baseline inspiratory stridor present.

Voice: mild dysphonia, slightly breathy speech.

(Continued)

CASE 44 (continued)

Flexible laryngoscopy with right TVC paresis/hypomobility.

For further anatomic assessment, you order a CT scan of the neck and chest. Image demonstrated below.

Question: Please describe the findings in the following figures (see Figures 44.1–44.3).

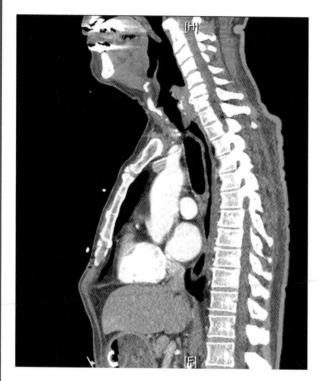

FIGURE 44.1   Sagittal CT.

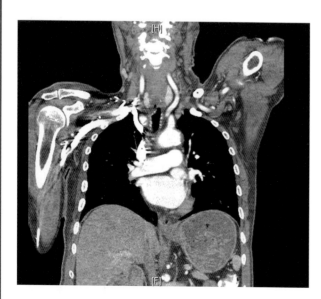

FIGURE 44.2   Coronal CT.

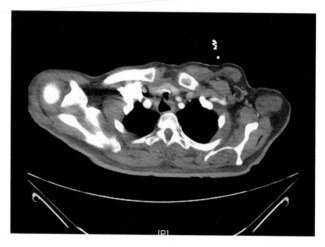

FIGURE 44.3   Axial CT.

Answer: Sagittal cut demonstrating a tracheoesophageal fistula (**TEF**) and segmental high-grade cervical tracheal stenosis (Figure 44.1).

Answer: Coronal cut demonstrating TEF and tracheal stenosis (Figure 44.2).

Answer: Axial cut at the root of the fistula site above stenotic segment (Figure 44.3).

Question: What is the most likely etiology of this patient's aerodigestive tract injury?

Answer: Post-traumatic. Given the history of prolonged intubation and start of symptoms directly following the first hospitalization, it is safe to believe this is a post-traumatic injury. It is likely that either a traumatic intubation or pressure necrosis from an inflated endotracheal tube (ETT) (within the trachea) and a nasogastric tube (within the esophagus) caused the injury. This case is particularly challenging in that there is both a TEF and a segment of tracheal stenosis.

Question: When discussing potential treatment algorithms regarding repair, what are important clinical aspects for a head and neck surgeon to consider?

Answer: Fully outline the extent, location, and consistency of the stenosis (location in relation to the subglottis and carina and the length and consistency of the stenosis). What is the patient's laryngeal and pulmonary function? Does the patient have medical, nutritional, or prior treatment history that would complicate surgical recovery? Patients who are not medically optimized for reconstructive surgery may be better served with conservative measures such as tracheostomy and gastrostomy tube placement. Select patients may be candidates for tracheal resection/anastomosis and esophageal reconstruction. Significantly large lesions may require assistance of

CASE 44   (continued)

cardiothoracic surgery for thoracotomy or extracorporeal membrane oxygenation (ECMO). Patients should be assessed for gastroesophageal reflux disease and managed aggressively. Poorly controlled reflux may impair healing and/or contribute to recurrent stenosis.

All treatment options (with respective risks and benefits) were discussed, and the patient and family wished to proceed with open surgical repair. The patient was taken to the operative room. A 3 cm segment of stenotic trachea (tracheal ring 2–5) was resected and primarily anastomosed. A suprahyoid release and anterior mediastinal pretracheal dissection was performed to facilitate the approximation. Additionally, a 1.3 cm TEF was identified which was closed in a multilayer fashion. A watertight seal was ensured for both the trachea and esophagus. A cervical collar was applied, and the patient's neck was placed in flexion for 7 days.

On postoperative day 7, the patient underwent repeat imaging and an esophagram (see Figure 44.4).

Figures 44.5a–c demonstrate the appearance of the area on postoperative CT.

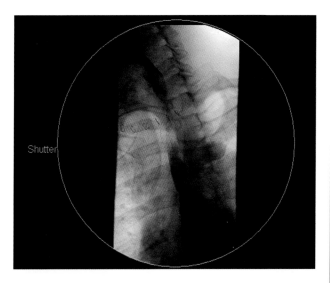

FIGURE 44.4   This image from the postoperative esophagram shows that no anastomotic leak was identified.

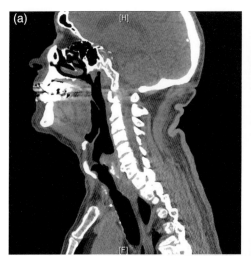

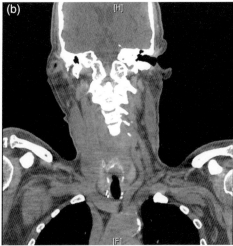

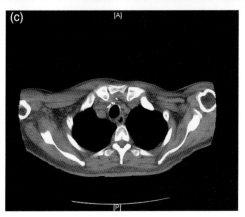

FIGURE 44.5   These images of the patient's postoperative neck CT, soft-tissue window in the sagittal (a), coronal (b), and axial (c) planes, show no further TEF is evident and the stenosis is improved.

(Continued)

Key Points

- Post-traumatic, idiopathic, and inflammatory etiologies are the most common causes of benign tracheal stenosis.
- In patients with persistent aspiration/pneumonia without a sensation of dysphagia, a tracheoesophageal fistula should be considered.
- For patients being considered for tracheal resection and re-anastomosis, proper screening for medical comorbidities and prior external beam radiation is important to minimize the risk of postoperative complications.

CASE 45

Yash Patil

Presentation

A 34-year-old female presents with an 11-month history of progressive dyspnea with exertion. She describes loud, noisy breathing with vigorous exercise that is worsening slowly. She was diagnosed with asthma by her primary care physician, but the medications she prescribed do not seem to be working. She denies any significant pain, odynophagia, aspiration, or dysphagia. She has no history of neck trauma or any recent surgeries but reports an uncomplicated cervical spine surgery 4 years ago. She reported no other systemic symptoms. Her primary care physician ordered an autoimmune panel demonstrating no obvious abnormality.

Physical Examination

General: Patient in no distress with very mild biphasic stridor detected only upon auscultation.

No retractions while breathing. Her voice is mildly hoarse.

The remainder of her head and neck examination is normal.

Question: What would be the next appropriate step in this patient's evaluation?

Answer: Flexible fiberoptic laryngoscopy and subsequent stroboscopy demonstrated a normal vibratory pattern and mucosal wave. The subglottis was visualized (see Figure 45.1).

Question: Given the above findings, what would be the most appropriate next step in the management of this patient?

Answer: The patient was scheduled for a microlaryngoscopy and bronchoscopy with biopsy and possible balloon dilation. A rigid zero-degree 4 mm Hopkins rod was used for evaluation of the airway. Both the supraglottis and glottis were found to be normal. The subglottis demonstrated a circumferential stenosis at the level of the cricoid cartilage and extending for 1.5 cm (see Figure 45.2). Given the patient's clinical stability, a CT of the neck and chest could also have been considered to further delineate the extent of stenosis.

The airway was sized with an uncuffed 4.5 endotracheal tube with a leak at 15 cm H_2O, indicating a high-grade 1 stenosis (Table 45.1). The remainder of the endoscopy was normal.

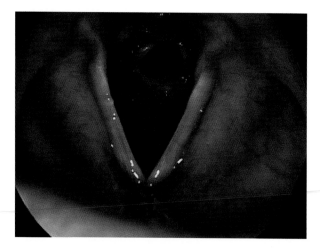

FIGURE 45.1   Subglottic stenosis viewed on stroboscopy. Notice the smooth nature of the abnormality as well as its relationship to the vocal folds.

The site of stenosis was injected with 0.5 ml of 40 mg ml^{-1} triamcinolone. Dilation was then performed using a 16 mm balloon. After dilation the airway was sized with a 7.0 endotracheal tube with a leak at 10 cm H_2O.

Question: Outline a differential diagnosis for this patient.

Answer:

1. Intubation, even of a short duration, can place a patient at risk for airway stenosis. Patients with idiopathic subglottic stenosis may be incidentally diagnosed at the time of or after an elective surgical procedure.

2. Inflammatory or infectious disorders should be evaluated as possible causes of laryngotracheal stenosis. Sarcoid (supraglottic), tuberculosis (glottis), Wegener granulomatosis (subglottic), and relapsing polychondritis are potential causes. Tests should be ordered based on history and physical exam. Routine screening for rare causes of subglottic stenosis is unnecessary.

CASE 45   (continued)

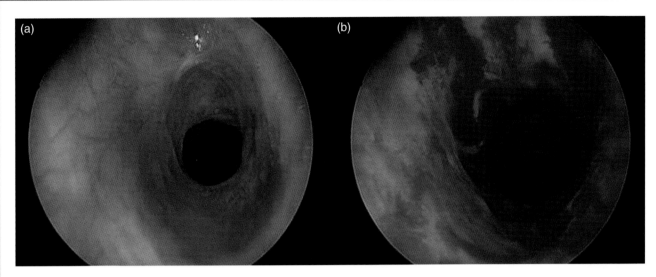

FIGURE 45.2   The idiopathic subglottic stenosis is seen prior to dilation (a), and immediately following dilation (b).

TABLE 45.1	Cotton–Myer classification of subglottic stenosis.[a]

Grade	Degree of stenosis
1	0–50%
2	51–70%
3	71–99%
4	100%

[a] *Source*: Based on Myer CM III, O'Connor DM, Cotton RT. Proposed grading system for subglottic stenosis based on endotracheal tube sizes. Ann Otol Rhinol Laryngol. 1994 Apr;103(4 Pt 1):319–23.

It is important to note that neck procedures, such as anterior cervical discectomy and fusion (ACDF) and thyroid surgery, place the recurrent laryngeal nerve at risk for temporary or permanent paralysis. It is important to evaluate this patient for vocal cord mobility given even a remote history of ACDF.

Question: What laboratory tests would be helpful in the evaluation of this patient?

Answer:

- Erythrocyte sedimentation rate (ESR) and C-reactive protein (CRP) levels were normal. These are important to check as they establish whether there is potentially an inflammatory etiology to the patient's stenosis.

- Cytoplasmic-staining anti-neutrophil cytoplasmic antibody (C-ANCA) and perinuclear-staining anti-neutrophil cytoplasmic antibody (P-ANCA) were both negative. P-ANCA antibodies target a protein called MPO, and C-ANCA antibodies target a protein called PR3. These are used in the workup and diagnosis of patients with suspected autoimmune vasculitis such as Wegener's disease (granulomatosis with polyangiitis), which can be a cause of subglottic stenosis.

- Angiotensin-converting enzyme (ACE) and calcium levels were normal. These can be elevated in patients with sarcoidosis, which can also cause subglottic stenosis.

Question: What is the most likely diagnosis for this patient?

Answer: Idiopathic subglottic stenosis.

Idiopathic subglottic stenosis is a diagnosis of exclusion in patients with airway stenosis. Antireflux therapy should be considered given that gastroesophageal reflux disease (GERD) may worsen subglottic stenosis, especially during treatment and recovery. Patients who are asymptomatic and have minimal airway stenosis may undergo observation alone.

Surgical Management

Patients may attain symptomatic relief with balloon dilation ± steroid injection. This may be performed on a repeated basis based on the patient's symptoms. Open surgical management is reserved for patients who fail endoscopic management or for patients who desire permanent surgical treatment. Cricotracheal resection (CTR) and tracheal resection (TR) are the two most commonly performed procedures. CTR is more effective in patients with idiopathic subglottic stenosis and patients with high-grade subglottic stenosis. Success rates for CTR are

(Continued)

CASE 45 (continued)

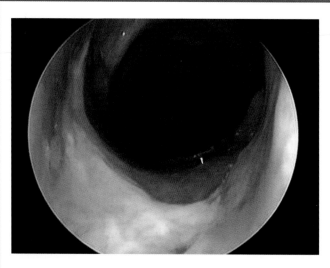

FIGURE 45.3 This bronchoscopic image was taken 3 months after the patient underwent a successful CTR with re-anastomosis.

often >95% for patients with idiopathic subglottic stenosis. In patients with idiopathic subglottic stenosis, removal of the diseased mucosa is crucial to long-term surgical correction and frequently necessitates removal of the anterior cricoid and all of the posterior cricoid mucosa. Tracheal resection alone is not adequate when disease involves the cricoid cartilage and mucosa. Often laryngotracheoplasty will fail in the long-term management of idiopathic subglottic stenosis, as the disease is not removed. Also, expansion surgery in adults may not heal as well as CTR or TR because of ossification of the tracheal and laryngeal framework.

The patient experienced immediate improvement after dilation, but the stenosis recurred after 6 weeks. She desired definitive treatment and underwent CTR. At 3 months, her airway appeared normal on endoscopy (see Figure 45.3).

Key Points

- Idiopathic tracheal and subglottic stenosis are diagnoses of exclusion and only should be made after evaluating for other potential causes of the pathology.
- Management of short segment airway stenosis is based on patient symptoms and can range from observation to endoscopic dilation with or without steroid injection or open surgical resection with repair.
- Aggressive management of acid reflux disease can help reduce the risk of recurrence of stenosis.
- In instances where there is significant subglottic stenosis, a formal CTR and reconstruction may be needed.

Multiple Choice Questions

1. Primary tumors of the trachea most frequently occur in all of the subsites *except*?

   a. Proximal third.

   b. Middle third.

   c. Distal third.

   d. Party wall.

   Answer: b. The majority of tracheal tumors arise from the proximal or distal third or the party wall between the trachea and esophagus.

2. Primary tumors of the trachea in adults are malignant what percentage of the time?

   a. 10%.

   b. 25%.

   c. 50%.

   d. 90%.

Answer: d. In adults, 90% of tracheal tumors are malignant. In children, 80% of tracheal tumors are benign.

3. The two most common primary tracheal tumors in adults are?

   a. Squamous cell carcinoma and adenoid cystic carcinoma.

   b. Adenoid cystic carcinoma and leiomyosarcoma.

   c. Granular cell tumor and mucoepidermoid.

   d. Squamous cell carcinoma and mucoepidermoid carcinoma.

Answer: a. Squamous cell carcinoma is the most common primary malignancy of the trachea. One-third of patients are unresectable at clinical presentation secondary to extent of local disease. Locoregional metastasis to mediastinal lymph nodes is common, and the 5-year survival for patients with mediastinal lymph involvement is 12.5% compared to 48% without node involvement.

Adenoid cystic carcinoma is the second-most common primary malignancy of the trachea. It is not associated with tobacco use. It has a predilection for perineural and submucosal spread, therefore microscopic clearance and negative margins can be difficult to achieve.

4. What are options that may be employed by the head and neck surgeon to decrease tension on the tracheal anastomosis site?

   a. Placement of a Grillo stitch.

   b. Preventing neck extension via continued postoperative mechanical ventilation.

   c. Cervical brace.

   d. Posterior plaster splint/upper body cast.

   e. Laryngosternopexy.

   f. All of the above.

   Answer: f. For all of these measures, the goal is to minimize tension across the anastomosis and therefore reduce the risk of postop dehiscence or stenosis. Potential life-threatening complications that can occur postoperatively include airway bleeding, restenosis, granulation tissue formation, mucous plug, anastomotic rupture, recurrent laryngeal nerve injury, aspiration pneumonia, mediastinitis, and pneumothorax/pneumomediastinum.

5. Which of the following would *not* be a contraindication to performing a tracheal resection and re-anastomosis?

   a. Diabetes mellitus.

   b. History of chronic G-tube dependence.

   c. Severe obstructive sleep apnea.

   d. History of prior neck irradiation.

   Answer: b. While dysphagia can be exacerbated by a tracheal resection and repair, a person with baseline chronic G-tube dependence may still be a reasonable candidate. In such an instance, less strain will be placed across the repair since patients will not be swallowing their nutrition. Diabetes as well as a history of prior external beam radiation can significantly impact healing of the trachea. In addition, severe obstructive sleep apnea is also a risk as these patients may need positive pressure ventilation after extubation, which would place additional stress on the reconstruction. While none of these factors are absolute contraindications to tracheal resection, their impact on outcomes should be used in decision making and patient counseling.

6. Surgical options for the treatment of idiopathic subglottic stenosis include all *EXCEPT* the following:

   a. Pericardial patch tracheoplasty.

   b. Cricotracheal resection.

   c. Laryngotracheoplasty.

   d. Observation.

   Answer: a. Pericardial patch tracheoplasty is a surgical technique used to correct tracheal stenosis rather than subglottic stenosis. Depending on the type and degree of stenosis, the other listed options are all accepted methods of managing subglottic stenosis.

7. What laboratory finding is usually seen in Wegener granulomatosis?

   a. Positive purified protein derivative.

   b. Increased ACE level.

   c. Increased C-ANCA.

   d. Increased antinuclear antibody (ANA) titers.

   Answer: c. Elevated C-ANCA titers suggest Wegener disease. A positive PPD test suggested tuberculosis. Increased ACE levels suggest sarcoidosis, while elevations in ANA titers can be seen in systemic lupus erythematosus.

8. In a patient with suspected laryngeal Wegener's, which study must be performed prior to operative intervention?

   a. Flexible fiberoptic laryngoscopy.

   b. Magnetic resonance imaging (MRI) of neck.

   c. CT of neck.

   d. Pulmonary function tests (PFTs).

   Answer: a. Flexible fiberoptic laryngoscopy allows for assessment of other upper airway pathology and for evaluation of vocal fold mobility. CT of the neck and chest may also be helpful but is not essential prior to bronchoscopy. MRI is not ideal due to the potential for motion artifact and the risk of airway complications while in the imaging machine. Pulmonary function tests would be of limited diagnostic utility in evaluating a patient with a known fixed upper airway obstruction.

Suggested Reading

Auchincloss, H.G. and Wright, C.D. (2016). Complications after tracheal resection and reconstruction: prevention and treatment. *J. Thorac. Dis.* 8 (Suppl. 2): s160–s167.

Bibas, B.J., Terra, R.M., Oliverira, A.L. Jr. et al. (2014). Predictors for postoperative complications after tracheal resection. *Ann. Thorac. Surg.* 98: 277–282.

Ching, H.H., Mendelsohn, A.H., Liu, I.Y. et al. (2015). A comparative study of cricotracheal resection and staged laryngotracheoplasty for adult subglottic stenosis. *Ann. Otol. Rhinol. Laryngol.* 124: 326–333.

Colice, G.L., Stukel, T.A., and Dain, B. (1989). Laryngeal complications of prolonged intubation. *Chest* 96 (4): 877–884.

El-Fattah, A.M., Kamal, E., Amer, H.E. et al. (2011). Cervical tracheal resection with cricotracheal anastomosis: experience in adults with grade III-IV tracheal stenosis. *J. Laryngol. Otol.* 125 (6): 614–619.

Gaissert, H.A., Grillo, H.C., Shadmehr, M.B. et al. (2004). Long-term survival after resection of primary adenoid cystic and squamous cell carcinoma of the trachea and carina. *Ann. Thorac. Surg.* 78 (6): 1889–1896.

Gaissert, H.A., Honings, J., and Gokhale, M. (2009). Treatment of tracheal tumors. *Semin. Thorac. Cardiovasc. Surg.* 21 (3): 290–295.

Gelbard, A., Francis, D.O., Sandulache, V.C. et al. (2015). Causes and consequences of adult laryngotracheal stenosis. *Laryngoscope* 125 (5): 1137–1143.

Lebovics, R.S., Hoffman, G.S., Leavitt, R.Y. et al. (1992). The management of subglottic stenosis in patients with Wegener's granulomatosis. *Laryngoscope* 102 (12 Pt 1): 1341–1345.

Myer, C.M.I.I.I., O'Connor, D.M., and Cotton, R.T. (1994). Proposed grading system for subglottic stenosis based on endotracheal tube sizes. *Ann. Otol. Rhinol. Laryngol.* 103 (4 Pt 1): 319–323.

Wang, H., Wright, C.D., Wain, J.C. et al. (2015). Idiopathic subglottic stenosis: factors affecting outcome after single-stage repair. *Ann. Thorac. Surg.* 100: 1804–1811.

Webb, B.D., Walsh, G.L., Roberts, D.B., and Sturgis, E.M. (2006). Primary tracheal malignant neoplasms: the University of Texas MD Anderson Cancer Center experience. *J. Am. Coll. Surg.* 202 (2): 237–246.

SECTION 11

Skull Base

Paul O'Neill

CASE 46

Kenneth Byrd

An 18-year-old female presents with unilateral nasal obstruction, increasing over the past 2 months. She was noted to have a visible mass in her left nasal cavity and was referred for further evaluation and treatment.

Question: What additional questions would you want to ask in the initial evaluation?

- Any allergic symptoms? Patient denies.
- Epistaxis? Occasional, self-limited.
- Hyposmia? Yes.
- Visual changes? Patient denies.
- Facial/palatal numbness? Patient denies.
- Constitutional symptoms (weight loss, nights sweats, fevers)? Patient denies.
- Lymphadenopathy? Patient denies.

Question: What additional questions regarding the patient's medical history would you ask?

- History of sinus surgery? Patient denies.
- History of childhood malignancy? Patient denies.
- History of radiation or toxin exposure? Patient denies.

Physical Examination

Skin: no obvious lesions.

Eyes: pupils round, equal, reactive. No limitations of extraocular movements. No proptosis.

Ears: TMs without retraction, no effusions.

Anterior rhinoscopy: beefy red lesion protruding into left nasal vestibule, nonpulsatile. Septum deviated to right.

Oral cavity: no lesions.

Neck: no lymphadenopathy.

Neurologic: no cranial nerve deficits.

Question: What is the next appropriate step in evaluation?

Answer: Rigid nasal endoscopy is performed. The right nasal cavity is without abnormal lesions. The septum is deviated to the right. The nasopharynx is clear. The nasal mass precludes endoscopy on the left.

Question: What would be the most appropriate next step in the patient's evaluation?

Answer: Unless the full lesion is seen on nasal endoscopy, imaging is the most appropriate next step to delineate the extent of the process and also to assess for any involvement of vascular structures and/or the skull base. With a large unilateral nasal mass, neoplasm should be strongly considered.

Computed tomography (CT) of the face/orbit/neck with and without contrast is performed (see Figure 46.1).

Question: What additional study would be beneficial in delineating the extent of the mass?

Answer: Magnetic resonance imaging (MRI) will provide information about the integrity of the dura and periorbita as well as distinguish between inspissated secretions and tumor (see Figure 46.2).

Imaging does not demonstrate any enlarged cervical lymph nodes.

A biopsy is performed in the office using cupped forceps and silver nitrate for hemostasis (see Figure 46.3). Another option would be biopsy under general anesthesia if significant vascularity is noted and there is concern for bleeding.

(Continued)

Essential Cases in Head and Neck Oncology, First Edition. Edited by Michael G. Moore, Arnaud F. Bewley, and Babak Givi.
© 2022 American Head and Neck Society. Published 2022 by John Wiley & Sons Ltd.

CASE 46 (continued)

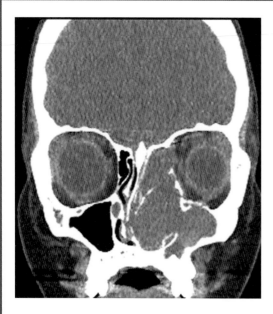

FIGURE 46.1 This noncontrasted coronal CT demonstrates opacification of the left nasal cavity, ethmoid sinuses, and maxillary sinus. The lamina papyracea is dehiscent.

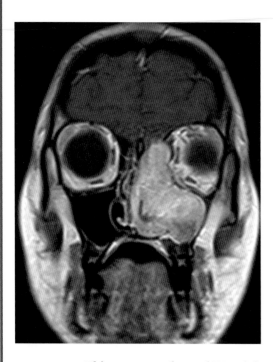

FIGURE 46.2 This contrast enhanced T1-weighted coronal MRI demonstrates an enhancing lesion of the left olfactory groove and nasal cavity. The dura and periorbita appear intact, and there is no intracranial extension.

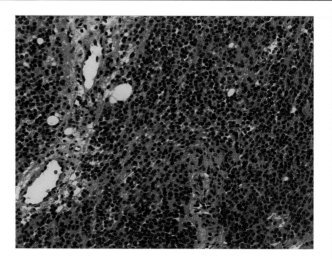

FIGURE 46.3 Biopsy reveals small, blue neoplastic cells with little cytoplasm. Additional stains are positive for chromogranin, S100; negative for cytokeratin.

Question: Given the above information, what is the most likely diagnosis?

Answer: Esthesioneuroblastoma or olfactory neuroblastoma.

Positron emission tomography (PET)/CT is performed to complete staging, which does not reveal hypermetabolic cervical nodes or distant metastases.

Question: What is the patient's AJCC 8th Edition stage?

Answer: The left-sided sinonasal tumor involves the medial orbit without invasion of anterior orbital contents or anterior cranial fossa. This therefore classified it as a T3N0M0 lesion (see Table 46.1).

Question: The Modified Kadish Staging System is an alternative approach to staging. How would this tumor be classified using the Modified Kadish Staging System?

Answer: This would be considered a Kadish C tumor as it extends into the medial orbit and narrowly involves the base of the skull. Table 46.2 outlines the Modified Kadish Staging System.

Treatment options are discussed with the patient after multidisciplinary tumor board discussion, including chemoradiation and surgery. Due to the proximity to the orbit and the patient's young age, she elects for surgical treatment.

Question: What would be the most appropriate surgical approach to pursue?

Answer: Due to the limited intracranial extension and lack of soft-tissue involvement, an endoscopic approach should be

CASE 46   (continued)

TABLE 46.1	**T-staging: nasal cavity and ethomoid sinus.**

T1: Tumor restricted to any one subsite, with or without bony invasion.

T2: Tumor invades two subsites in a single region or extending to involve an adjacent region within the nasoethmoidal complex, with or without bony invasion.

T3: Tumor extends to invade the medial wall or floor of the orbit, maxillary sinus, palate, or cribriform plate.

T4a: Moderately advanced local disease. Tumor invades any of the following: anterior orbital contents, skin of nose or cheek, minimal extension to anterior cranial fossa, pterygoid plates, sphenoid or frontal sinuses.

T4b: Very advanced local disease. Tumor invades any of the following: orbital apex, dura, brain, middle cranial fossa, cranial nerves other than V_2, nasopharynx, or clivus.

TABLE 46.2	**Kadish staging of olfactory neuroblastoma.**

Kadish A: Tumor is confined to the nasal cavity.

Kadish B: Tumor involves the nasal cavity and paranasal sinuses.

Kadish C: Tumor spreads beyond the nasal cavity/paranasal sinuses including involvement of the cribriform plate, anterior skull base, orbit, or intracranial cavity.

Kadish D: Tumor has metastasized to cervical lymph nodes and/or distant sites.

considered by a team capable of performing endoscopic skull base surgery. A transfacial approach can also be considered but would increase morbidity due to the associated facial scarring and the increased potential for soft-tissue seeding.

The patient undergoes endoscopic resection of the anterior skull base. The tumor is initially debulked to its sites of attachment on the superior lamina papyracea and septum. Mucosal margins are assessed after resection of the sites of attachment. The lamina papyracea is noted to be thin in the area of attachment, but the underlying periorbita is normal in appearance.

Question: What is the next appropriate step?

Answer: Resection of the periorbita with margin assessment.

The periorbita is resected and margins assessed, which are clear. The underlying fat and ocular musculature are not involved, as suggested by preoperative MRI. Orbital exenteration in the setting of skull base malignancy is controversial, but evidence suggests that it is not necessary in the absence of gross involvement of intraconal structures.

Frozen section margins are cleared at the contralateral olfactory mucosa. A Draf 3 frontal sinusotomy is performed, and the ipsilateral cribriform and ethmoid roof are drilled to expose the ipsilateral dura. Dural resection including the olfactory bulb and tract is performed. Dural margins and proximal olfactory tract are free of tumor. Reconstruction is performed with a collagen underlay and right nasoseptal flap.

Question: Five days later when packing is removed, the anterior portion of the graft is noted to be displaced with leakage of cerebrospinal fluid (CSF). What is the most appropriate step in management?

Answer: Operative repair. Because the graft is displaced, operative repair should be performed immediately. Lumbar drainage alone is unlikely to result in a water-tight seal. Options for surgical repair include fascia lata graft, tunneled extracranial pericranial flap, fat, acellular dermis, or other biologic graft. In this case, the previously raised nasoseptal flap was placed over fascia lata without lumbar drainage with successful closure of the CSF leak.

Question: Final pathology reveals olfactory neuroblastoma (Hyams grade II) with clear margins, including periorbita, medial lacrimal sac, and dura. What additional treatment should be recommended?

Answer: Postoperative adjuvant radiation therapy. Due to close margins in the orbit and T3 stage, postoperative radiation therapy should be recommended. Elective radiation to the neck is an area of controversy but should be considered in patients with Kadish C and Hyams grade III/IV (see Table 46.3).

Question: After treatment, What type of follow-up imaging is appropriate, and when?

Answer: Post-treatment imaging should be performed within 6 months. The imaging modalities used may vary by institution and provider. MRI has superior resolution for the orbit and dura to assess the primary site. MRI of the neck or contrasted CT neck may be used to assess the regional nodes. PET/CT is used at many institutions to assess the primary site, regional nodes, and for distant metastases but should not be performed prior to 12 weeks post-treatment due to increased false positives because of treatment effect.

(Continued)

CASE 46   (continued)

TABLE 46.3   Hyams grading system for esthesioneuroblastomas.

	Grade I	Grade II	Grade III	Grade IV
Architecture	Lobular	Lobular	Variable	Variable
Fibrillary matrix	Prominent	Present	Minimal	Absent
Mitosis	Absent	Present	Prominent	Marked
Necrosis	Absent	Absent	May present	Common
Nuclear pleomorphism	Absent	Moderate	Prominent	Marked
Rosettes	Homer Wright	Homer Wright	Flexner–Wintersteiner	Flexner–Wintersteiner

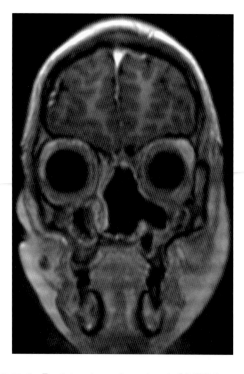

After radiation therapy, a 12-week post-treatment MRI demonstrates no recurrent disease (see Figure 46.4). The patient should then be followed according to the National Comprehensive Cancer Network Guidelines, every 1–3 months for year 1, 2–6 months in year 2, 4–8 months in years 3–5, and yearly after 5 years. Of note, patients with esthesioneuroblastoma should be counseled that they may develop delayed nodal metastasis even 10–20 years post-treatment.

FIGURE 46.4   Post-treatment contrasted MRI demonstrating nasoseptal flap along left skull base.

Key Points

- All patients presenting with a unilateral nasal mass should be assessed for the possibility of a sinonasal neoplasm.
- After a history, physical examination, and nasal endoscopy, imaging should be obtained prior to biopsy to avoid a CSF leak and/or significant bleeding from an encephalocele or highly vascular lesion.
- CT imaging and MRI with and without contrast are indicated as they have complementary roles in evaluating the extent of the primary tumor with regards to bone erosion and orbital and skull base/intracranial involvement.
- Commonly used staging systems for esthesioneuroblastomas include the AJCC and Kadish Systems.
- Upfront surgical resection is the preferred management of nonmetastatic esthesioneuroblastomas.
- Endoscopic resections should be considered in these tumors, but open approach may be needed for tumors with significant orbital involvement, anterior tumor extension, or superolateral extension.
- The Hyams grading system provides insight into the aggressiveness of the tumor with elective treatment of the neck being considered for grade III/IV tumors.

CASE 47

Zoukaa Sargi

History of Present Illness

A 74-year-old male is referred for evaluation of bilateral neck swelling and a mass in the right side of the nose. His symptoms started 2 months ago, first with a lump noted in the upper neck, then with intermittent bleeding from the right side of the nose.

Question: What additional questions would you want to ask as part of the initial evaluation?

- Any prior history of sinonasal problems or surgeries? Patient denies. Of particular interest would be a history of inverting papilloma.
- Any associated nasal symptoms? Minimal congestion on the right side. Sinonasal tumors often result in sinus obstruction, causing symptoms that mimic inflammatory sinonasal disease, often resulting in a delay in diagnosis.
- Any visual symptoms, such as double vision or decreased vision? Patient denies. Diplopia suggests orbital involvement or significant pressure on the orbit causing orbital dystopia. Diplopia could also be the result of involvement of the cavernous sinus affecting one of the oculomotor nerves. Decreased visual acuity could result from pressure on the optic nerve or direct involvement of the nerve by malignancy.
- Any headaches? Just minimal right-sided facial pressure, no major headaches. Headaches could suggest associated sinus infection, skull base involvement, or significant intracranial disease. However, significant obstructive sinonasal disease and significant skull base and intracranial involvement could be present without headaches.
- Any right ear pain or drainage? Minimal ear pressure, no drainage, no hearing loss. Ear pain could occur because of referred otalgia or Eustachian tube obstruction caused by sinonasal or nasopharyngeal lesions. This could result in otorrhea if the tympanic membrane is not intact. Conductive hearing loss could result from otitis media with effusion.
- Any numbness or pain of the cheek, palate, or upper teeth? Patient denies. Involvement of branches of the maxillary division (V2) of the trigeminal nerve in the posterior nasal cavity (greater palatine nerve), in the maxillary sinus (infraorbital nerve), or in the pterygomaxillary fossa could result in pain or numbness in the corresponding territories. With significant disease, there can also be tumor extension along other trigeminal nerve branches, the ophthalmic (V1) and mandibular (V3) divisions.
- Any sore throat or difficulty swallowing? Patient denies. Significant involvement of the palate, the lateral nasopharyngeal wall, and the oropharynx from tumors arising in the nasal cavity could result in sore throat and dysphagia.
- Have the neck masses enlarged significantly since they were first noted? There has been increase in the size of the right neck node and, more recently, development of left upper cervical lymphadenopathy. The history suggests significant growth over a short period of time.
- Any systemic symptoms such as fever, night sweats, chills, fatigue, or unintentional weight loss? The patient reports having lost 15 pounds in 2 months without changes in diet or activity. Systemic symptoms could suggest hematologic malignancies or systemic spread of nonhematologic malignancies arising in the sinonasal cavity.

Question: What additional aspects of the history are important?

- Smoking history. Could predispose to sinonasal malignancies.
- Occupation and professional exposure. Sinonasal cancer is associated with exposure to wood dust, leather dust, formaldehyde, nickel/chromium compounds, organic solvents, welding fumes, and arsenic.
- Family history. This may be relevant for certain types of sinonasal malignancies.
- Ethnicity. Certain ethnic groups are more vulnerable to developing Epstein-Barr Virus (EBV)-related malignancies.

Physical Examination

Well-nourished male in no distress.

Orbital exam shows no dystopia, normal visual acuity and fields, normal function of extraocular muscles, and no reported diplopia.

Facial sensation is subjectively normal.

Anterior rhinoscopy is unremarkable except for left-sided septal deviation prior to vasoconstriction.

Examination of the oral cavity and oropharynx is unremarkable.

Palpation of the neck reveals suspicious 2.5 cm nodes at level II bilaterally with some smaller suspicious adjacent nodes in level III.

After topical anesthesia and vasoconstriction, nasal endoscopy is performed and shows a mass of the posterior right lateral nasal wall extending into the nasopharynx. The lesion is partially ulcerated but does not appear hypervascular. There is no evidence of active bleeding. The remaining upper aerodigestive tract is normal beyond the nasopharynx.

Question: What would be the next step in the management of this patient?

Answer: There is a high concern for a sinonasal malignancy. As a result, it is important to obtain imaging and a tissue

(Continued)

CASE 47   (continued)

diagnosis. Imaging should be done first to avoid the mistake of biopsying an encephalocele or a highly vascular tumor in the clinic (see Figure 47.1).

Question: What would be your next step in the evaluation of this patient?

Answer: Given that the lesion is accessible and does not appear to be very vascular, and after gentle manipulation and application of topical anesthetics with pledgets, a biopsy is performed in the office using a rigid telescope and through cutting forceps. Depending on the patient, the location of the tumor, and the setting, biopsy sometimes is best performed in an operating room setting. Histopathology is demonstrated in Figure 47.2.

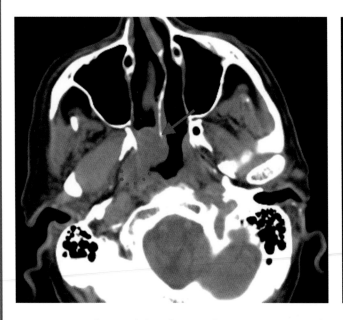
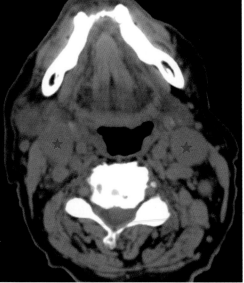

FIGURE 47.1   These axial CT images demonstrate a mass in the posterior nasal cavity and bilateral enlarged cervical lymph nodes. The CT images are limited by lack of intravenous contrast but show the lesion in the right posterior nasal cavity (red arrow) with some extension into the nasopharynx as well as bilateral bulky lymphadenopathy (red stars) in the upper neck. There does not appear to be bone erosion on the CT scan.

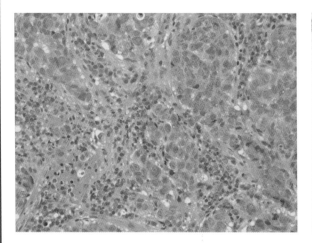
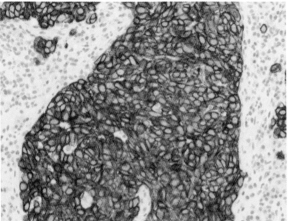

FIGURE 47.2   Pathology shows a poorly differentiated invasive carcinoma, formed of tumoral nests composed of large round cells with high nuclear to cytoplasmic ratio and significant mitotic activity. The tumor cells are positive for CK7 and negative for CK5/6, p40, p16, EBER, synaptophysin, and HLA DR by immunohistochemistry.

CASE 47 (continued)

Question: What is the diagnosis?

Answer: Sinonasal undifferentiated carcinoma (**SNUC**). While differences can be seen on H&E stained tissue, the diagnosis of poorly differentiated sinonasal tumors rests on immunohistochemical staining profile. Differential diagnosis is broad and includes, in addition to epithelial neoplasms, mucosal melanoma, esthesioneuroblastoma, NK T-cell lymphoma, extraosseous Ewing sarcoma, and rhabdomyosarcoma. By definition, on microscopic pathology, the diagnosis of SNUC requires an absence of differentiated foci without either squamous or glandular differentiation as well as absence of neural-type rosettes. With immunohistochemical staining, reaction to keratins is often strong and diffuse, as seen above with CK7, which is strongly and diffusely positive (membranous).

Question: What additional tests would your order at this point?

Answer: SNUC is staged using either TNM (AJCC) staging for nasal cavity malignancies or modified Kadish Staging. High-quality MRI of the paranasal sinuses and skull base with and without contrast is needed to determine the extension of the primary tumor beyond the nasal cavity, which will determine T stage and resectability of the primary tumor. This could also detect metastatic retropharyngeal lymph nodes, which are commonly involved with disease (see Figure 47.3).

Given the high incidence of distant metastases, especially in the presence of bulky nodal disease, PET/CT is needed to complete the workup. Most patients with SNUC have advanced-stage disease, and up to 10% could have distant metastatic disease at presentation.

PET-CT images show significant activity at the primary site and in bilateral neck nodes (see Figure 47.4). In addition, significant metabolic activity is noted in retropharyngeal nodes with no evidence of distant metastatic disease.

Question: In the absence of distant metastases, how would you treat this patient?

Answer: There is debate here. SNUC is a rare aggressive tumor often presenting with advanced stage, which carries a poor prognosis. SNUC should always be managed with a multidisciplinary team of providers. Traditionally, for early local disease, surgical resection usually followed by adjuvant therapy offers patients the best chance of cure. Chemotherapy in addition to radiation in the adjuvant setting could be considered, although reports in the literature on triple therapy in that setting show mixed results. For locally advanced and/or those with regional metastatic disease, however, data have shown improved efficacy when patients are managed with induction chemotherapy (**IC**) followed by definitive chemoradiation therapy (**CRT**). In a series out of

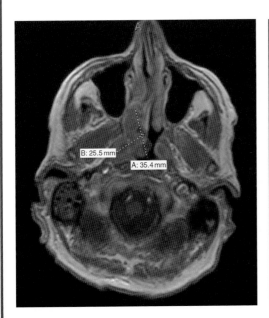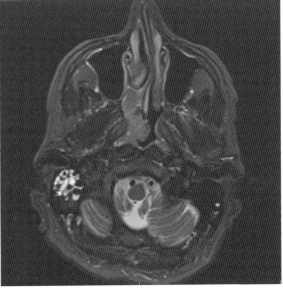

FIGURE 47.3 This T1-weighted image (left) shows a tumor extending from the posterior lateral nasal wall into the nasopharynx, spreading laterally along the Eustachian tube. T2-weighted images with contrast and fat suppression (right) show the tumor well and are helpful to assess tumor spread into fat-containing spaces and to determine tumor spread versus secretions in obstructed paranasal sinus cavities. Intracranial extension is not seen on the MRI. Only retained secretions are noted in the sphenoid sinus, and fluid is seen in the left mastoid.

(Continued)

CASE 47 (continued)

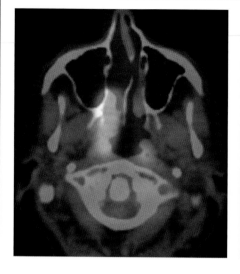
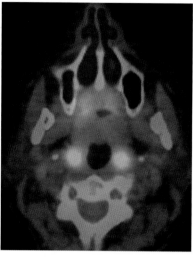
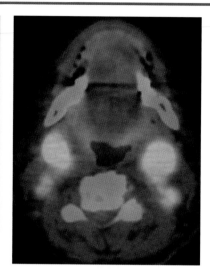

FIGURE 47.4 These fused axial images from the patient's 18-FDG PET/CT shows a hypermetabolic lesion of the posterior right sinonasal cavity along with bilateral retropharyngeal and cervical lymphadenopathy.

MD Anderson, patients without distant metastases were treated with IC. In those who had partial or complete response, an 81% 5-year disease-specific survival (**DSS**) was observed when treated with subsequent definitive CRT, compared to 54% in those who underwent surgical resection followed by adjuvant therapy. However, in nonresponders to IC, those treated with CRT had a 0% DSS compared to 39% in those treated with salvage surgery followed by adjuvant therapy. This approach therefore appears to stratify treatment based on responsiveness to IC. Additional research is on-going looking at genetic and molecular aspects of tumors that could shed light on specific molecular targets and novel therapeutic interventions.

Key Points

- Sinonasal undifferentiated carcinoma is an aggressive small round blue cell tumor.
- Workup includes initial history, physical exam, imaging, and tissue biopsy.
- Metastatic workup is critical as up to 10% of patients with SNUC present with distant metastases on initial assessment.
- For patients without metastatic disease, consideration should be made for induction chemotherapy followed by definitive chemoradiation therapy for responders. For nonresponders or for those with early stage local disease, surgery with adjuvant therapy should be considered.

CASE 48

Carl H. Snyderman

History of Present Illness

A 76-year-old male with a history of skin cancer of the scalp presents with a 1-year history of progressive numbness of the right cheek.

Question: What additional history would you want?

- Location of previous skin cancers: right parietal scalp.
- Prior treatment of skin cancers: local excision by dermatologist; no radiation therapy.

- Swelling or mass: firm swelling of cheek tissues below right eye.
- Other areas of numbness: none.
- Headaches/pain/pressure: none.
- Sinus or nasal problems: no sinus symptoms or treatment. No nasal obstruction.
- Epistaxis: none.
- Eye symptoms: increased tearing of right eye. No diplopia or loss of vision.
- Difficulty chewing: no problems with eating.

CASE 48   (continued)

Physical Examination

Examination of the face revealed firm induration of the subcutaneous tissues of the right cheek below the infraorbital rim with a poorly defined mass measuring 5 × 2 cm. There was some scarring from prior surgery but no skin lesion.

There was no proptosis and eye movements were normal without diplopia.

Ear exam was normal.

Exam of the nose (including nasal endoscopy), oral cavity, pharynx, and neck was normal. Cranial nerves were intact except for hypesthesia of the infraorbital nerve.

Question: What additional information do you want? (Choose all that apply.)

- Biopsy of right cheek: **yes**/no. It demonstrates invasive squamous cell carcinoma.

- CT scan of the face and neck with contrast: **yes**/no (see Figure 48.1).
- MRI: **yes**/no. An MRI will show superior soft-tissue delineation and may also be helpful in assessing for perineural invasion and/or skull base involvement.

MRI scan was obtained to better differentiate tumor from orbital tissues and detect perineural invasion (see Figure 48.2).

Question: What is the most likely source of this cancer?

Answer: Perineural recurrence of a cutaneous skin cancer. Although this cancer may have originated in the maxillary sinus, skin cancers are much more frequent. A subcutaneous mass or cranial neuropathy may be the initial presentation of a skin cancer, and more than 20% of patients can have perineural spread without an obvious primary tumor of the skin. Most commonly, the facial or trigeminal nerves are affected by perineural invasion. The median duration of symptoms is 6 months.

(a)

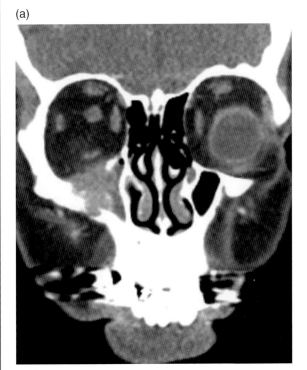

(b)

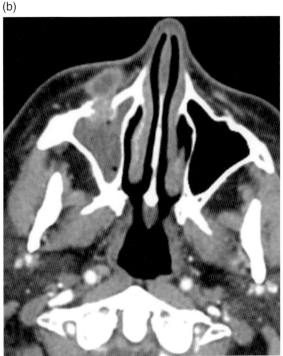

FIGURE 48.1 These contrast-enhanced coronal (a) and axial (b) images show a right maxillary mass involving the infraorbital rim and extending along the infraorbital canal posteriorly, with tumor involvement of the pterygopalatine fossa on the right. There was bony erosion of the orbital floor but no frank intraorbital involvement. There is no evidence of any cervical lymphadenopathy.

(Continued)

CASE 48 (continued)

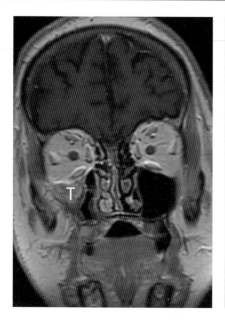 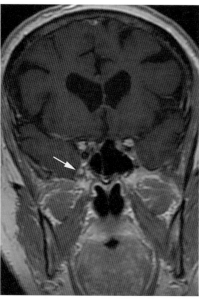

FIGURE 48.2 MRI (coronal T1-weighted with contrast) demonstrated separation of tumor (T) and extraocular muscles. In comparison to the contralateral side, the maxillary nerve enhances and is slightly enlarged at foramen rotundum (arrow).

Question: What would be the recommended treatment for this patient?

Answer: In the absence of medical comorbidities that preclude surgery, surgery followed by radiation therapy offers the best chance for cure. If the patient is treated nonsurgically, radiation therapy needs to include the pterygomaxillary space and skull base.

Question: What surgery would you perform?

Answer: Excision of skin of right cheek with partial maxillectomy, resection of orbital floor, endoscopic endonasal skull base resection. The inferior maxilla is not involved, and a total maxillectomy can be avoided. Based on MRI, the orbit can be spared. An endoscopic endonasal transpterygoid approach provides access to the contents of the pterygomaxillary space and Meckel's cave (see Figure 48.3).

An endoscopic endonasal transpterygoid approach was performed with removal of the posterior wall of the maxillary sinus, ligation of the internal maxillary artery, and resection of the contents of the pterygomaxillary space. The infraorbital nerve was followed to foramen rotundum. The vidian nerve was identified within the pterygoid canal and sacrificed (see Figure 48.4). The base of pterygoid was drilled circumferentially around foramen rotundum to expose Meckel's cave, and proximal margins of the maxillary and vidian nerves were obtained. The dura remained intact without evidence of a CSF leak.

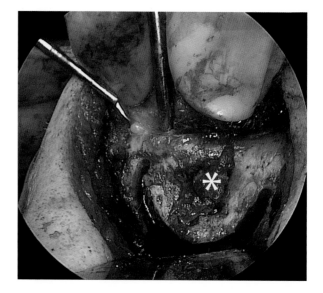

FIGURE 48.3 This intraoperative image shows a wide excision of the right cheek mass was performed with transection of the tumor-involved infraorbital nerve (*). A plane of dissection was developed between the periorbita and tumor, and the anterior maxilla and inferior orbital rim were then removed en bloc. All tumor-involved periorbita was resected.

CASE 48   (continued)

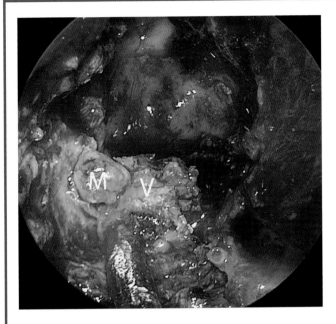

FIGURE 48.4 This intraoperative endoscopic image shows the view of the maxillary (M) and vidian nerves (V) after the pterygoid plates have been removed.

Question: What is the most important landmark for locating the petrous segment of the internal carotid artery?

Answer: The pterygoid (vidian) canal. The vidian nerve is formed by the greater superficial petrosal nerve and deep petrosal nerve and leads to the petrous segment of the internal carotid artery. Drilling the bone between the pterygoid canal and foramen rotundum (lateral recess of sphenoid sinus) exposes Meckel's cave.

Reconstructive Considerations

Reconstruction of the skull base was not necessary since the dura remained intact and the internal carotid artery was not exposed. The soft tissues of the masticator space were covered with fibrin glue. Reconstruction of the orbital floor was not necessary since the majority of the periorbita remained intact. Due to the risks of exposure following radiation therapy, the orbital rim was not reconstructed with hardware. The soft-tissue defect was reconstructed with a paramedian forehead flap. This provided an excellent color match and adequate thickness of tissue. A cervicofacial advancement flap would not have provided adequate thickness of soft tissue (see Figure 48.5.).

The patient had no postoperative complications. Orbital function was intact with no diplopia. Three weeks postoperatively,

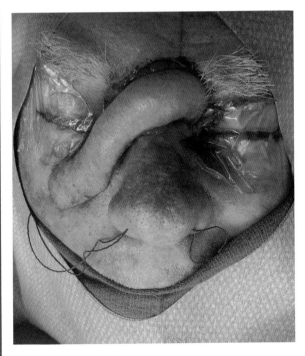
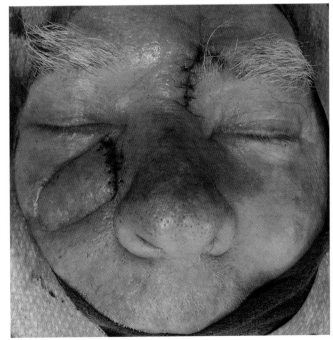

FIGURE 48.5 Soft-tissue reconstruction of the right cheek with staged paramedian forehead flap following resection of recurrent cutaneous squamous cell carcinoma.

(Continued)

CASE 48 (continued)

the second stage of reconstruction was performed with release of the forehead flap pedicle. Postoperative radiation therapy to the surgical field (including the skull base and pterygomaxillary space) was delivered once healing was complete. Chemotherapy has unproven benefit in this situation. Depending on the molecular profile of the tumor, immunotherapy (checkpoint inhibitor) may be considered as an adjunct after radiation therapy.

Key Points

- Recurrent head and neck cutaneous squamous cell carcinomas often present with findings of a cranial neuropathy.
- History, physical exam, and imaging with MRI are critical to assess the extent of disease.
- If surgically resectable, ideal management includes surgical resection followed by adjuvant radiation therapy.
- Consideration of the proximal margin of involved nerves is important in treatment planning (as part of surgical resection and in designing adjuvant radiation therapy fields).
- Combined open and endoscopic techniques can be used to aid in tumor resection and reconstruction.

Multiple Choice Questions

1. You are evaluating a 12-year-old male who presents with right-sided epistaxis and nasal blockage. On office exam, you identify a right-sided red/purple nasal polypoid lesion. Which of the following would be an appropriate next step for this patient?

   a. Treatment with nasal steroids and follow-up in 4 months.

   b. In-office nasal endoscopic biopsy of the lesion.

   c. Trip to the operating room for an excisional biopsy of the mass.

   d. MRI of the paranasal sinuses with and without gadolinium.

   Answer: d. In this patient where there is a concern for a juvenile nasal angiofibroma, imaging would be an appropriate next step. In children, MRI is often preferred to minimize radiation exposure. Nasal steroids would not have a role here. In-office biopsy before imaging should be avoided as the lesion could be highly vascular and/or have a connection to the CSF space. While a trip to the operating room for resection may be needed, imaging would be important before this procedure to assist with counseling and operative planning.

2. Which of the following would be a contraindication to consideration of an endoscopic resection of a sinonasal malignancy?

   a. Erosion of the lamina papyracea.

   b. Erosion the nasal bones.

   c. Erosion of the cribriform plate.

   d. Extension of the tumor into the lower aspect of the pterygoid plates.

   Answer: b. With advances in nasal endoscopic techniques for tumor resection and anterior skull base reconstruction, this approach has become a mainstay in the management of both benign and malignant sinonasal tumors. Contrain-

dications include significant anterior extension that can't be accessed using nasal endoscopic instruments, frank involvement of intraconal orbital contents (while orbital exenteration has been described endoscopically, a combined open and endoscopic approach is often recommended), and superolateral extension of the tumor involving the lateral frontal sinus or orbital roof beyond the optic nerve axis. By using endoscopic drills, tumor extension into the pterygoid plates can often safely be addressed endoscopically.

3. When available, what is the preferred method for anterior skull base reconstruction following an orbit-sparing extended endoscopic anterior skull base tumor resection of a tumor involving the left ethmoid roof?

   a. Free fascia lata graft.

   b. A layered repair including a vascularized nasoseptal flap.

   c. A layered repair including a free abdominal fat graft.

   d. Anterolateral thigh free flap.

   Answer: b. The nasoseptal flap is a vascularized mucoperichondrial flap fed by the posterior septal branch off of the sphenopalatine artery. Its use has greatly expanded the field of endoscopic skull base surgery as it allows for repair of large defects, including those with high-flow CSF leaks. For free grafts such as abdominal fat and fascia lata, given the lack of a vascularized component, there is a higher leak rate for larger defects. The anterolateral thigh free flap, while helpful for skull base reconstruction when there is a large associated dead space from a concomitant maxillectomy/orbital exenteration, would be too large for the defect described.

4. Which of the following would not be considered a small round blue cell tumor?

   a. Well-differentiated squamous cell carcinoma.

   b. Lymphoma.

c. Sinonasal undifferentiated carcinoma.

d. Mucosal melanoma.

Answer: a. Small round blue cell tumors are a group of diseases that are characterized by their appearance on H&E histopathologic assessment. These tumors have a high nuclear to cytoplasmic ratio with the majority of the cells making up the tumor having a similar appearance. Immunohistochemical staining is needed to further characterize these tumors. Well-differentiated squamous cell carcinoma would not fall into this category.

5. Which of the following is true regarding the management of nonmetastatic sinonasal undifferentiated carcinoma?

   a. Definitive surgical resection is often adequate to provide disease control.

   b. Management of cervical lymphatics is often not necessary as these tumors rarely spread.

   c. These tumors are largely radioresistant.

   d. Response to induction chemotherapy may play a role in guiding therapy.

   Answer: d. Recent data suggest that responders to induction chemotherapy should be considered for definitive CRT. Those who do not respond or who progress should be offered salvage surgery, when possible, followed by adjuvant therapy. Due to the high risk of regional spread, management of the neck is critical to avoid regional recurrence.

6. Which of the following patients would not be a candidate for surgical resection of recurrent skin cancer of the right cheek?

   a. Patient with evidence of involvement of the inferior oblique muscle.

   b. Patient with evidence of tongue numbness and abducens nerve palsy.

   c. Evidence of widening of the infraorbital canal on CT imaging.

   d. Evidence of right-sided perifacial pathologic lymphadenopathy.

   Answer: b. In a patient with tongue numbness and cranial nerve VI palsy, there is a concern for involvement of the cavernous sinus and Meckel's cave. In such an instance, the ability to clear the proximal margin with surgery would be compromised, and often nonsurgical routes of therapy should be considered.

7. What is the blood supply to a paramedian forehead flap?

   a. Superficial temporal artery.

   b. Supraorbital artery.

   c. Supratrochlear artery.

   d. Anterior ethmoidal artery.

   Answer: c. Supratrochlear artery.

Suggested Reading

Amit, M., Abdelmeguid, A.S., Watcherporn, T. et al. (2019). Induction chemotherapy response as a guide for treatment optimization in sinonasal undifferentiated carcinoma. *J. Clin. Oncol.* 37 (6): 504–512.

Bell, D., Saade, R., Roberts, D. et al. (2015). Prognostic utility of Hyams histological grading and Kadish-Morita staging systems for esthesioneuroblastoma outcomes. *Head Neck Pathol.* 9 (1): 51–59.

Binazzi, A., Ferrante, P., and Marinaccio, A. (2015). Occupational exposure and sinonasal cancer: a systematic review and meta-analysis. *BMC Cancer* 15: 49.

de Bonnecaze, G., Verillaud, B., Chaltiel, L. et al. (2018). Clinical characteristics and prognostic factors of sinonasal undifferentiated carcinoma: a multicenter study. *Int. Forum Allergy Rhinol.* 8 (9): 1065–1072.

Fortes, F.S.G., Sennes, L.U., Carrau, R.L. et al. (2008). Endoscopic anatomy of the pterygopalatine fossa and the transpterygoid approach: development of a surgical instruction model. *Laryngoscope* 118 (1): 44–49.

Gamez, M.E., Lal, D., Halyard, M.Y. et al. (2017). Outcomes and patterns of failure for sinonasal undifferentiated carcinoma (SNUC): the Mayo Clinic experience. *Head Neck* 39 (9): 1819–1824.

Gardner, P.A. and Snyderman, C.H. (2015). Suprapetrous approach to Meckel's cave and the middle cranial fossa. In: *Master Techniques in Otolaryngology – Head and Neck Surgery: Skull Base Surgery* (eds. C.H. Snyderman and P.A. Gardner), 277–284. Philadelphia: Wolters Kluwer.

Komotar, R.J., Starke, R.M., Raper, D.M. et al. (2013). Endoscopic endonasal compared with anterior craniofacial and combined cranionasal resection of esthesioneuroblastomas. *World Neurosurg.* 80: 148–159.

Kuan, E.C., Arshi, A., Mallen-St Clair, J. et al. (2016). Significance of tumor stage in sinonasal undifferentiated carcinoma survival: a population-based analysis. *Otolaryngol. Head Neck Surg.* 154 (4): 667–673.

Kuo, P., Manes, R.P., Schwam, Z.G. et al. (2017). Survival outcomes for combined modality therapy for sinonasal undifferentiated carcinoma. *Otolaryngol. Head Neck Surg.* 156 (1): 132–136.

Morand, G.B., Anderegg, N., Vital, D. et al. (2017). Outcome by treatment modality in sinonasal undifferentiated carcinoma (SNUC): a case-series, systematic review and meta-analysis. *Oral Oncol.* 75: 28–34.

Patel, S.G., Singh, B., Stambuk, H.E. et al. (2012). Craniofacial surgery for esthesioneuroblastoma: report of an international collaborative study. *J. Neurol. Surg. B Skull Base* 73 (3): 208–220.

Reyes, C., Mason, E., Solares, C.A. et al. (2015). To preserve or not to preserve the orbit in paranasal sinus neoplasms: a meta-analysis. *J. Neurol. Surg. B Skull Base* 76 (2): 122–128.

Warren, T.A., Nagle, C.M., Bowman, J., and Panizza, B.J. (2016). The natural history and treatment outcomes of perineural spread of malignancy within the head and neck. *J. Neurol. Surg. B* 77: 107–112.

SECTION 12
Cutaneous Malignancies
Charley Coffey

CASE 49

Arnaud Bewley

History of Present Illness

A 57-year-old male presents with an area of nodularity at the medial aspect of his left brow. He has a history of prior basal cell carcinoma (BCC) of the brow excised via Mohs 2.5 years prior. He notes a tingling sensation radiating over the left forehead. He has a history of type II diabetes and hypertension. He has a history of heavy alcohol use but is sober now, and 40+ pack-year smoking but has quit recently.

Question: What are additional important points in history taking?

Answer: it is important to ask about vision changes in any patient with skin cancers near the orbit given risk for perineural invasion with advanced cutaneous malignancies. Although BCCs rarely metastasize to the neck, it is still important to consider and examine the nodal basins and ask about neck or parotid masses. Immunosuppression is a known risk factor for a wide variety of skin malignancies.

Physical Examination

A 1 cm, mobile, nodular lesion with raised edges is seen on the medial side of the left brow, as shown in Figure 49.1. Left forehead and brow sensations are diminished. Cranial nerves are otherwise intact. Extraocular motions are intact, vision grossly normal. No parotid or neck masses are identified.

Question: What would you recommend next?

Answer: Considering the history and physical exam, a punch biopsy of the lesion is the most appropriate next step.

A punch biopsy is performed. A representative slide of the histologic specimen is shown in Figure 49.2. The histopathologic slide demonstrates detached islands of basaloid cells with

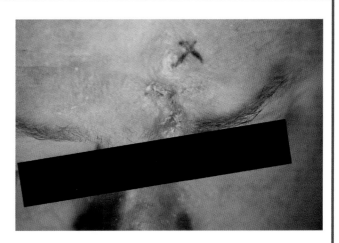

FIGURE 49.1 This clinical photo demonstrates the patient's ulcerative skin lesion with surrounding ill-defined induration. It is mobile from the underlying bone.

peripheral palisading, with an artifactual cleft formed between some islands and the surrounding stroma, consistent with BCC.

Question: What would you recommend next?

Answer: Considering the history of BCC and exam findings of sensory changes, further imaging to determine the extent of the disease is appropriate and recommended.

Question: What imaging modality would you choose?

Answer: Computed tomography (CT) scan is a good low-cost method for assessing any head and neck tumor. It allows for evaluation of the soft tissue extent of a tumor, delineation of underlying bone involvement, and determination of presence of lymphadenopathy. However, in the setting of symptoms concerning for perineural invasion, magnetic resonance

(Continued)

CASE 49   (continued)

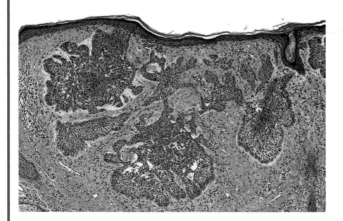

FIGURE 49.2   Histopathology slide of the punch biopsy. Copyright © 2012 Michael Bonert, MD, FRCPC (https://commons.wikimedia.org/wiki/User:Nephron). You are free to share and adapt this image as per the CC BY-SA 3.0 (https://creativecommons.org/licenses/by-sa/3.0/legalcode).

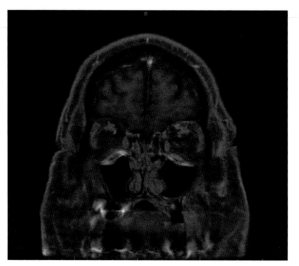

FIGURE 49.3   This is a T1 weighted contrast-enhanced MRI of the face.

imaging (MRI) is essential for delineating any involvement of the supraorbital branch of the trigeminal nerve and evaluating for extent into the orbit or trigeminal ganglion.

Although ultrasound can be useful in looking for evidence of lateral neck disease it has limited ability to delineate the extent of a primary tumor. Positron emission tomography (PET) scan or PET/CT is useful for ruling out metastatic disease in the setting of any advanced head and neck malignancy. However, in this case of a BCC where regional and distant spread would be of very low risk, a PET/CT would be of limited use.

MRI with contrast is obtained. A single representative coronal image is shown below.

Question: Can you identify the critical finding on the Coronal T1 weighted MRI depicted in Figure 49.3?

Answer: This is a contrast enhanced T1 coronal MRI. It demonstrates thickening and enhancement of the supraorbital nerve within the left orbit consistent with the tumor's retrograde invasion toward the skull base. On more posterior coronal cuts, the trigeminal ganglion does not demonstrate any enhancement.

Question: What treatment modality, if any, would you recommend? What is the basis for this recommendation?

Answer: Given the evidence of localized disease without invasion of the skull base, primary surgical resection of the tumor has the best chance of cure. Since the likelihood of resection with negative margins and acceptable functional and oncologic outcome is high, primary surgical treatment is the preferred method of treatment.

Question: What is the extent of your recommended surgery?

Answer: Retrograde invasion along the supraorbital nerve beyond the supraorbital foramen typically requires orbital exenteration to clear microscopic disease. Orbitotomy with excision of

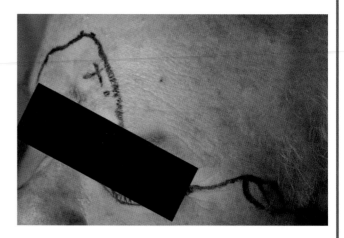

FIGURE 49.4   This intraoperative photo demonstrates the proposed incisions used at the time of the tumor resection. Note that an orbital exenteration is planned. In this instance, the temple incision was carried over to join a preauricular incision to allow for an ipsilateral parotidectomy for clearance of an involved facial nerve branch.

the nerve and preservation of the orbital contents will most likely leave disease along distal branches of the nerve that arise within the orbit. Neck dissection and parotidectomy are unnecessary, given the very low risk of metastatic spread with BCC. However, these basins will likely be exposed and could be sampled at no increased morbidity if free-flap reconstruction is planned.

You plan a wide excision with orbital exenteration and soft-tissue reconstruction with a radial forearm free flap. The planned incision for the resection of the primary tumor is depicted in Figure 49.4.

CASE 49   (continued)

The pathologic specimen demonstrates a morpheoform BCC with perineural invasion. You were able to clear the left supraorbital nerve at the orbital apex, however, there is a positive margin at the contralateral right supratrochlear nerve. Patient has an uncomplicated postoperative course and returns for follow-up.

Question: What would you recommend next?

Answer: The National Comprehensive Cancer Network (NCCN) recommends consideration of adjuvant radiation therapy for patients with positive margins or extensive perineural invasion, which includes invasion of named nerves. These features are associated with a high rate of local recurrence that may be reduced with radiation, though there is limited evidence to demonstrate a survival advantage with adjuvant radiation therapy. A recommendation of adjuvant radiotherapy in this patient is justified.

The patient elects to undergo adjuvant radiotherapy. Unfortunately, at his 1-year postoperative visit he is noted to have a subcutaneous nodule at the periphery of the flap on the right. A contrast enhanced MRI demonstrates enhancement of the right supraorbital nerve extending to the skull base. A punch biopsy of the nodule confirms recurrent BCC.

Question: What are his treatment options at this time?

Answer: Reirradiation of the right orbit would likely result in permanent vision loss, and neither this nor exenteration of the only seeing eye is appropriate. While hospice may be appropriate in the future, at present there are therapeutic options available and due to the time course of this disease, imminent death is not likely. Vismodegib is a Hedgehog pathway inhibitor that is approved for patients with metastatic or unresectable BCC. In a randomized prospective trial, 65% of patients demonstrate some improvement with up 20% achieving a complete response.

Key Points

- MRI is essential in the setting of an advanced cutaneous malignancy with symptoms concerning for perineural invasion.
- Morpheoform, infiltrative, and micronodular BCC are all subtypes associated with a more irregular invasive front that is associated with a higher rate of local recurrence.
- Retrograde invasion along the supraorbital nerve beyond the supraorbital rim typically requires orbital exenteration to clear microscopic disease.

- The NCCN recommends consideration of adjuvant radiation therapy for patients with positive margins or extensive perineural invasion that includes invasion of named nerves.
- Vismodegib is a Hedgehog pathway inhibitor that should be considered in patients with unresectable or metastatic disease, or on instances where a patient is not willing to pursue definitive surgical or non-surgical treatment.

CASE 50

Vasu Divi

History of Present Illness

A 75-year old patient presents to your clinic with a cutaneous lesion of the right temple (below). He has a history of significant sun exposure throughout life and rarely uses sunscreen.

Question: What are important points in history taking about this lesion?

Answer: Rate of growth, presence of numbness, changes in movements of the face, pain, and presence of facial or neck masses are all important points that need to be investigated.

Patient reports that it enlarged from 5 mm to 2 cm over a few weeks, he only experiences mild pain, no numbness or facial movement changes or masses have been noticed.

Question: What are the important points to elicit in past medical history?

Answer: Any history of skin cancers, hematologic malignancies, transplant and immunosuppression are important to identify. Smoking history in addition to sun exposure is also a risk factor.

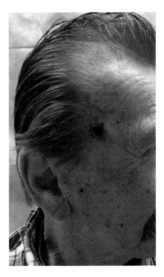

FIGURE 50.1   This photograph demonstrates the patient's right temple cutaneous lesion.

(Continued)

CASE 50 (continued)

Patient in the above Figure 50.1 has had two BCCs removed from forehead and nasal tip and was diagnosed with chronic lymphocytic leukemia (CLL) 3 years ago. He is a former smoker who quit 10 years ago and has a 30 pack-year history of smoking.

Question: What are the important characteristics to identify in the physical examination?

Answer: Lesion size, appearance ulceration, assessment of depth, mobility, and character of borders (clear versus indistinct) are important in the examination of the primary lesion. Careful examination of the cranial nerves and determining the presence of numbness, motor deficit, and parotid or neck masses are important. Complete examination to identify other lesions is essential.

This lesion is 3 cm, ulcerated with indistinct borders, and appears thick. The lesion is mobile over the underlying tissue. No neural deficit or parotid or neck masses are identified. No additional lesions are found.

Question: What would be the most appropriate next step?

Answer: A biopsy is the most appropriate next step. While good for superficial lesions, shave biopsies may not give a full histologic picture for deep or pigmented lesions. For large, thick lesions such as this, a punch biopsy is the best choice. Unlike a shave biopsy, punch biopsy would establish the lesion thickness and potentially allow identification of other high-risk features. A punch biopsy is also less disruptive than an incisional biopsy.

An incisional biopsy can induce inflammation and disrupt gross assessment of tumor and is not recommended. While ideal for pigmented lesions, an excisional biopsy, in a large lesion like this is not practical.

A punch biopsy is performed. The pathology report shows: SCC, poorly differentiated. Depth of invasion: 6.5 mm into subcutaneous fat. Perineural invasion: not identified.

Question: According to the AJCC 8th Edition staging, what is the current T category of the lesion?

Answer: T3. Since depth of invasion is greater than 6 mm, without evidence of underlying bone involvement or obvious cranial neuropathy, the tumor is clinically staged as T3.

Question: In addition to having an advanced stage, what are the additional high-risk features in this patient?

Answer: Size greater than 2 cm, history of CLL, and poorly differentiated histology have been demonstrated to have strong association with regional metastatic spread and local recurrence. In addition, location on ear or lip, perineural invasion, lymphovascular invasion, and recurrent lesions have also been identified as high-risk features of cutaneous SCC.

Question: What would you recommend next?

Answer: The role of imaging for high-risk cutaneous SCC is not well established. For lesions that are suspected to have deep invasion, or lesions with multiple high-risk clinical features, preoperative imaging may help to better evaluate the extent of invasion at the primary site and the status of at-risk regional lymphatics. Contrasted MRI is preferred if perineural disease or deep soft-tissue involvement is suspected, while CT will better assess suspected bone invasion. Considering multiple high-risk features, ordering imaging is reasonable.

You elect to obtain imaging. MRI of the neck is shown in the below Figure 50.2:

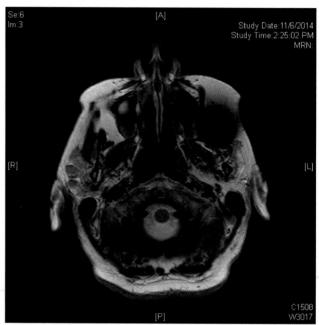

FIGURE 50.2 This T2 weighted axial MRI demonstrates two suspicious lesion in the right parotid gland. The remainder of the neck imaging is normal with no evidence of perineural invasion or involvement of deeper structures.

Two suspicious lesions are noted in the parotid gland, The remainder of the neck imaging is normal. No evidence of perineural invasion or invasion into deeper structures is seen.

Question: What would you recommend next?

Answer: Considering the high-risk nature of the disease and patient comorbidity, further investigation to complete metastatic workup is reasonable. At minimum, CT scan of the chest is indicated to determine if there is any distant metastatic disease. PET/CT could alternatively be used for staging, but would be considerably more expensive than chest CT, while providing limited additional information to guide therapy. Fine needle aspiration of the parotid gland lesions could confirm the cytopathologic diagnosis of regional metastatic disease. However, in this setting the clinical suspicion for nodal disease is high enough to warrant treatment without requiring preoperative cytopathologic assessment, particularly as a negative or indeterminate FNA result in this context would not "override" the recommendation for surgery. Early dental evaluation is important if adjuvant radiation therapy proves necessary. Completing dental evaluation before surgery is not required, but is good practice to optimize avoidance of treatment delay.

CASE 50   (continued)

CT scan of the chest does not show any evidence of distant disease.

Question: What treatment, if any, do you recommend?

Answer: Wide local excision of primary site with appropriate reconstruction and parotidectomy and neck dissection is the most effective treatment in this case. To adequately manage regional lymphatic disease the entire involved and high-risk nodal basins should be surgically addressed. In this instance, that includes the parotid gland and upper neck nodes (levels Ib, II, and III).

Mohs micrographic excision provides intraoperative assessment of the entire tumor margin and is an excellent option for many high-risk cutaneous SCC. It can be offered to this patient but will require two stage operation in most scenarios (Mohs, followed by parotidectomy, neck dissection and reconstruction). There is evidence that regional lymphatics can be adequately staged with sentinel lymph node biopsy (SLNB). Rates of detection of sub-clinical nodal metastases with SLNB appear to be between 12 and 17% based upon current evidence. However, it remains unclear whether SLNB (followed by completion lymph node dissection or adjuvant RT) improves oncologic outcomes for cutaneous SCC. Since there is clinical suspicion for nodal involvement and advanced T-stage, sentinel node biopsy would be inappropriate.

Definitive radiation is not considered first-line therapy for advanced-stage cutaneous SCC. However, it may be considered for patients deemed poor surgical candidates or those who refuse surgery.

The final pathology from the resection demonstrates:

4 cm, poorly differentiated SCC with 7 mm depth of invasion & negative margins. Perineural invasion is present. 5 parotid nodes are positive, while 0 of 22 neck nodes are involved. There is no evidence of extracapsular extension.

Question: What is the next step in management?

Answer: Adjuvant radiotherapy is indicated in this case. The pathologic features indicate a high-risk tumor with significant risk of disease relapse. There is no high-level evidence that adding systemic therapy to radiation therapy confers survival benefits. A recent Phase III trial of concurrent carboplatin did not show survival benefit when given in the adjuvant setting. However, critics note that single-agent carboplatin is inferior to cisplatin and that the study was powered to detect a larger survival benefit than should have been anticipated. Some retrospective case series suggest a survival benefit for adjuvant systemic therapy. Therefore, many institutions continue to treat advanced cutaneous SCC similar to mucosal SCC, including addition of systemic therapy for positive margins and extracapsular extension. Recently the FDA approved cemiplimab, an anti-PD-1 antibody, for use in metastatic and unresectable disease. Use in the adjuvant setting is currently being investigated.

Key Points

- Patients with underlying immunosuppression are at higher risk for development of cutaneous cancers, especially invasive SCC.
- Evaluation of patients with suspected SCC includes a history, a physical exam, and a punch biopsy of the lesion of concern.
- In instances where there is suspicion of deep invasion and/or regional metastatic disease, further imaging such as CT and/or MRI should be performed.
- The parotid gland is the most common site for regional metastases for cutaneous cancers of the head and neck.

Management of patients with pathologic parotid lymphadenopathy should include a wide resection of the primary tumor along with a subtotal/total parotidectomy and ipsilateral neck dissection.
- Postoperative adjuvant radiation therapy should be considered for lesions that are advanced, recurrent, have perineural invasion of named nerves, close margins, and/or evidence of regional metastatic disease.
- Treatment with cemiplimab can be considered for unresectable or metastatic cutaneous SCC or in patients who refuse or who are unfit for surgery.

CASE 51

David Neskey

History of Present Illness

A 74-year-old male presents with recurrent irritation of the left eye over the past 2 years, which was previously diagnosed as a recurring chalazion. More recently, the longstanding yellowish papule developed ulceration, leading to diffuse swelling of the left lower eyelid.

Question: What additional questions would you want to ask?

Answer: Asking about visual changes is important in any patient with skin lesions near the orbit, given the risk for perineural invasion with advanced cutaneous malignancies. Systemic immunosuppression is also a known risk factor for aggressive skin malignancies.

Patient does not report any visual changes. He has a history of CLL.

(Continued)

CASE 51   (continued)

Physical Examination

There is a 1 cm lesion on the left lower eyelid with some associated scleral injection. No other cutaneous lesions are appreciated. The remainder of the head and neck exam is normal, except for some tenderness overlying the mandible. There are no palpable parotid or cervical masses.

Management

Question: What would you include in your differential diagnosis?

Answer: A variety of benign or malignant lesions could be considered in the differential diagnosis. Benign lesions include:

- Stye: they tend to be painful, and most resolve with warm compresses.
- Chalazion: blockage of a sebaceous gland that causes the eyelid to swell. Typical chalazion will resolve with warm compresses.
- Conjunctivitis is an infection of the conjunctiva that can lead to scleral injection. Treatment with ophthalmic antibiotics will clear the infection.
- Blepharitis: typically bilateral and not likely in this scenario.

   None of these benign lesions are likely here.

Malignant Lesions

- BCC should be considered here but is less likely given that the lesion seemed to start below the epidermis.
- SCC could also be considered, but it is less likely given that the lesion seemed to start below the epidermis.
- Melanoma also could be considered but is less likely since the lesion is not pigmented.
- Merkel cell carcinoma (MCC) is in the differential diagnosis, considering advanced age and history of immunosuppression.
- Lymphoma: this would be an unusual presentation for a lymphoma, although it still should be considered.
- Sebaceous carcinoma: for lesions starting around the eyelid, sebaceous adenocarcinoma should always be considered.

Question: What would you do next?

Answer: Given the longstanding nature of the lesion and the 3-month history of pain overlying the mandible further imaging is reasonable. CT scan is an affordable and helpful first step. However, considering the length and high suspicion of a malignant process, a biopsy should be performed.

   Review of the CT scan reveals an enlarged perifacial node (<3 cm) adjacent to the left mandible without any other adenopathy appreciated in the parotid or lateral neck. Biopsy of the eyelid lesion reveals finely vacuolated cytoplasm consistent with sebaceous carcinoma. Subsequent PET/CT does not show any distant metastatic disease. In general, the risk of distant disease is low and most consider imaging beyond neck and chest CT optional.

Question: What is the clinical stage?

Answer: The staging of this tumor is based on the TNM staging for eyelid carcinoma. Since the tumor is 1 cm and appears not to invade the tarsal plate or the eyelid margin, it could be staged: T2a. Any abnormal lymphadenopathy is equivalent to N1. The overall stage is T2aN1M0, stage: IIIb.

Question: What treatment would you recommend?

Answer: The treatment of sebaceous carcinoma is surgical. In these cases, collaboration with oculo-oncology and oculoplastic specialists is important. A thorough ophthalmic examination is necessary. In this case, since the globe or conjunctiva do not appear to be involved, there is no need for orbital exenteration. Wide local excision and reconstruction of the eyelid with parotidectomy and ipsilateral neck dissection is the appropriate treatment.

   Definitive surgical resection with frozen section margin assessment was performed. The conjunctiva was minimally involved but the lesion did involve the tarsal plate. Negative margins were achieved without exenteration given the minimal conjunctival involvement. The defect was reconstructed with a Tenzel rotational flap. Parotidectomy and left neck dissection (levels I–IV) was also performed.

Question: How might initial surgical management have been altered to decrease the risk of local recurrence?

Answer: Intraoperative frozen section evaluation for residual tumor may not be completely reliable due to the propensity of sebaceous carcinoma to demonstrate patchy epithelial involvement with skip areas. Several cases have been reported in which surgical margins were deemed free of disease, but residual carcinoma was still detected in the paraffin-embedded permanent sections. Staged reconstruction of the primary surgical defect can help avoid this pitfall.

   The reconstructed surgical defect healed well. Patient recovered from surgery without complications. The surgical pathology report described a 9 mm sebaceous carcinoma resected with negative margins. Involvement of the tarsal plate was noted. There was also metastatic carcinoma present in 1 of 38 lymph nodes, without extracapsular extension.

Question: What is the pathologic stage?

Answer: Since there is involvement of the tarsus, the clinical stage is upstaged to T2b. The overall stage is T2bN1M0, stage IIIb.

Question: What would be the most appropriate next step in this patient's management?

Answer: Due to the close surgical margins and lymph node involvement, this patient should be considered for adjuvant radiation therapy. Currently, no data exist to support adjuvant chemotherapy or immunotherapy.

Key Points

- The majority of sebaceous carcinomas arise from the eyelid and periorbital region because this location has the greatest number of sebaceous glands.
- The most frequent sites of regional metastases from head and neck sebaceous carcinoma are preauricular, parotid, and ipsilateral cervical lymph nodes.
- Intraoperative frozen section evaluation for residual tumor may not be completely reliable due to the propensity of sebaceous carcinoma to demonstrate patchy epithelial involvement with skip areas.
- At present, while adjuvant external beam radiation is recommended for high-risk lesions and those with evidence of nodal metastases, there are no data to show improved outcomes with combined chemoradiation therapy or immunotherapy.

CASE 52

Bharat Yarlagadda

History of Present Illness

A 68-year-old white male presents with a left preauricular skin lesion, which has been present for several months and is increasing in size. He has a history of multiple prior nonmelanoma skin lesions that have been treated with cryotherapy and Mohs surgical excision. The lesion of concern has been oozing and bleeding periodically. He has not had other head and neck complaints or symptoms. He reports significant sun exposure throughout childhood and young adulthood. He has no other history of head and neck surgery or radiation exposure.

Question: What additional questions would you want to ask?

Answer: Asking about facial numbness or tingling is important in any patient with skin lesions given risk for perineural invasion with advanced cutaneous malignancies. Immunosuppression is a known risk factor for aggressive skin malignancies. Asking about any recent facial or neck masses is important.

   The patient does not have any history of immunosuppression and does not report any numbness or neck mass.

Physical Examination

Fitzpatrick type II, with evidence of diffuse photodamage. There is a 1.5 cm exophytic mass on the left ear that appears mobile relative to the root of the helix and tragus. External auditory canal is clear (see Figure 52.1). The rest of the exam is within normal limits.

Question: What would you recommend next?

Answer: The suspicion for a malignant lesion is high in this scenario. The best first step is a punch biopsy. Incisional and excisional biopsies are best to be avoided as the first step

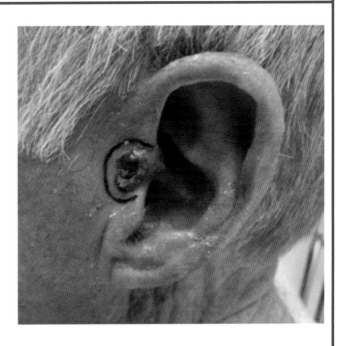

FIGURE 52.1   This photo demonstrates the lesion of the patient's preauricular skin.

especially when a differential diagnosis of MCC or SCC is possible.

   A punch biopsy of the lesion was performed; histopathologic findings are shown in Figure 52.2.

Question: What is the most likely diagnosis in this patient?

(*Continued*)

CASE 52 (continued)

(a)   (b)

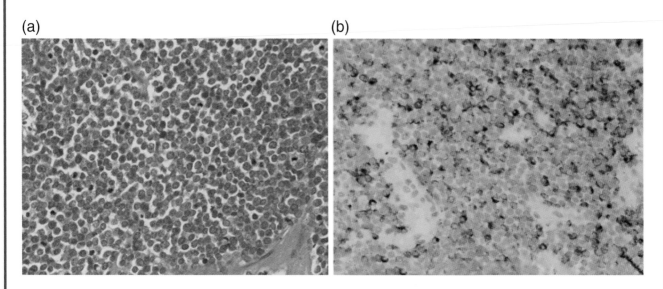

FIGURE 52.2 This is a small blue cell tumor seen on H&E (a). Stain for CK20 is positive (b), while TTF-1 and HMB45 are negative (not shown). Source: Image courtesy of Bharat Yarlagadda MD and Lisa Serra MD.

Answer: MCC is considered a small round blue cell tumor (Figure 52.2a). However, routine histopathology with H&E staining has a high rate of misdiagnosis, and immunohistochemistry is often required. CK20 is a sensitive marker for MCC and is positive in 75–100% of tumors (Figure 52.2b). TTF-1 is never positive in MCC, but is usually present in other small blue cell tumors (lung origin, e.g.). Neuroendocrine markers such as chromogranin, synaptophysin, and neuron-specific enolase are not specific for MCC but are usually positive and can assist in diagnosis when CK20 is negative. HMB 45 is used to diagnose malignant melanoma. Infection with the Merkel cell polyomavirus is also a risk factor for development of these tumors.

MCC is considered a clinically aggressive disease with propensity for regional metastatic spread and a high rate of death from distant metastatic disease. It is relatively rare in comparison to other cutaneous malignancies with an incidence of 0.32/100 000 in the United States.

Question: What would you recommend next?

Answer: Since the risk of regional and distant metastases is high, further workup is indicated. A PET/CT would be an appropriate next step. If the cost or availability is a limiting factor, neck and chest CT could be considered.

The patient had a PET/CT completed, which demonstrated no evidence of regional or distant metastatic disease.

Question: What is the stage of the disease?

Answer: Based on the AJCC 8th Edition, the clinical stage is cT1N0M0, stage I.

Question: What treatments, if any, would you recommend?

Answer: Since the disease is resectable with acceptable functional and cosmetic outcomes, wide local excision with concurrent sentinel node biopsy and appropriate reconstruction is the preferred choice. One to two centimeter margins are recommended. Though there is some controversy regarding the role of elective nodal dissection for MCC, current NCCN guidelines recommend SLNB rather than elective lymphadenectomy. A positive sentinel node has a significant impact on prognosis and predicts a higher rate of locoregional recurrence. SNLB has been reported to identify micro-metastatic disease in up to 1/3 of early stage MCC patients, and is thus offered routinely to these patients. Ideally, SLNB is performed at the time of wide local excision to prevent alteration of the lymphatic drainage patterns.

Wide local excision and SLNB were performed. The tragal and helical root cartilages were resected to provide an adequate deep margin. The sentinel node was found at the tail of the parotid gland, anterior to the great auricular nerve (see Figure 52.3). Methylene blue was used to aid in localization of the node. The wound was closed with cheek skin advancement with a near-linear closure.

Final pathologic analysis indicates a 1.5 cm tumor resected with negative margins, no lymphovascular invasion or perineural invasion, and a negative sentinel lymph node.

CASE 52 (continued)

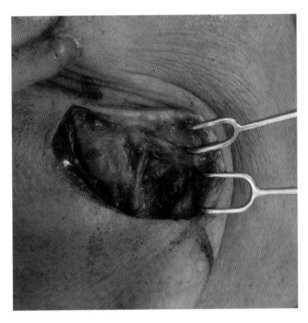

FIGURE 52.3   This intraoperative photo shows the methylene blue dye localized to a sentinel lymph node in the tail of the left parotid gland.

Question: What is the final stage?

Answer: The pathologic stage remains the same as the clinical stage: pT1N0M0, stage I.

Question: What would you recommend to this patient?

Answer: This patient is noted to have early stage disease. Radiation therapy is offered in the adjuvant setting for both early and advanced stage disease, and has been shown to improve locoregional control, although not necessarily improve overall survival in early stage patients. Radiation can be considered primary treatment in patients ineligible for surgery. In the setting of positive margins, definitive radiation can be considered if re-resection is not feasible. Radiation to the primary site may be withheld for select tumors <1 cm with no adverse pathologic features, in immune-competent patients. Nodal irradiation is offered if the SLNB is positive or at risk of being false-negative, and if nodal dissection yields multiple involved nodes or demonstrates extracapsular extension. Definitive nodal irradiation is offered for clinically evident disease when nodal dissection is not possible. In this case, considering a primary tumor larger than 1 cm, in spite of early stage disease and negative margin resection, adjuvant radiotherapy is recommended.

The role of systemic therapy is less clear. Platinum-based chemotherapy regimens are offered concurrently with radiation for patients ineligible for surgery. Concurrent bimodality regimens are also reported in the adjuvant setting, although the benefit to the addition of chemotherapy is not clear, and is currently not a part of the NCCN guidelines. Checkpoint immunotherapy may be offered to patients with disseminated metastatic disease but often are in the context of a clinical trial.

Key Points

- MCC is a small round blue cell tumor that is typically CK20 positive and TTF-1 negative.
- MCC is considered a clinically aggressive disease with a propensity for regional metastatic spread and a high rate of death from distant metastatic disease.
- Both UV exposure and immunosuppression are considered risk factors for MCC, as is infection with Merkel cell polyomavirus.
- Current NCCN guidelines recommend SLNB rather than elective lymphadenectomy.
- Radiation therapy is offered in the adjuvant setting for both early and advanced-stage disease and has been shown to improve locoregional control.

CASE 53

Rizwan Aslam

History of Present Illness

A 75-year-old male presents with a cutaneous lesion of the left temple. The patient has noted the lesion for approximately the past 3–4 months. There has been a noticeable change in the growth of the lesion and its color. He has no history of skin lesions, no significant past medical history.

Physical Examination

A solitary skin lesion is noted, as shown in Figure 53.1. The lesion measures about 9 mm. There is no palpable lymphadenopathy and no other findings.

Question: What would you recommend next?

Answer: Although the lesion is small and appears superficial, any pigmented, asymmetric lesion with a history of change

(Continued)

CASE 53 (continued)

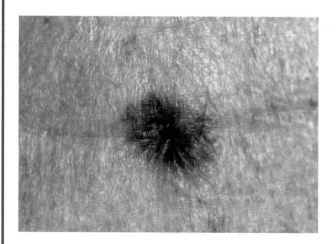

FIGURE 53.1 **This clinical photograph shows the lesion. It is approximately 9 mm in maximal dimension.**

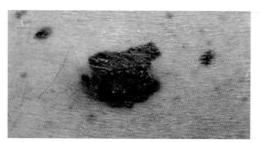

FIGURE 53.2 **This clinical photo shows the primary lesion with new evidence of ulceration and surrounding noncontiguous pigmented lesions.**

and growth needs to be investigated. The most appropriate first step is a punch biopsy.

Punch biopsy of the lesion shows: Malignant melanoma, 1.5 mm thick with no ulceration, <1 mitosis/mm2. No lymphovascular invasion or tumor regression is noted.

Question: What is the stage of the disease?

Answer: According to AJCC 8th Edition staging, this is a cT2aN0M0, stage IB melanoma. Although tumor thickness is the primary determinant of T stage, the presence or absence of ulceration is also a critical prognostic factor and is thus incorporated into TNM and overall staging. Though mitotic rate remains a predictor of survival, it is no longer included in AJCC staging. Staging of the nodal basis and metastatic status may be considered more accurate following radiographic and/or histopathologic assessment. Still, clinical assessment by careful head and neck exam alone is sufficient to assign initial clinical staging.

Question: What other tests do you recommend in your workup?

Answer: Routine imaging or lab tests are not indicated for stage I-II disease unless there are clinical concerns based upon specific signs or symptoms. Therefore, in this case no other tests are indicated.

Question: What treatment would you offer?

Answer: For invasive melanoma of the head and neck, the primary lesion should be widely excised with 1–2 cm circumferential margins. SLNBx should be considered standard of care for all patients with cN0, M0 disease, except for very thin T1a lesions.

You plan a wide excision with SLNB. However, at the preoperative visit you notice multiple new pigmented lesions adjacent to the original biopsy site, all within 2 cm of the primary lesion (see Figure 53.2).

Question: How would you describe the findings above?

Answer: This picture is most consistent with satellite lesions. Regional spread of tumor via lymphatic vessels in the dermis or subcutaneous tissue outside of nodal basins is a poor prognostic factor. This is reflected in AJCC staging of nodal disease, with N1c, N2c, or N3c corresponding to the presence of satellite or in-transit disease in association with zero, one, or multiple involved nodes, respectively. Satellite lesions are defined as within 2 cm of the primary tumor, while in-transit metastases are >2 cm from the primary lesion.

Question: What would you recommend at this point?

Answer: Since satellite lesions upstage the disease to stage III, further workup is recommended. Baseline imaging and BRAF mutation testing are recommended. If the disease is resectable with acceptable functional and cosmetic outcome, it is recommended that an excision is done to clear margins. If all final margins are clear and there is no evidence of regional disease, observation could be considered, but most would recommend systemic therapy with PD1 blockade. Agents such as nivolumab or pembrolizumab are considered the first line of treatment. In patients with BRAF activating mutations, dabrafenib/trametinib could be used. If the disease is too advanced for local excision, biopsy to prove satellite lesions is recommended and then systemic therapy.

Key Points

- Melanoma has two growth phases: radial and vertical. Melanoma in situ and microinvasive melanoma demonstrate predominantly radial growth.
- Although melanoma accounts for only about 1% of cutaneous malignancies, it is responsible for the majority of skin cancer deaths.
- The lifetime risk of developing melanoma is much higher for whites (2.6%) than blacks (0.1%), and fair-skinned whites are at particularly elevated risk.
- Nodular melanoma is the second most common melanoma and the most aggressive and rapidly growing subtype.
- For invasive melanoma of the head and neck, the primary lesion should be widely excised with 1–2 cm circumferential margins.
- SLNB should be considered standard of care for all patients with cN0, M0 disease, with the exception of very thin T1a lesions.
- Systemic therapy is the mainstay of treatment in advanced disease (stage III and above).

CASE 54

Lucy Shi and Stephen Kang

History of Present Illness

A 63-year-old man with biopsy-proven melanoma of the right forehead presents for evaluation. The patient is a farmer and has sustained significant sun damage over the years. He first noticed the forehead lesion several months ago. The lesion continued to progress in size during this time frame, and he was referred to a dermatologist who performed a punch biopsy. Pathology revealed a superficial spreading melanoma with a Breslow thickness of 2.1 mm with ulceration and clear deep margins. He was subsequently referred for further evaluation. No other significant points in history.

Physical Examination

There is a pigmented lesion of the forehead with irregular borders and central ulceration. It is about 1.5 cm in diameter. No neuropathy, no facial or cervical masses identified.

Question: What stage do you assign to this lesion following your initial evaluation?

Answer: T3bN0M0, stage IIB. A lesion between 2.01–4.0 mm thick with ulceration and no clinical evidence of nodal or distant disease is stage cT3N0M0, stage IIB according to AJCC 8th Edition staging guidelines.

Management

Question: What would you recommend next?

Answer: Imaging is not required to evaluate the nodal basin in the absence of symptoms concerning for gross metastatic spread. However, baseline imaging should be considered, particularly for thicker tumors, such as that described here, especially in individuals at high risk for disease spread to the parotid gland or obese individuals where pathologic nodes may avoid palpation. A contrast enhanced CT neck would be the best choice to evaluate the regional nodal basin.

The CT is performed and does not show any evidence of lymphadenopathy.

Question: What would you recommend next?

Answer: The initial management of early stage, resectable melanoma is surgical. Lesion thickness is strongly predictive of sentinel node positivity. Any patient with a lesion of greater than 1.0 mm thickness or of greater than 0.75 mm with ulceration and/or mitotic rate > 1 mm² should be offered SLNB.

Neck dissection is reserved in melanoma for patients with gross regional disease either on clinical workup or demonstrated a positive SLNB. There is no role for elective radiation of the nodal basin in melanoma. Adjuvant radiation can be considered to improve regional control after therapeutic or completion neck dissection in certain instances.

Question: What is the most appropriate margin of normal tissue that should be resected around the lesion for this patient?

Answer: 2.0 cm. According to the NCCN guidelines on cutaneous melanoma, melanoma lesions of depth 2.1–4.0 mm should be excised with a 2.0 cm margin, although in anatomically challenging areas, a slightly smaller margin is still acceptable. These recommendations are based on a number of large trials that found no survival advantage between 1 and 2 cm margins and >3 cm margins.

(Continued)

CASE 54 (continued)

Question: When performing SLNB, what node(s) should be removed?

Answer: All nodes that have >10% of the highest SLN count should be removed. SLN identification is based on a combination of preoperative lymphoscintigraphy followed by gamma probe detection of labeled lymph nodes and intraoperative use of methylene or isosulfan blue dye. Per the NCCN guidelines, all nodes with gamma probe activity of greater than 10% that of the highest sentinel node or that are blue in color should be removed.

The patient undergoes a wide local excision of the primary lesion and SLNB. Pathology reveals negative margins and two positive micrometastatic sentinel lymph nodes in level IB and IIA, respectively.

Question: What is the next appropriate step?

Answer: Prior to the completion of the Multicenter Selective Lymphadenectomy Trial-II (MSLT-II), a completion lymph node dissection (CLND) was recommended following a positive SLNB. However, this trial demonstrated that while CLND improved regional disease control, it did not improve melanoma-specific survival. Regional control significantly impacts quality of life, though surgical sequelae such as lymphedema may also impact quality of life. Thus, the current recommendations per the NCCN and the American Society of Clinical Oncology (ASCO) state that for all anatomical subsites, if a SLNB were positive, a CLND should be offered to the patient following full discussion of the risks and benefits of the procedure as well as the alternative of observation.

Question: If one sentinel lymph node is found to be positive, what is the risk of another nonsentinel lymph node being positive in the head and neck?

Answer: Two large single-institution reviews of melanoma in the head and neck have quoted the rate of nonsentinel lymph node positivity to be 22–25%. Thus, a full discussion of the benefits and risks of completion neck dissection is indicated following a positive SLNB.

Question: What is the appropriate initial treatment option for this patient if there were clinically positive nodes at the time of presentation?

Answer: In patients with clinically apparent lymphadenopathy, the patient should undergo upfront therapeutic lymphadenectomy in addition to wide local excision of the primary (2 cm margins).

Question: The patient undergoes completion lymphadenectomy without complications. The final pathology report does not show additional positive nodes. What would you recommend?

Answer: Since the disease is completely removed, observation is an option. However, most patients are offered systemic immunotherapy with PD1 pathway blockers such as Nivolumab or Pembrolizumab. A multidisciplinary discussion and referral to a melanoma medical oncology specialist is warranted. Regardless, close surveillance is recommended.

Key Points

- Any patient with a lesion of greater than 1.0 mm thickness or of greater than 0.75 mm with ulceration and/or mitotic rate >1 mm^2 should be offered SLNB.
- All nodes with gamma probe activity of greater than 10% that of the highest sentinel node or that are blue in color should be removed.
- SLNB is the most important prognostic factor for disease progression and disease-specific survival.
- If an SLNB is positive, a CLND should be offered to the patient following a full discussion of the risks and benefits of the procedure as well as the alternative of observation.
- In patients with clinically apparent lymphadenopathy, the patient should undergo upfront therapeutic lymphadenectomy.
- Compared to other anatomic subsites, melanoma of the head and neck has a lower rate of SLN identification, higher rates of false-negative SLNB, and a higher risk of regional recurrence and mortality.

Multiple Choice Questions

1. Which of the following is/are considered aggressive subtype(s) of BCC?
   a. Superficial.
   b. Nodular.
   c. Microndular.
   d. Pleomorphic.

Answer: c. Nodular, pleomorphic, and superficial subtypes are considered less aggressive and less likely to recur. Morpheoform, infiltrative, and micronodular BCC are all subtypes associated with a more irregular invasive front that is associated with a higher rate of local recurrence. Basosquamous BCC demonstrates a more squamous differentiation pattern including keratin pearls and is considered an aggressive subtype.

2. What is the mechanism of action of vismodigib?

   a. Inhibition of MAP kinase pathway.

   b. Inhibition of hedgehog signaling pathway.

   c. Inhibition of BRAF V600E mutation.

   d. Programmed death pathway blockade.

   Answer: b. Vismodigib is a small molecule inhibitor of hedgehog signaling. It inhibits SMO, thereby inactivating GL1 and the downstream factors involved in hedgehog signaling.

3. What is the most common site of disease for sebaceous carcinoma?

   a. Eyelid.

   b. The nasal dorsum.

   c. The nasal vestibule.

   d. The occipital scalp.

   Answer: a. The majority of sebaceous carcinomas arise from the eyelid and periorbital region because this location has the largest number of sebaceous glands.

4. Which subtype of melanoma is the most aggressive?

   a. Nodular.

   b. Superficial spreading.

   c. Desmoplastic.

   d. Acral lentiginous.

   Answer: a. Nodular melanoma is the second most common melanoma and the most aggressive and rapidly growing subtype. It is characterized by early progression to a vertical growth phase. Less common variants of melanoma include nevoid, desmoplastic, clear cell, and solitary dermal melanoma.

5. Based on findings of the Multicenter Selective Lymphadenectomy Trial-I (MSLT-I), sentinel node biopsy

   a. Improves disease-specific survival in patients with nodal disease.

   b. Does not affect disease-free survival.

   c. Represents an important tool for staging and prognostication.

   d. Improves overall survival.

   Answer: c. MSLT-I confirmed what had been shown by many previous retrospective trials: SLNB is the most important prognostic factor for disease progression and disease-specific survival (DSS). The trial also demonstrated higher disease-free survival rates in the SLNB group across all subgroups. Importantly, in intermediate thickness melanoma (1.2–3.5 mm Breslow depth), patients with positive SLNB and immediate neck dissection had superior melanoma-specific survival than those who were observed and had a delayed neck dissection when metastases were clinically apparent. SLNB would not have a role in patients with cN+ disease.

6. Compared to melanoma of other anatomic sites, melanoma of the head and neck

   a. Has a lower likelihood of positive surgical margins following resection.

   b. Has lower rates of SLN identification.

   c. Has lower false-negative rates on SLNB.

   d. Has a lower risk of regional recurrence.

Answer: b. Compared to other anatomic subsites, melanoma of the head and neck has a lower rate of SLN identification, higher rates of false-negative SLNB, and a higher risk of regional recurrence and mortality.

Suggested Reading

Basal Cell Carcinoma

Asgari, M.M., Moffett, H.H., Ray, G.T. et al. (2015). Trends in basal cell carcinoma incidence and identification of high-risk subgroups, 1998–2012. *JAMA Dermatol.* 151 (9): 976–981.

Sekulic, A., Migden, M.R., Oro, A.E. et al. (2012). Efficacy and safety of vismodegib in advanced basal-cell carcinoma. *N. Engl. J. Med.* 366 (23): 2171–2179.

Van Loo, E., Mosterd, K., and Krekels, G.A. (2014). Surgical excision versus Mohs' micrographic surgery for basal cell carcinoma of the face: a randomized clinical trial with 10-year follow-up. *Eur. J. Cancer* 50 (17): 3011–3020.

Melanoma

American Academy of Dermatology Ad Hoc Task Force for the ABCDEs of Melanoma, Tsao, H., Olazagasti, J.M. et al. (2015). Early detection of melanoma: reviewing the ABCDEs. *J. Am. Acad. Dermatol.* 72: 717.

Faries, M.B., Thompson, J.F., Cochran, A.J. et al. (2017). Completion dissection or observation for sentinel-node metastasis in melanoma. *N. Engl. J. Med.* 376 (23): 2211–2222.

Gillgren, P., Drzewiecki, K.T., Niin, M. et al. (2011). 2-cm versus 4-cm surgical excision margins for primary cutaneous melanoma thicker than 2 mm: a randomised, multicentre trial. *Lancet* 378 (9803): 1635–1642.

Morton, D.L., Thompson, J.F., Cochran, A.J. et al. (2014). Final trial report of sentinel-node biopsy versus nodal observation in melanoma. *N. Engl. J. Med.* 370 (7): 599–609.

Wong, S.L., Faries, M.B., Kennedy, E.B. et al. (2018). Sentinel lymph node biopsy and management of regional lymph nodes in melanoma: American Society of Clinical Oncology and Society of Surgical Oncology clinical practice guideline update. *Ann. Surg. Oncol.* 25 (2): 356–377.

Cutaneous Squamous Cell Carcinoma

Ahmed, M., Moore, B.A., and Schmalbach, C.E. (2014). Utility of sentinel node biopsy in head & neck cutaneous squamous cell carcinoma: a systematic review. *Otolaryngol. Head Neck Surg.* 150 (2): 180–187.

Durham, A.B., Lowe, L., Malloy, K.M. et al. (2016). Sentinel lymph node biopsy for cutaneous squamous cell carcinoma on the head and neck. *JAMA Otolaryngol. Head Neck* 142 (12): 1171–1176.

Migden, M.R., Rischin, D., Schmults, C.D. et al. (2018). PD-1 blockade with cemiplimab in advanced cutaneous squamous-cell carcinoma. *N. Engl. J. Med.* 379 (4): 341–351.

Porceddu, S.V., Bressel, M., Poulsen, M.G. et al. (2018). Postoperative concurrent chemoradiotherapy versus postoperative radiotherapy in high-risk cutaneous squamous cell carcinoma of the head and neck: the randomized phase III TROG 05.01 trial. *J. Clin. Oncol.* 36: 1275–1283.

Merkel Cell Carcinoma

Chen, M.M., Roman, S.A., Sosa, J.A. et al. (2015). The role of adjuvant therapy in the management of head and neck Merkel cell carcinoma: an analysis of 4815 patients. *JAMA Otolaryngol. Head Neck Surg.* 141 (2): 137–141.

Jouary, T., Leyral, C., Dreno, B. et al. (2012). Adjuvant prophylactic regional radiotherapy versus observation in stage I Merkel cell carcinoma: a multicentric prospective randomized study. *Ann. Oncol.* 23 (4): 1074–1080.

Schmalbach, C.E., Lowe, L., Teknos, T.N. et al. (2005). Reliability of sentinel lymph node biopsy for regional staging of head and neck Merkel cell carcinoma. *Arch. Otolaryngol. Head Neck Surg.* 131 (7): 610–614.

Sebaceous Carcinoma

Gaskin, B.J., Fernando, B.S., Sullivan, C.A. et al. (2011). The significance of DNA mismatch repair genes in the diagnosis and management of periocular sebaceous cell carcinoma and Muir-Torre syndrome. *Br. J. Ophthalmol.* 95 (12): 1686–1690.

Shields, J.A., Demirci, H., Marr, B.P. et al. (2005). Sebaceous carcinoma of the ocular region: a review. *Surv. Ophthalmol.* 50 (2): 103–122.

Song, A., Carter, K.D., Syed, N.A. et al. (2008). Sebaceous cell carcinoma of the ocular adnexa: clinical presentations, histopathology, and outcomes. *Ophthal. Plast. Reconstr. Surg.* 24 (3): 194–200.

SECTION 13

Salivary

Antoine Eskander

CASE 55

Michael G. Moore

History of Present Illness

A 50-year-old female presents for evaluation of a slowly growing left cheek mass. She was seen by her primary care physician and promptly sent to you. She has had no additional workup to date.

Question: What additional questions would you want to ask in the initial evaluation? (Choose all that apply.)

- Any other symptoms from it? Pain? Patient denies.
- Any other adjacent lumps that have been noticed? Patient denies.
- Any prior skin tumors removed? Patient denies.
- Any heat or cold intolerance? Incorrect. Would be relevant for thyroid pathology.
- Any weakness or twitching of the face? Patient denies.
- Any family history of facial tumors? Not applicable. There is no known inheritance pattern of salivary tumors.
- Any numbness of the face? Patient denies.
- Any change in hearing? Patient denies.
- Any difficulty opening and closing the mouth? Patient denies.

Question: What additional aspects of the history are important?

- Any prior surgery or trauma to the area? Patient denies.
- Do you smoke? Patient denies. Can predispose to

Warthin's tumors.
- Any dry mouth or other systemic conditions such as Sjogren's disease? Patient denies. Can predispose to parotid lymphoma.

Physical Examination

Skin/scalp: Fitzpatrick 3, no obvious lesions or scars.

Ears: within normal limits, bilaterally.

Anterior rhinoscopy is normal.

Oral cavity exam shows no lesions. Normal salivary flow. No obvious stones.

Neck exam shows a firm, mobile mass in the left preauricular area.

No palpable lymphadenopathy.

Cranial nerves II–XII grossly within normal limits.

Question: What would be your next step in the evaluation of this patient?

Answer: Magnetic resonance imaging (MRI) of the neck with and without gadolinium was ordered. For salivary lesions, MRI provides excellent soft-tissue detail and can also assess for perineural invasion and/or skull base involvement. A representative T2-weighted axial image is displayed in Figure 55.1.

Computed tomography (CT) would be another good option but would not be needed if an MRI is already being performed. A neck ultrasound can be helpful in imaging and guiding biopsies of salivary lesions but can be limited for tumors with extension into the deep lobe.

(Continued)

Essential Cases in Head and Neck Oncology, First Edition. Edited by Michael G. Moore, Arnaud F. Bewley, and Babak Givi.
© 2022 American Head and Neck Society. Published 2022 by John Wiley & Sons Ltd.

CASE 55 (continued)

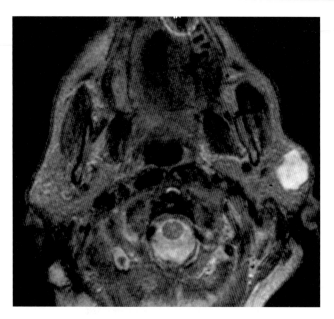

FIGURE 55.1 This is an axial T2-weighted image showing the middle portion of the left parotid mass. Notice the hyperintense T2 signal as well as the lobulated (bosselating), well-circumscribed edges of the tumor.

Question: Based on the history, physical examination, and imaging characteristics, what is the most likely diagnosis for this patient?

Answer: While this lesion could be indicative of any parotid tumor, it has the characteristic appearance of a pleomorphic adenoma (hyperintense on T2 images, well-defined borders, and bosselating edges). If this were a lymph node, it would be obviously pathologic based on size and morphology.

Question: What would be an appropriate next step in the evaluation/management of this patient?

Answer: Fine needle aspiration (FNA) would be the appropriate next step in an effort to obtain a tissue diagnosis. Ultrasound guidance may be helpful in an effort to optimize the yield of the biopsy. Incisional biopsies should universally be avoided for salivary tumors due to the risk of tumor seeding.

Question: FNA was performed showing mixed rests of epithelial cells as well as a background of chondromyxoid matrix. What would be the most appropriate option for management?

Answer: This biopsy result is characteristic of a pleomorphic adenoma, the most common salivary neoplasm. Management involves resection of the lesion with a cuff of surrounding normal salivary tissue, when possible. Intracapsular enucleation leads to an unacceptably high risk of recurrence; however, careful extracapsular dissection can allow for complete tumor removal and may be appropriate for experienced surgeons in select cases.

Question: The patient undergoes a superficial parotidectomy with facial nerve preservation and has an uneventful recovery. Six months later, she presents to your office with a complaint of her cheek skin "leaking" around the time of meals. What is the most likely cause of his symptoms?

Answer: This patient has developed Frey syndrome, which is fairly common and results from regeneration of postsynaptic parasympathetic nerves that are cut during parotidectomy to sweat glands in the overlying skin. The rate of Frey syndrome may be reduced by placing a barrier between the cut parotid parenchyma and the overlying skin through different parotid bed reconstructive techniques. While a salivary fistula can develop resulting in swelling or incisional drainage, it would be expected to manifest much sooner than 6 months.

Key Points

- The majority of parotid masses are benign, with pleomorphic adenoma being the most common neoplasm.
- Initial evaluation of parotid masses involves a history, physical examination, and imaging, with MRI providing excellent soft-tissue detail of the tumor.
- While not absolutely necessary, FNA is often helpful to achieve a tissue diagnosis and to help guide in counseling the patient prior to treatment.
- Appropriate treatment of benign salivary tumors involves complete tumor excision with preservation of surrounding cranial nerve branches. For parotid neoplasms, this often involves a partial or complete superficial parotidectomy with facial nerve dissection, but extracapsular dissection may be appropriate for select lesions.
- Frey syndrome occurs as a result of aberrant regeneration of postganglionic parasympathetic fibers to the sweat glands in the overlying skin. Approaches to prevent this phenomenon center around the creation of a barrier between the cut parotid parenchyma and the overlying skin.

CASE 56

Chris Rassekh

History of Present Illness

A 69-year-old white male presents with a right salivary gland "blockage." The patient has no pain but has a spot under his jaw that is tender to touch. The patient also endorses dry mouth at night. He feels he has swelling and has a sensation of numbness along the right jaw line.

Past Medical History

Prostate cancer status postsurgery 2 years ago.

Question: What additional history would you like to obtain? (Choose all that apply.)

- Any history of tongue numbness? Good question. He has none.
- Any chewing problems or difficulty opening the mouth? He denies.
- Any swelling of the area with eating? He denies.
- Any abnormal taste of saliva? He denies.

Physical Examination

Well-developed middle-aged male in no distress with a normal voice.

Normal dentition.

Right submandibular gland is firm and tender. No flow from the right submandibular duct. Other major salivary ducts with scant saliva but appear to have flow. No floor of mouth lesion. There is some tenderness over the gland and also the right mandible to palpation. No lip or chin numbness, normal facial nerve function. He does have numbness of the some of the skin overlying the right submandibular gland.

No lymphadenopathy.

No other cranial nerve abnormalities.

The remainder of the head and neck exam is normal.

Question: What further workup should be considered in this patient?

Answer: Imaging should be done first here. In this instance, a CT was chosen due to the desire to evaluate for a stone and/or a neoplasm (see Figure 56.1). An MRI would be a reasonable option, as would an ultrasound.

Question: What would be the appropriate next step in the evaluation of this patient?

Answer: At this point, there is no evidence of a tumor, however, the patient's numbness is concerning. An ultrasound can be helpful in further evaluation of the gland for lesions and ductal dilation and also to assess the adjacent nodes. An MRI can also assist in this assessment, and an MR sialogram was performed in this patient.

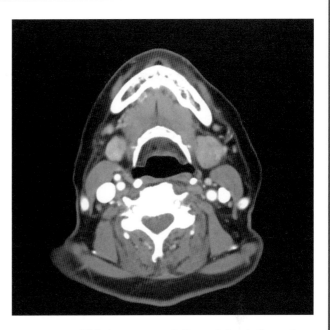

FIGURE 56.1 This is a representative axial cut of a neck CT with IV contrast. The right submandibular gland is diminutive and slightly hyperdense, possibly on the basis of chronic sialadenitis. There is a small adjacent lymph node. No mass is seen in that region. No evidence of radiopaque sialolith. The aerodigestive tract is normal in appearance, without mass. There is no adenopathy by imaging criteria. The other salivary glands are normal in appearance.

Neck Ultrasound Report

Within the right submandibular gland there is a tubular hypoechoic soft-tissue lesion that traverses the gland, extending beyond the gland into the adjacent subcutaneous tissues through which facial vessels are noted, without underlying displacement. There is no evidence of ductal dilatation or calculi seen within the submandibular gland. The shape of the lesion and the perivascular distribution are more suggestive of an infiltrating process rather than a focal primary tumor. The findings could be related to an inflammatory process, such as chronic inflammation, or an infiltrative process including both neoplastic and non-neoplastic conditions, for example, IgG4 sclerosing disease. The contralateral left submandibular gland and the parotid glands bilaterally are unremarkable, noting expected fatty replacement of the parotids bilaterally.

An MRI was also performed (see Figure 56.2).

MRI Report

There is an incompletely characterized mass in the right inferior submandibular gland measuring approximately $18 \times 12 \times 20\,\text{mm}$ (AP×TR×CC). The right submandibular gland is smaller in size than the left. No associated submandibular duct dilatation. No periglandular inflammatory changes.

(Continued)

CASE 56 (continued)

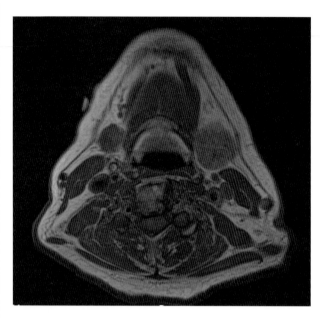

FIGURE 56.2 **This is a contrast-enhanced T1-weighted MRI in the axial plane. The right submandibular gland is small and more heterogeneous in intensity than the left.**

No focal abnormality of the remaining visualized salivary glands.

No pathologic cervical lymph nodes by imaging criteria.

Question: Given the ultrasound and MRI findings, what would be the appropriate next step for this patient?

Answer: In this instance, there is concern for a neoplasm in the gland, and as a result, a tissue diagnosis is needed to help guide the next steps in management. An ultrasound-guided FNA would be appropriate.

Cytology Report

Submandibular gland, right, 2.1 cm, US-FNA: salivary gland neoplasm with basaloid features. Note: The differential diagnosis includes basal cell adenoma, cellular pleomorphic adenoma, and less likely basal cell adenocarcinoma and adenoid cystic carcinoma.

Question: Given the above information, what is the most appropriate next step in management?

Answer: This patient should have submandibular gland excision and should be consented for level I neck dissection in this case because given the history, the FNA report should be viewed as highly suspicious for adenoid cystic carcinoma. However, this must be proven histologically, and it is still possible this is a benign tumor. As a result, patient counseling is critical.

This is a very unusual case that initially presented resembling inflammatory disease but from the beginning had symptoms suggestive of malignancy and specifically adenoid cystic carcinoma with perineural invasion. In this situation, the submandibular gland was atrophic because of perineural invasion involving the submandibular ganglion. There was also extensive perineural invasion involving the facial vasculature, but no evidence of cervical metastases. The decision to preserve the lingual nerve (and certainly the hypoglossal) was made with the thought that the morbidity of nerve resection would outweigh the potential oncologic benefit of additional resection. It should be noted that intraoperatively there was no evidence of invasion of the lingual nerve but rather only the submandibular ganglion. If the lingual nerve was grossly invaded, this would have also been resected.

Question: What would be the next step in this patient's management?

Answer: Given the diagnosis of adenoid cystic carcinoma, chest imaging is indicated to rule out pulmonary metastases. In this patient, a chest CT revealed no nodules. Moreover, this patient with extensive perineural invasion of adenoid cystic carcinoma is at very high risk for microscopic residual disease, as in nearly all patients with adenoid cystic carcinoma. As a result, referral for adjuvant radiation therapy is appropriate. As opposed to most other salivary malignancies, further nerve resection to achieve microscopic margin clearance is not thought to result in an improvement in disease control if adjuvant radiation is implemented. In this instance, tumor board consensus was that no further surgery should be done to address the primary tumor or adjacent cervical lymphatics as adenoid cystic cancers rarely develop cervical lymph node metastases. Given the risk of distant metastatic spread to the lungs, a contrast enhanced of the CT of the chest should be performed to complete his work-up.

Key Points

- Evaluation of patients with submandibular gland pathology starts with a detailed history and physical examination.
- Additional workup for submandibular gland pathology may include CT, MRI, and/or ultrasound, with an ultrasound-guided FNA being recommended if a discrete lesion is identified.
- Adenoid cystic carcinoma is the most common malignancy of the submandibular gland.
- Presentation of adenoid cystic carcinoma can be subtle and often is highlighted by deficits in sensory, motor, or even autonomic nerve functions.
- Treatment of submandibular gland tumors typically involves a level I dissection. This is done to allow for nodal clearance and assessment and because revision level I dissection carries a very high risk to the marginal mandibular, lingual, and hypoglossal nerves.
- Treatment of adenoid cystic carcinoma involves surgical resection with postoperative radiation therapy. In instances where resection of major cranial nerves is needed to achieve microscopically negative margins, it is not clear that aggressive nerve resection provides increased disease control when adjuvant radiation therapy is instituted.

CASE 57

Michael G. Moore

History of Present Illness

A 62-year-old female presents for evaluation of a left cheek mass. She states that it started initially around 2 months ago as a sore lump under her ear and has progressed fairly rapidly since then. She now has noticed a small amount of drainage from the skin below her ear. She has no fevers or systemic symptoms. She denies any prior surgery or radiation in the area. No prior skin cancers removed. She has no history of any rheumatologic conditions.

Past Medical History

Hypertension and diet-controlled type II diabetes mellitus.

Past Surgical History

None.

Medications

Hydrochlorothiazide.

Allergies: none.

Physical Examination

Patient is a middle-aged female in no acute distress.

She has normal function in cranial nerves II–XII.

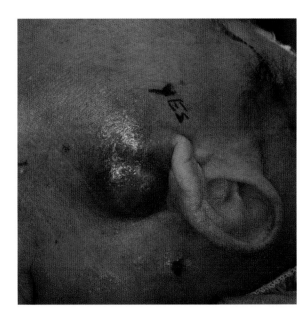

FIGURE 57.1 This clinical photo shows the patient's left parotid mass with involvement of the infra-auricular skin.

Right ear has a normal EAC and TM.

Neck exam shows a firm, hypomobile (but not fixed) mass in the left infra-auricular area. The overlying skin is violaceous with scant drainage. There are no obvious palpable pathologic lymph nodes in the other portions of her neck (see Figure 57.1).

On the left, there is mild mass effect on the lower aspect of the pinna and cartilaginous EAC. TM appears normal.

Nasal and oral cavity exam are normal.

Question: What would be your next step(s) in evaluation of this patient? (Choose all that apply.)

CT of the neck with IV contrast: **yes**/no. In this patient, there is concern for malignancy with involvement of the adjacent temporal bone and possibly the mandible. As a result, a CT of the neck would be a good next step. This will also provide information on any regional nodal involvement (see Figure 57.2).

FNA: **yes**/no. Obtaining a tissue diagnosis is critical here. Since it is involving the overlying skin, a derm punch biopsy could also be used. Here, FNA demonstrates a poorly differentiated cancer of the left parotid gland, possibly high-grade mucoepidermoid cancer.

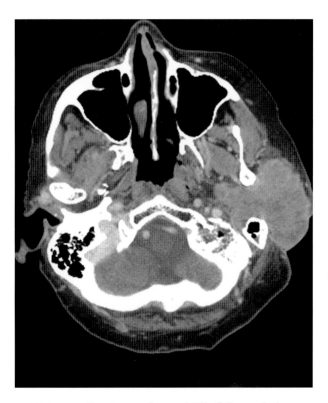

FIGURE 57.2 Contrast-enhanced CT of the neck demonstrates a large lesion filling the left parotid gland with extension to the overlying skin and encasement of the contents of the stylomastoid foramen.

(Continued)

CASE 57   (continued)

Question: What would be an appropriate next step for this patient?

Answer: This patient appears to have an aggressive malignant process of the left parotid gland with involvement of the overlying skin. For high-grade tumors that are stage III or IV, a workup for distant metastatic disease is warranted, and positron emission tomography (PET)/CT is one option for this. Another option would be to get a CT of the chest with IV contrast. The patient should also be presented at a multidisciplinary tumor board. MRI may provide additional information related to perineural and/or skull base invasion, but in this instance with normal facial and trigeminal nerve function, it may not change the treatment approach.

Question: What would be the appropriate oncologic management for this patient's cancer?

Answer: In this instance, the patient has a locally advanced high-grade malignancy with extension to surround the facial nerve at the stylomastoid foramen. As a result, despite normal facial nerve function, facial nerve resection will likely be required. Due to the close association with the external auditory canal and mastoid tip, a lateral temporal bone resection will be needed to achieve a clear margin in these locations. An ipsilateral neck dissection was performed in this patient despite being cN0 due to the patient's advanced high-grade primary tumor.

The patient ultimately underwent a left-sided radical parotidectomy with facial nerve sacrifice, left-sided modified radical neck dissection, wide resection of overlying skin, resection of the posterior mandible ramus, and a left-sided lateral temporal bone resection. Intraoperatively, there was a small cerebrospinal fluid leak noticed from the dura overlying the tegmen mastoidi (see Figure 57.3).

Question: Given the associated defect, what would be an appropriate option for reconstruction?

Answer: An anterolateral thigh free flap would be an appropriate option to replace both soft-tissue loss as well as the overlying skin. Due to the large dead space created by the resection, a radial forearm free flap or lateral arm free flap would not be appropriate, unless the patient was morbidly obese. Other large soft-tissue free flaps such as a latissimus dorsi or rectus abdominus flap could be used. Moreover, depending on the body habitus, an ipsilateral supraclavicular flap may also be an option.

Question: The patient's final pathology demonstrated a T4aN0M0 high-grade mucoepidermoid carcinoma of the left parotid gland with close but negative margins at the

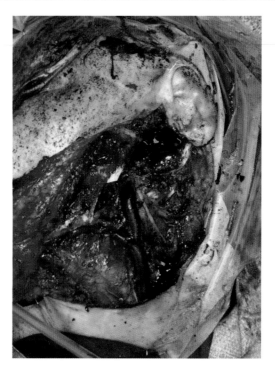

FIGURE 57.3   This is an intraoperative photo following a left-sided radical parotidectomy with facial nerve resection, left modified radical neck dissection preserving the internal jugular vein and spinal accessory nerve, resection of the posterior mandible ramus, and left lateral temporal bone resection.

jugular foramen. What would be the most appropriate next course of action?

Answer: The use of adjuvant therapy following surgical resection of salivary cancers is still in evolution. However, given the advanced stage of the tumor, the high-grade histology, and close margins, the patient would definitely be a candidate for adjuvant radiation therapy assuming there were no other contraindications. Close observation would yield a much higher risk of locoregional failure. The use of adjuvant chemotherapy is not indicated as a sole treatment, and adding it to radiation therapy is typically done in the context of a clinical trial. Due to the morbidity of a jugular foramen resection and the fact that it would not be for residual gross disease, it typically would not be recommended in this situation. For individuals where there truly is an involved margin, their multidisciplinary team must weigh the potential risks versus benefits of repeat resection.

Key Points

- Signs and symptoms concerning for salivary cancer include rapid growth, pain, drainage from the overlying skin, and weakness, twitching, or numbness of the face.
- In patients where there is concern for an advanced high-grade malignancy, PET/CT is helpful to complete staging.
- In patients with intact preoperative facial nerve function, the goal is typically to preserve the nerve at the time of surgery. An exception would be in instances where there is complete encasement of the nerve with a high-grade neoplasm and/or obvious gross tumor involvement of the nerve.
- Indications for neck dissection include high-grade histopathologies, T3/T4 primary tumors, or evidence of regional lymph node involvement at the time of presentation.

- Indications for adjuvant radiation therapy include stage III or IV salivary cancers (includes T3/T4 tumors and pN+ disease), high-grade histopathologies, involved or close surgical margins, or significant perineural or lymphovascular invasion.
- In instances where the parotid gland and surrounding structures have to be resected as part of the tumor ablation, reconstruction may be necessary to optimize wound healing, function, and cosmesis. In many instances, soft-tissue flaps such as anterolateral thigh free flaps or lateral arm flaps are used. However, regional flaps such as the submental or supraclavicular flaps may be implemented in certain instances.

CASE 58

Michael G. Moore

History of Present Illness

A 57-year-old male presents for evaluation of progressive snoring. He states he was in the usual state of health until around 6 months ago, when his wife started to tell him that his snoring was worsening. Over the past month, he has had much more daytime fatigue. His primary care physician ultimately referred him to you for evaluation.

Past Medical and Surgical History

Unremarkable.

Physical Examination

Middle-aged male in no acute distress. He has slightly muffled speech but is breathing comfortably.

His ears and nose are normal.

Figure 58.1 shows a view of the exam of his oropharynx, where there is a bulge in the left soft palate. It is nonindurated and somewhat firm to palpation, but the overlying mucosa appears spared. He has no trismus and his cranial nerves II–XII are intact bilaterally.

Fiberoptic exam shows a bulge medially of the left lateral pharyngeal wall but no other lesions. The vocal folds move symmetrically, and the hypopharyngeal and laryngeal components of the airway are normal.

Question: What would be your next step in evaluation and management of this patient?

Answer: The concern in this individual is that he has a mass involving the left parapharyngeal space. As a result, cross-sectional imaging would be appropriate. A CT or an MRI would be recommended in this instance (see Figure 58.2). Given the time course of the process, lack of pain, fever, or other signs/symptoms such as induration of the area and trismus, a pharyngitis or peritonsillar abscess are unlikely.

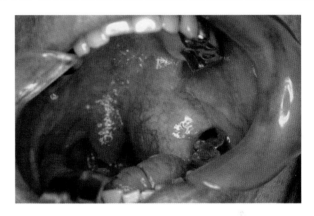

FIGURE 58.1   This is a transoral view of the oropharynx demonstrating a nonindurated bulge of the left soft palate. The patient has no significant trismus.

Question: A transoral FNA shows the lesion is likely a pleomorphic adenoma. What would be the most appropriate surgical approach to remove this lesion?

Answer: This appears to be a tumor of the left prestyloid parapharyngeal space. On the current image, it is difficult to determine the extent of attachment to the deep lobe of the left parotid gland, but it is possible the tumor originated from a minor salivary gland rest within the parapharyngeal space. For such tumors, gentle blunt dissection after removal of the styloid process often allows for tumor delivery without tumor spill and without the need for more invasive approaches such as a transmandibular approach. The styloid process is usually removed or outfractured during the resection prior to fully mobilizing the tumor as otherwise rocking the tumor in the parapharyngeal space with blunt dissection for delivery can sometimes lead to the tumor leaning into the tip of the styloid and rupturing the tumor capsule. Transoral excision of parapharyngeal space tumors has been described but is not considered the standard of care and may introduce the risk of

(Continued)

CASE 58 (continued)

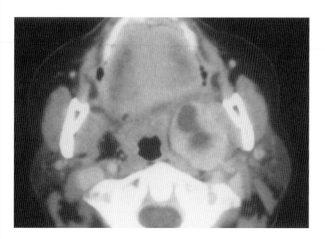

FIGURE 58.2 **This is a representative axial slice from this patient's CT of the neck with IV contrast. A mass can be identified in the left parapharyngeal space. Note that the fat has been displaced medially while the carotid artery and internal jugular vein have been pushed posteriorly.**

infection as well as injury to major neurovascular structures. He is a young, healthy individual with progressive symptoms that likely are resulting from tumor growth. As a result, observation would not be an ideal choice.

Question: This patient underwent a successful transcervical approach to resect the left parapharyngeal space mass. A few months after surgery, he presents with a complaint of sharp pain along the left jawline soon after he starts eating that usually subsides over time. What is the likely cause of these symptoms?

Answer: This patient appears to be experiencing first bite syndrome, which is a phenomenon that can occur following extensive surgery within the parapharyngeal space and infratemporal fossa. It is thought to be related to disruption of the sympathetic nerves in this region, thus resulting in unopposed parasympathetic input upon initiation of a meal. The resulting forceful contraction of the parotid tissue can be quite painful.

Key Points

- Salivary neoplasms are the most common tumors of the prestyloid parapharyngeal space and can either arise from rests of salivary tissue or from the extension from the deep lobe of the adjacent parotid gland.
- Many patients will be asymptomatic from these tumors, but larger tumors can start to exert mass effect on the pharynx, resulting in oropharyngeal obstructive symptoms such as snoring.
- History and physical exam are important to differentiate parapharyngeal space masses from oropharyngeal infections such as tonsillitis or a peritonsillar abscess. In infections, induration is often seen, leading to trismus and progressive pain.
- Imaging is critical in evaluating parapharyngeal space tumors. MRI and CT can be used to assess the extent of the tumor, as well as its relationship with the deep lobe of the parotid. Moreover, the deviation of the parapharyngeal fat and the carotid sheath contents will provide insight into the lesion's location in the prestyloid or poststyloid space.
- Treatment of parapharyngeal space masses, especially those that are symptomatic, is surgical excision. The approach to resection typically depends on tumor extent, location, size, and type of pathology. Typically, a transcervical approach is used with a transparotid approach instituted in instances where there is significant involvement of the parotid gland.

CASE 59

Jessica Yesensky

History of Present Illness

An 86-year-old female presents to clinic for evaluation of rapidly enlarging right neck mass over the past 2–3 months. The mass was initially painless but now is somewhat tender. She notes noisy breathing with difficulty lying flat over the past few weeks and endorses dysphagia with solids and a 10 lb weight loss in the past 2 months.

Past Medical History

History of Sjogren's disease and rheumatoid arthritis.

CASE 59   (continued)

Past Surgical History

She denies any prior head and neck surgeries and has not had any prior skin cancers of the head and neck.

Social History

Patient has no smoking or alcohol history. (Smoking history can predispose to Warthin's tumor.)

Review of Symptoms

The patient denies any night sweats or fevers. The rest of her nine-point review of systems is noncontributory.

Physical Examination

Patient is an elderly female with muffled, "hot potato" voice. Unlabored respirations, but audible stertor.

She has an approximately 10×8 cm firm hypomobile mass extending from tail of parotid/angle of mandible to submandibular region (see Figure 59.1).

No cervical lymphadenopathy is appreciated. Her oral cavity and oropharynx exam show no obvious trismus or mucosal lesions, but she does have a bulge of the right lateral pharynx (see Figure 59.2). Her cranial nerve exam is intact bilaterally.

Flexible laryngoscopy demonstrates a bulge on the lateral pharyngeal wall extending from nasopharynx to oropharynx. The hypopharynx and larynx appear normal.

Question: What would be an appropriate next step in the evaluation/management of this patient?

Answer: This patient has what appears to be a rapidly progressive mass of the right parotid gland. While a tissue diagnosis is an important step, it is important to first obtain imaging.

For this patient, an MRI of the neck, with and without gadolinium, was obtained (see Figure 59.3).

Question: Based on the history, physical exam, and imaging, what remains highest on your differential diagnosis?

Answer: This patient has an enlarging mass, originating from the parotid, that has extended into neck and parapharyngeal space over the span of a couple of months. Despite the size and extent, there was no evidence of bony destruction, infiltration surrounding soft tissue, or nerve deficits to suggest infiltrative or invasive tumor, which may be seen with aggressive primary salivary gland malignancies. MRI demonstrates a solid, homogeneous mass, without necrosis or cystic components. These features are most suggestive of rapidly evolving lymphoma.

Question: What about the patient predisposes her the most to this diagnosis?

Answer: Sjogren's disease represents an autoimmune disease characterized by immune-mediated destruction of exocrine glands, predominately lacrimal and salivary glands. The

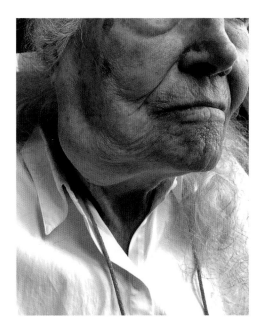

FIGURE 59.1   This photo demonstrates the patient's enlarged right parotid gland.

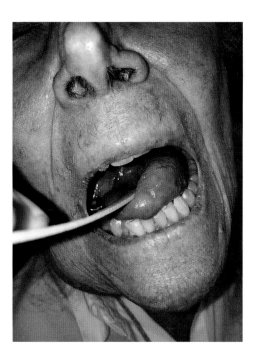

FIGURE 59.2   This transoral photograph of the oropharynx shows medial displacement of the right tonsil and soft palate with deviation of uvula to left.

(Continued)

CASE 59 (continued)

disease consists of heavy lymphocytic infiltration of the salivary glands, and these patients have five to nine times the risk of developing lymphoma. Lymphoma should be considered in patients with Sjogren's who present with a parotid mass.

Primary lymphoma of the parotid is rare and represents about 2–3% of parotid neoplasms and <1% of all parotid masses. The peak age of occurrence is between 50 and 80 years, and the sex distribution is about equal.

Question: What is your next step in the workup/management of this patient?

Answer: A transcervical open incisional biopsy was performed to obtain tissue for diagnosis. In most instances of parotid tumors, open incisional biopsies should be avoided. However, in this instance, where lymphoma is a likely diagnosis and the extent of the disease would preclude definitive resection, an open biopsy is appropriate. Here, a sample was sent for frozen histologic examination to rule out pathologies other than lymphoma. The tissue was sent fresh for lymphoma workup according to our pathology protocol.

If your suspicion for lymphoma is high, FNA will often not provide sufficient information for diagnosis, and incisional/excisional biopsy is necessary. Most parotid lymphomas are amenable to excision and require superficial lobectomy for definitive diagnosis. Large tumors, as seen with our patient, are not amenable to total excision. Therefore, it is recommended to perform either an incisional biopsy or image-guided core biopsies to permit adequate histopathologic evaluation.

Treatment consists of nonsurgical therapies, and it is not necessary to remove the entire mass.

The procedure was done in the operating room under local anesthesia given the patient's airway involvement. There is little data evaluating the effects of acute steroid use on accuracy of biopsy results. Data has suggested that use of steroids can potentially cause secondary histologic changes and obscure diagnosis.

Question: This patient most likely has what type of lymphoma?

Answer: Diffuse large B-cell lymphoma (DLBCL), a type of non-Hodgkin's lymphoma, is the most common lymphoma encountered in the parotid (and the most common in the head and neck in general). Most patients have Ann Arbor stage I or II at time of diagnosis. It has been suggested that patients with lymphoma in the setting of Sjogren's have worse prognosis. This patient was in fact diagnosed with DLBCL and started on chemotherapy.

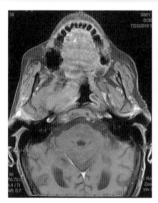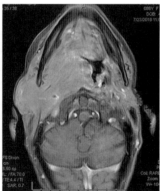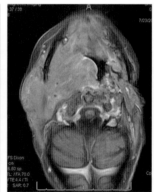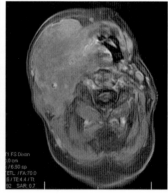

FIGURE 59.3 These are representative T1-weighted cuts of an axial MRI of the neck with contrast demonstrating a large mass of the right parotid gland with significant mass effect on the oropharyngeal airway.

Key Points

- Lymphoma of the parotid gland is rare but should be considered in individuals with large, rapidly enlarging masses.
- A history of Sjogren's disease is common, and this accompanying diagnosis may predispose to a worse prognosis.
- Evaluation of patients with rapidly enlarging parotid masses includes a thorough history and physical exam followed by imaging with CT and/or MRI of the neck.

- FNA can be considered but is often nondiagnostic, and therefore, an open biopsy or core biopsy is needed. This should be sent as a fresh sample (in saline, not in formalin) and sent for lymphoma protocol.
- If an incisional biopsy is performed, it should be in an area that minimizes the risk to the facial nerve and also where the entire surgical tract could be resected if definitive mass removal is found to be needed.

CASE 60

Michael G. Moore

History of Present Illness

An 82-year-old male presents to your office with a chief complaint of a left-sided cheek mass.

Question: What additional questions would you like to ask?

- How long has it been there? It has been there for 2 months and is slowly enlarging.
- Is it painful? Important to know as pain may suggest the presence of malignancy or infection. He states it is causing him a little pain.
- Does he have any history of facial weakness or twitching? Important to ask this. He denies any facial weakness or twitching and states he has no other lumps in his head and neck.
- Any history of skin cancers? He has a history of numerous cutaneous malignancies (primarily small squamous cell carcinomas) that have been removed by dermatology. Most recently, he had a Merkel cell carcinoma removed with clear margins from his left preauricular region. At that time, no sentinel lymph node biopsy was performed.

Past Medical History/Past Surgical History

He has a history of chronic obstructive pulmonary disease (COPD), chronic renal insufficiency related to poorly controlled hypertension, renal transplant in 2008, coronary artery disease with prior ischemic cardiomyopathy, s/p cardiac transplant in 2012.

Current Medications

Prednisone, tacrolimus, albuterol, aspirin, furosemide, metoprolol, ipratropium inhaler.

   Allergy to penicillin.

Review of Systems

He admits to some dyspnea with walking two blocks but is ambulatory, mild baseline dysphagia, multiple areas of superficial skin changes. Current renal and cardiac function are satisfactory. Otherwise is noncontributory.

Family Medical History

Noncontributory.

Social History

He is a former smoker but not a current smoker.
   He is married and denies any significant alcohol abuse.

Physical Examination

Alert, elderly male in no acute distress.

Skin: diffuse actinic changes. No obvious active malignant lesion on the skin of the head and neck. He has a well-healed scar in the left preauricular region.

Ears: external ears, external auditory canals, and tympanic membranes are within normal limits.

Nose: anterior rhinoscopy is normal.

Oral cavity/oropharynx: no lesions.

Neck: has a firm, mobile mass in the tail of the left parotid that is slightly tender to palpation. No other obvious pathologic lymphadenopathy.

Cranial nerve exam is intact bilaterally, including all branches of the facial nerve.

Question: Based on the above findings, what would be your next step in the diagnostic workup?

Answer: Given this patient's medical and surgical history, he is at high risk for regional recurrence of his Merkel cell carcinoma or another previously removed cutaneous cancer. Patients with prior solid organ transplants are at particular risk due to the chronic immunosuppression. This would be most appropriately assessed through an ultrasound-guided FNA.

Question: His FNA suggests carcinoma with neuroendocrine features. What would be your next course of action?

Answer: This appears to be a regional recurrence of the patient's Merkel cell cancer. It is important to note that the standard of care at the time of the original primary tumor resection would have been to include a sentinel lymph node biopsy. This would have likely identified this disease prior to the development of a macroscopic metastasis. Regardless, given the patient's current presentation, prior to determining the appropriate treatment plan, his staging should be completed. A PET/CT would be a reasonable next step, along with presentation at a multidisciplinary tumor board. Given the patient's challenging disease course as well as his underlying health status, careful consideration must be given to the goals of care, the treatment options that exist, and what the relative rates of disease control and treatment-related morbidity are with these choices.

   Figure 60.1 shows images from the patient's CT and fused PET/CT scan, respectively.

Question: After multidisciplinary tumor board discussion, thorough medical evaluation, and a lengthy discussion with the patient about options for therapy, the patient underwent a left-sided subtotal parotidectomy and level I–V selective neck dissection with a resection of a small amount of overlying neck skin. Final

(Continued)

CASE 60 (continued)

(a)

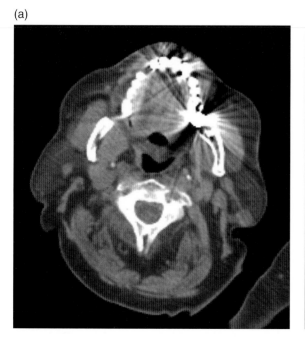

(b)

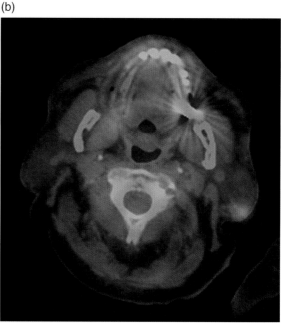

FIGURE 60.1 (a) The noncontrasted axial CT image shows a small lesion in the superficial left parotid gland with apparent extension to the overlying skin. No other obvious pathologic lymphadenopathy was seen. (b) This axial fused PET/CT image demonstrates hypermetabolism of this lesion. Of note, there was no evidence of other regional or distant disease seen on the whole-body scan.

pathology demonstrated a 2 cm focus of metastatic Merkel cell carcinoma to the left parotid gland with extracapsular spread. Margins were clear, and there were no other positive nodes in the parotid or neck dissection specimen. Postoperatively, the patient was noted to have weakness of the lower lip depressor muscles on the left side. Intraoperatively, the patient was noted to have an anatomically intact nerve. What would be the most appropriate course of action for this patient?

Answer: Given the fact that the nerve appeared anatomically intact, the decreased function likely represents nerve paresis. As a result, with time, some or all of the nerve function should recover. This can occur over the course of a few weeks to months for mild injury, or it can take from 12 to 18 months for more severe insults. In this patient, he underwent a parotidectomy and neck dissection. When parotidectomy is combined with a level I/perifacial nodal dissection, paresis of the marginal mandibular nerve is common, even when the nerve is left anatomically intact.

Key Points

- All adult patients with parotid masses should be asked about a history of skin cancers of head and neck.
- Patients with a history of immune suppression following prior solid organ transplant and/or lymphoma treatment are at increased risk for cutaneous malignancies.
- FNA, with or without ultrasound guidance, is the preferred method for obtaining a tissue diagnosis.
- If confirmed to be a regional recurrence of cutaneous cancer or a stage III or IV salivary cancer, further imaging with either PET/CT or a neck and chest CT is indicated to complete staging.
- Management of regionally metastatic cutaneous cancer typically involves surgery with adjuvant therapy.

- For patients with evidence of parotid gland metastases and no other involved cervical nodes, it is recommended to also perform a level II–IV neck dissection as a part of the surgery to address potential subclinical disease. For patients with facial skin or scalp skin primaries anterior to the external auditory canal, dissection of level Ib and the perifacial nodes should be considered. For scalp primaries posterior to the coronal plane of the external auditory canal, the suboccipital nodes also should be included.
- For patients with evidence of additional cervical node involvement, and in parotid cancers that are cN+, a level I–V neck dissection should be performed.

Multiple Choice Questions

1. Which of the following would be an appropriate candidate for extracapsular dissection of a parotid tumor?

   a. A 2 cm high-grade mucoepidermoid cancer of the midparotid gland.

   b. A 4 cm pleomorphic adenoma of the deep lobe of the parotid gland.

   c. A 3 cm Warthins tumor of the inferior aspect of the parotid tail.

   d. None of the above.

   Answer: c. Extracapsular dissection can be beneficial for select benign/low-grade tumors that are in favorable locations such as the parotid tail. The effectiveness of this approach is greatly dependent on patient selection and surgeon experience. It is not recommended for high-grade malignancies as it may compromise the margin of resection and also does not address the intraparotid lymphatics.

2. A 45 year-old male patient develops Frey syndrome following excision of a left parotid pleomorphic adenoma. Which of the following may have placed the patient at higher risk for this complication?

   a. The use of a facelift approach.

   b. Performance of a superficial parotidectomy.

   c. Placement of an abdominal fat graft for reconstruction after tumor excision.

   d. Performance of extracapsular dissection.

   Answer: b. Frey syndrome results from postganglionic parasympathetic fibers re-innervating to the sweat glands in the overlying skin, resulting in gustatory sweating. As a result, increasing the amount of cut surface of the parotid tissue will place a patient at higher risk. Extracapsular dissection and the use of parotid bed reconstruction as a barrier can help reduce the rate of this complication.

3. For a patient undergoing resection of a T2N0M0 submandibular gland adenoid cystic carcinoma, all of the following risks of surgery should be discussed except:

   a. Lower lip numbness.

   b. Asymmetry to the smile.

   c. Tongue numbness.

   d. Dysarthria.

   Answer: a. Lip numbness would result from resection of the mental or inferior alveolar nerve and would not be expected from this surgery. Injury or need to resect the lingual, hypoglossal, or marginal mandibular branch of the facial nerve should all be discussed.

4. Which of the following salivary tumors are not found in the submandibular gland?

   a. Pleomorphic adenomas.

   b. Acinic cell carcinomas.

   c. Salivary duct carcinoma.

   d. Warthins tumors.

   Answer: d. Warthins tumor.

5. What is the most common type of salivary cancer?

   a. Adenoid cystic carcinoma.

   b. Ex-pleomorphic carcinoma.

   c. Mucoepidermoid carcinoma.

   d. Acinic cell carcinoma.

   Answer: c. Mucoepidermoid carcinoma is the most common parotid cancer, while adenoid cystic carcinoma is the most common in the submandibular gland, sublingual gland, and minor salivary glands. Due to the larger parenchyma of the parotid gland and thus the higher frequency of parotid cancers relative to the other glands, mucoepidermoid cancer is the most common salivary cancer overall.

6. Which of the following patients would be a good candidate for facial nerve preservation at the time of surgery?

   a. Patient with a 3 cm ex-pleomorphic carcinoma of the superficial lobe of the parotid gland with normal facial nerve function.

   b. A 5 cm high-grade mucoepidermoid carcinoma extending from the deep lobe of the parotid gland to the overlying skin in a patient with normal facial nerve function and left cheek pain.

   c. A 2 cm superficial lobe parotid adenoid cystic carcinoma with 6 months of complete facial paralysis.

   d. A 4 cm regional recurrence of cutaneous squamous cell carcinoma with 4 weeks of progressive weakness of the upper and lower face.

   Answer: a. In patients with normal facial nerve function preoperatively, the goal of the operation should be to preserve the facial nerve unless it is encased or grossly involved with high-grade cancer. Preoperative pain, tumor extension involving both the deep and superficial lobes, and pre-existing facial weakness all predict the need for facial nerve resection.

7. Which of the following is not typically seen in the prestyloid parapharyngeal space?

   a. Lipoma.

   b. Vagal nerve schwannoma.

   c. Pleomorphic adenoma.

   d. Lymphoma.

   Answer: b. The parapharyngeal space is divided into the prestyloid from the post-styloid space by the stylopharyngeal fascia. The contents of the prestyloid parapharyngeal space include fat, minor salivary rests, extension of the deep lobe of the parotid gland, and, occasionally, lymph nodes. As a result, neoplasms of these tissues of origin are most common in this space. The post-styloid parapharyngeal space contains neurovascular structures and, as a result, tumors such as nerve sheath tumors and paragangliomas are most common in this location.

8. Which of the following techniques may prove helpful in removing a 4 cm parapharyngeal space pleomorphic adenoma?

   a. Transnasal intubation.

   b. Combined transmastoid and transcervical facial nerve transposition.

   c. Enucleation.

   d. Preoperative embolization.

   Answer: a. When performing a transcervical approach to the parapharyngeal space, it is important to optimize exposure through upward retraction of the mandible. Transnasal intubation assists with this as it avoids having the endotracheal tube between the teeth or gums. Additional maneuvers that can be helpful include careful outfracture of the styloid tip to avoid puncture of the tumor during dissection, removal of the submandibular gland (for large tumors), and division of the stylomandibular ligament. Transmastoid mobilization of the main trunk of the facial nerve would not be necessary for this tumor and would place the facial nerve at unnecessary risk. Enucleation, or intracapsular dissection, has fallen out of favor for pleomorphic adenomas due to the unacceptable recurrence rates associated with this technique. Preoperative embolization may be helpful for certain vascular lesions such as large upper neck paragangliomas, but it would not be needed for a salivary tumor.

9. A 52-year-old female patient presents to your office for discussion of management options of an incidentally found lesion in her right parapharyngeal space (see figure). FNA of the lesion is consistent with a pleomorphic adenoma. After discussion of management options, the patient elects to pursue surgical excision. What would be the most appropriate approach to surgery?

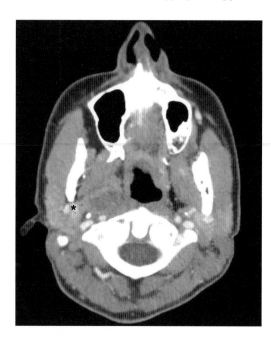

a. Transcervical resection with finger dissection of the mass.
b. Transmandibular.
c. Transoral.
d. Transcervical/transparotid.

Answer: d. In this patient, the lesion has a lateral extension that abuts the retromandibular vein (*). While parapharyngeal space tumors that develop from salivary rests of tissue are often removed successfully with finger/blunt dissection, this mass appears to have a broader source of origin in the deep lobe of the right parotid gland. The most superficial aspect of the mass is at the level of the retromandibular vein, which likely means that the tumor is closely associated with the facial nerve. As a result, blunt dissection without formal identification of the

facial nerve would not only risk nerve injury but also could lead to tumor fragmentation and spillage.

10. A patient presents for evaluation of dry mouth. Which of the following would *not* be the most suggestive of the diagnosis of Sjogren disease?

a. A positive blood rheumatoid factor.
b. A lower lip minor salivary gland biopsy showing lymphocytic infiltrate.
c. A positive serum angiotensin-converting enzyme (**ACE**) level.
d. An elevated SSA/Ro and SSB/La titer.

Answer: c. Sjogren disease is an autoimmune condition characterized by dry mouth and dry eyes, with potential injury also being seen in the skin, other mucous membranes, and even organs such as the liver, pancreas, and kidneys. Diagnosis is typically made with blood serologies (such as elevated SSA/SSB, RF, and ANA). Biopsy of the lower lip minor salivary tissue showing high densities of lymphocytic infiltrates around salivary tissue. Elevated ACE levels are seen in patients with sarcoid disease.

11. A 70-year-old patient presents with evidence of a left parotid recurrence from a left cheek cutaneous squamous cell carcinoma. Exam shows a mobile 3 cm left parotid mass with normal facial nerve function. PET/CT shows a 3 cm superficial parotid lobe mass that is a hypermetabolic mass along with a similar 2 cm mass in left level II of the neck. No evidence of distant metastatic disease. Multidisciplinary tumor board discussion yields a recommendation of up-front surgical management with adjuvant therapy to be dictated by pathologic findings. What would be the most appropriate surgical management of this patient?

a. A left partial superficial parotidectomy to remove the parotid mass and a left level II–III selective neck dissection.
b. A left subtotal parotidectomy with a left level I–V modified radical neck dissection.
c. A left radical parotidectomy with facial nerve sacrifice and left radical neck dissection levels I–V.
d. Patient should be managed with nonsurgical therapy.

Answer: b. In this patient with regional metastases in the left parotid and neck, it is necessary to not only remove the gross disease but also the adjacent at-risk parotid and cervical lymphatics. As a result, a subtotal parotidectomy and a comprehensive neck dissection is needed. Given that the patient has normal preoperative facial nerve function, facial nerve resection would not be appropriate. Of note, in instances where there is evidence of nodal metastatic disease in the neck, the risk of microscopic disease within level V has been shown to be 40% or higher. As a result, a comprehensive level I–V neck dissection would be recommended here.

12. A 53-year-old male patient presents with a painful right parotid mass. The mass is mobile and around 2 cm in size in the superficial lobe of the gland. Facial nerve function is normal. FNA is consistent with salivary duct carcinoma, and imaging shows the primary tumor with no evidence of regional or distant disease. What would be the appropriate surgical management of this patient?

a. A right partial superficial parotidectomy.

b. A right subtotal parotidectomy with right level II–IV selective neck dissection.

c. A right subtotal parotidectomy with right level I–V modified radical neck dissection.

d. A right radical parotidectomy with right level I–V modified radical neck dissection.

Answer: b. In this patient with a high-grade parotid cancer, there is no evidence of regional metastatic disease. Due to the high risk of occult metastasis, it is recommended to remove the lymph nodes within the parotid (using a subtotal or total parotidectomy) as well as the most at-risk nodes in the neck through a level II–IV selective neck dissection. It has been shown that in patients with cN+ disease, there is a high risk of disease in level V, so in these patients a comprehensive neck dissection is recommended. Again, for patients with preoperative normal facial nerve function, facial nerve resection is only recommended if the nerve is found to be encased or grossly involved by tumor.

Suggested Reading

Ali, S., Palmer, F.L., DiLorenzo, M. et al. (2014). Treatment of the neck in carcinoma of the parotid gland. *Ann. Surg. Oncol.* 21 (9): 3042–3048.

Andreasen, S. et al. (2016). Pleomorphic adenoma of the parotid gland 1985–2010: a Danish nationwide study of incidence, recurrence rate, and malignant transformation. *Head Neck* 38 (Suppl 1): E1364–E1369.

Barnes, L., Myers, E., and Prolopakis, E. (1998). Primary malignant lymphoma of the parotid gland. *Arch. Otolaryngol. Head Neck Surg.* 124: 573–577.

Deschler, D.G. and Eisele, D.W. (2016). Surgery for primary malignant parotid neoplasms. *Adv. Otorhinolaryngol.* 78: 83–94.

Fasolis, M., Zavattero, E., Iaquinta, C., and Berrone, S. (2013). Dermofat graft after superficial parotidectomy to prevent Frey syndrome and depressed deformity. *J. Craniofac. Surg.* 24: 1260–1262.

Herman, M.P., Werning, J.W., Morris, C.G. et al. (2013). Elective neck management for high-grade salivary gland carcinoma. *Am. J. Otolaryngol.* 34 (3): 205–208.

Hirshoren, N., Ruskin, O., McDowell, L.J. et al. (2018). Management of parotid metastatic cutaneous squamous cell carcinoma: regional recurrence rates and survival. *Otolaryngol. Head Neck Surg.* 159 (2): 293–299.

Kato, H. et al. (2014). Salivary gland tumors of the parotid gland: CT and MR imaging findings with emphasis on intratumoral cystic components. *Neuroradiology* 56 (9): 789–795.

Kokemeuller, H., Eckardt, A., Bachvogel, P., and Hausamen, J.-E. (2004). Adenoid cystic carcinoma of the head and neck – a 20 year experience. *Int. J. Oral Maxillofac. Surg.* 33 (1): 25–31.

Lewis, A.G., Tong, T., and Maghami, E. (2016). Diagnosis and management of malignant salivary gland tumors of the parotid gland. *Otolaryngol. Clin. North Am.* 49: 343–380.

Lim, C.M., Gilbert, M., Johnson, J.T. et al. (2015). Is level V neck dissection necessary in primary parotid cancer? *Laryngoscope* 125 (1): 118–121.

Liu, Y., Li, J., Tan, Y. et al. (2015). Accuracy of diagnosis of salivary gland tumors with the use of ultrasonography, computed tomography, and magnetic resonance imaging: a meta-analysis. *Oral Surg. Oral Med. Oral Pathol. Oral Radiol.* 119 (2): 238–245. e2.

Liu, C.C., Jethwa, A.R., Khariwala, S.S. et al. (2016). Sensitivity, specificity, and posttest probability of parotid fine-needle aspiration: a systematic review and meta-analysis. *Otolaryngol. Head Neck Surg.* 154 (1): 9–23.

Mehta, V. and Nathan, C.A. (2015). Extracapsular dissection versus superficial parotidectomy for benign parotid tumors. *Laryngoscope* 125: 1039–1040.

Mydlarz, W.K. and Agrawal, N. (2014). Transparotid and transcervical approaches for removal of deep lobe parotid gland and parapharyngeal space. *Oper. Tech. Otolaryngol. Head Neck Surg.* 25 (3): 234–239.

Nishishinya, M.B., Pereda, C.A., Munox-Fernandez, S. et al. (2015). Identification of lymphoma predictors in patients with primary Sjogren's syndrome: a systematic literature review and meta-analysis. *Rheumatol. Int.* 35 (1): 17–26.

Ruoboalho, J., Mäkitie, A.A., Aro, K. et al. (2017). Complications after surgery for benign parotid gland neoplasms: a prospective cohort study. *Head Neck* 39 (1): 170–176.

Sheahan, P. (2014). Transcervical approach for removal of benign parapharyngeal space tumors. *Oper. Tech. Otolaryngol. Head Neck Surg.* 25 (3): 227–233.

Shum, J.W., Emmerling, M., Lubek, J.E., and Ord, R.A. (2014). Parotid lymphoma: a review of clinical presentation and management. *Oral Surg. Oral Med. Oral Pathol. Oral Radiol.* 118 (1): 1–5.

Tanvetyanon, T., Qin, D., Padhya, T. et al. (2009). Outcomes of postoperative concurrent chemoradiotherapy for locally advanced major salivary gland carcinoma. *Arch. Otolaryngol. Head Neck Surg.* 135: 687–692.

Xiao, C.C., Zhan, K.Y., White-Gilbertson, S.J. et al. (2016). Predictors of nodal metastasis in parotid malignancies: a National Cancer Database study of 22,653 patients. *Otolaryngol. Head Neck Surg.* 154 (1): 121–130.

Yoo, S.H., Roh, J.L., Kim, S.O. et al. (2015). Patterns and treatment of neck metastases in patients with salivary gland cancers. *J. Surg. Oncol.* 111 (8): 1000–1006: https://doi.org/10.1002/jso.23914.

Zeng, X.T., Tang, X.J., Wang, X.J. et al. (2012). AlloDerm implants for prevention of Frey syndrome after parotidectomy: a systematic review and meta-analysis. *Mol. Med. Rep.* 5 (4): 974–980.

SECTION 14

Reconstruction

Rizwan Aslam

CASE 61

Avinash Mantravadi

History of Present Illness

A 52-year-old female presents with a painful oral lesion. She states that she first noted irritation in the region of the left gingivobuccal sulcus 3 months ago. Over time, this has become increasingly painful, and she recently noted loosening of several teeth in this area. She has been taking primarily liquids by mouth due to the pain and has lost approximately 20 pounds unintentionally over this period of time. She also noticed tightening of the skin under her chin in recent weeks.

She denies numbness of the lip or chin, respiratory difficulty, or voice changes.

She recently underwent a biopsy in the office on initial evaluation with one of your colleagues, which returned positive for moderately differentiated squamous cell carcinoma (SCC). Metastatic workup was negative for distant disease. She is scheduled for upfront surgical management and has been referred to you to discuss reconstructive options.

She has no medical problems and takes no medications on a daily basis. She has a history of right rotator cuff surgery and has had limitation of range of motion and strength since that time. She denies any history of trauma to the lower extremities. She is left-hand dominant.

Review of systems is otherwise negative.

Physical Examination

The patient is emaciated but awake and alert and in no acute distress.

Nasal cavity and microscopic ear examinations are normal.

Oral cavity examination demonstrates a 7 × 5 cm ulcerative lesion that appears epicentered in the left gingivobuccal sulcus. The tumor involves the left buccal space and extends medially across the entire floor of mouth and ventral tongue,

the oral vestibule, and mandibular alveolar ridge to the right retromolar trigone. The lesion is adherent to the mandible and deeply invasive through the anterior floor of mouth. There is direct extension of tumor inferiorly to the submental and chin skin. The lower lip is preserved.

Cranial nerves II–XII are intact and symmetric bilaterally.

She has no evidence of prior scars of the upper and lower extremities.

Question: What would be appropriate next steps in the evaluation of this patient?

- Computed tomography (CT) of the neck with IV contrast: **yes**/no. This would be an excellent next step. This will help evaluate the extent of the primary lesion and look for metastatic lymphadenopathy. CT also provides a good assessment of the underlying mandible.

  Representative CT imaging is demonstrated in Figure 61.1.

- Positron emission tomography PET/CT: **yes**/no. This would be appropriate to complete staging in this patient with evidence of stage IV disease.
- Ultrasound of the neck: yes/**no**. While this could be helpful in evaluating for cervical lymphadenopathy and to assist with biopsies, it would add little here since a tissue diagnosis has already been obtained. Ultrasound is also not able to provide accurate assessment of bone erosion.

Question: Based on the initial physical examination and imaging findings, which of the following reconstructive options would be most appropriate to discuss with the patient for the anticipated defect?

- Reconstruction bar with anterolateral thigh free-flap soft-tissue coverage: yes/**no**.
- Fibula osteocutaneous flap: yes/**no**.

(Continued)

Essential Cases in Head and Neck Oncology, First Edition. Edited by Michael G. Moore, Arnaud F. Bewley, and Babak Givi.
© 2022 American Head and Neck Society. Published 2022 by John Wiley & Sons Ltd.

CASE 61 (continued)

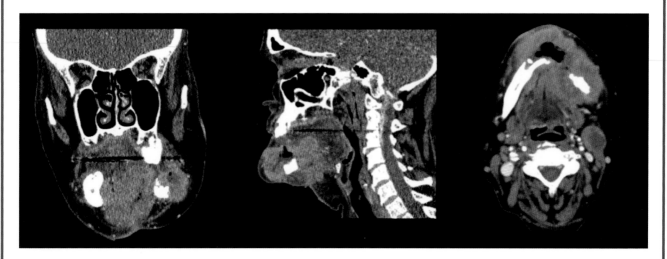

FIGURE 61.1 Contrasted CT imaging with representative coronal, sagittal, and axial slices. There appears to be evidence of cortical erosion of the left mandible with extension across the midline. There also appears to be pathologic lymphadenopathy in the left neck.

- Scapula/latissimus osteocutaneous flap: **yes**/no
- Radial forearm osteocutaneous free flap: yes/**no**

The patient has very locally advanced disease that will result in a defect involving multiple subsites and surfaces. Based on the physical examination and imaging, the resection will include the buccal mucosa, oral vestibule, entire floor of mouth and ventral tongue, alveolar ridge, and through-and-through resection of the chin and submental skin, as well as the mandible from approximately the left ramus to the right midbody. In an emaciated and malnourished patient, the skin paddle associated with fibula and radial forearm free flaps is suboptimal as this will not be adequate to reconstruct all soft-tissue subsites. The iliac crest has substantial donor site morbidity including pain and decreased mobility in the postoperative period. In this patient with pre-existing morbidity involving the right shoulder from prior rotator cuff surgery, the right scapula/latissimus combined flap provides adequate bone and soft tissue to reconstruct all subsites while using a donor site with pre-existing limitations that the patient has already grown accustomed to.

To assess all options for reconstruction, a lower extremity CT angiogram is obtained, which demonstrates one-vessel runoff to the foot bilaterally. The patient is taken to the operating room for a composite resection of the mandible, floor of mouth, ventral tongue, buccal space, chin and submental skin, as well as tracheostomy and bilateral modified radical neck dissections.

Question: Which method would you use to maintain preoperative mandibular anatomic position and dental occlusion during tumor resection and reconstruction? (Choose all that apply.)

- Exposure of the mandible and preplating prior to mandibular resection: yes/**no**
- Application of external fixator device prior to mandibular resection and plate bending to an appropriate mandibular shape: **yes**/no
- Free hand plating across defect after mandibular resection: yes/**no**
- Three-dimensional virtual surgical planning with design and use of custom cutting guides and custom mandibular reconstruction plate: yes/**no**

Based on preoperative imaging and clinical characteristics, exposure of the mandible and preplating cannot be accomplished without violation of tumor with associated risks of tumor spillage. After mandibular resection is completed with associated loss of pterygoid attachments on the left-hand side, free-hand plate bending risks inaccurate positioning of the condyle in the glenoid fossa, which can result in altered mouth opening or closing postoperatively. Three-dimensional surgical planning and the design of a custom plate may be considered; however, given the far advanced nature of the patient's disease, it is unclear of the exact location of planned mandibular cuts. In addition, a long segment of bone is likely required, such that the placement of a custom plate may result in a gap too far to span with existing bone stock from the planned donor site of bone harvest. Application of an external fixator device prior to tumor resection will preserve premorbid occlusion and anatomic position in space while preserving the option to design a reconstruction bar that is appropriate for a new mandibular projection and allows for the available bone stock to span the length of the bar.

At the conclusion of tumor resection, the defect is as noted in Figure 61.2.

CASE 61   (continued)

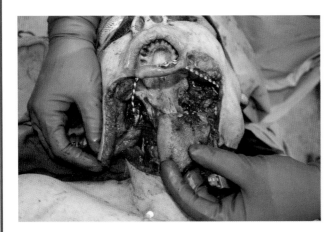

FIGURE 61.2   **This is an intraoperative photo of the composite bone, soft tissue, and skin defect after resection of far-locally advanced oral cavity SCC.**

Question: Approximately 15 cm of bone will be required for mandibular reconstruction. What is the optimal flap design for reconstruction of this defect?

- Latissimus dorsi/serratus-rib flap based on thoracodorsal artery and vein: yes/**no**
- Scapular/parascapular osteocutaneous flap based on circumflex scapular artery and vein: yes/**no**
- Latissimus dorsi/scapular tip flap based on thoracodorsal artery and vein: yes/**no**
- Combined scapular/parascapular osteocutaneous and latissimus dorsi/scapular tip flaps ("megaflap") based on subscapular artery and vein: **yes**/no

Based on the defect, the patient requires reconstruction of soft-tissue defects to include the buccal space, floor of mouth, oral vestibule, and chin/submental skin. An extended length of bone is required for mandibular reconstruction. There is inadequate length of rib available for reconstruction of this defect based on the serratus branch of the thoracodorsal artery. The skin paddles of the scapular/parascapular osteocutaneous flap will likely be adequate for intraoral reconstruction; however, they will likely be inadequate for reconstruction of the external soft-tissue defect. In addition, the lateral border of the scapula based on the circumflex scapular artery and vein alone can provide 10–14 cm of bone, depending on the patient's anatomy. As a result, the lateral border alone based on the circumflex scapular artery and vein is unlikely to be adequate or reliable at its distal extent. The scapular tip alone based on the thoracodorsal artery and vein will not provide enough length for reconstruction of this mandibular defect. The combined scapular/parascapular osteocutaneous and latissimus dorsi/scapular tip flap ("megaflap") will provide adequate soft tissue for reconstruction of all soft-tissue defects as well as reliable vascularized bone length adequate to span

this defect. This will require dissection and preservation of the angular branch of the thoracodorsal artery as well as dissection of all pedicles up to the subscapular artery and vein to its takeoff from the axillary vessels. It is possible, that even this amount of bone may not provide a complete replacement of the length of resected bone. In these instances, the patient's projection may need to be brought back slightly and/or a small gap may need to be left on the posterolateral aspect of the repair. In such instances, it is critical to use a load-bearing plate to avoid hardware failure.

A composite scapular/parascapular osteocutaneous and latissimus dorsi/scapular tip flap is harvested with all skin paddles and bone segments demonstrating signs of healthy perfusion at the conclusion of flap elevation. The subscapular artery and vein are anastomosed to the left facial artery and vein in the standard fashion uneventfully. The scapular and parascapular skin paddles are inset into the oral mucosal defect, and the latissimus skin paddle will be used for submental and chin skin coverage.

Question: During flap inset, it is noted that the scapular and parascapular skin paddles are not adequately perfused. However, the scapula bone and latissimus are healthy and well perfused, with bright red bleeding. The arterial and venous pedicles are examined and remain patent with no evidence of thrombosis or spasm. What is the next best step in management?

- Check to ensure that there is no compression or twisting of the circumflex scapular artery branches to the skin: **yes**/no

In a composite free flap with multiple skin paddles and bone segments, perfusion may be compromised by a number of factors. After establishing that the primary anastomoses are patent, it is important to confirm if all components of the flap are compromised, which would indicate a circulatory issue at the level of the primary anastomoses, including thrombosis or spasm. If some components are well perfused while others are not, it is then critical to evaluate the vascular supply to the compromised components. The cutaneous branches of the circumflex scapular artery may be compressed and twisted after bone is plated and the pedicle is delivered to the neck, which may decrease perfusion to the skin. The best initial step is to ensure that there is no obstruction, compression, or twisting of the branches supplying the skin. This is a simple maneuver and can be performed visually without any additional equipment.

- Intraoperative fluorescence angiography to assess flap perfusion: yes/**no**

After confirmation is obtained that there is no external compression of the skin paddle vessels, fluorescence angiography may be performed to better delineate the nature of the issue. However, this should not be used as an initial step in interrogating the flap.

(*Continued*)

CASE 61 (continued)

- Administration of IV heparin: yes/**no**
- Administration of tissue-plasminogen activator (tPA): yes/**no**

As both arterial and venous anastomoses are established to be patent with no evidence of thrombosis, there is no role for systemic administration of heparin or tissue plasminogen activator.

The flap is explored and there is no external compression or twisting of the circumflex scapular artery branches to the skin paddles. Intraoperative fluorescence angiography is performed, which demonstrates patent arterial and venous anastomoses and excellent perfusion of the latissimus skin paddle and lateral border/scapula tip bone segments. However, poor perfusion of the skin of the scapular/parascapular skin paddles is noted. After an extended period of waiting, the condition does not improve.

Question: What is the next best step in management?

- Removal of scapular skin paddles and harvest of a second fasciocutaneous or myocutaneous free flap with microvascular anastomosis: **yes**/no

In reconstructing this defect, the intraoral closure is most critical at sealing off the oral cavity and saliva from the soft tissues of the neck. Use of a compromised flap for the most important aspect of the closure is not appropriate and will inevitably lead to flap loss, dehiscence, fistula formation, and salivary contamination of the neck with possible compromise of the remaining healthy components of the flap. It has been confirmed that there are no concerns for thrombosis or spasm at the main pedi-

cle and that the latissimus and bone segments are well perfused with no signs of compromise. Therefore, these components of the flap can be retained and used as originally planned. The poor perfusion to the scapular skin paddles may be caused by a number of other factors including microcirculatory spasm, hypothermia, or unreliability in the patient's microvascular anatomy.

- Removal of all skin paddles and bone segments and harvest of a second contralateral scapula/latissimus combined flap: yes/**no**

In selecting a second flap after partial or total failure of scapular system free flap, the contralateral scapula should be avoided as there is typically not enough remaining soft-tissue laxity to achieve primary closure. Radial forearm or anterolateral thigh free flaps are better options.

- Continued use and inset of the existing skin paddles as originally planned: yes/**no**
- Placement of packing with plans to return to the operating room the following day: yes/**no**

While packing and staging the reconstruction can be considered in instances of patient instability or extreme fatigue of the surgical team, it is best avoided unless absolutely necessary. Flap revision is best accomplished as soon as possible in order to minimize contamination of the wound, which may result in failure of additional reconstructive efforts. Can be considered in the setting of patient instability of fatigue of the surgical team; however, flap revision or salvage reconstruction is best accomplished as early as possible.

Key Points

- For segmental mandibulectomy defects extending across the midline, reconstruction with an osseous free flap is recommended to avoid plate extrusion and contraction of the anterior soft-tissue envelope.
- Selection of the ideal bone donor site is determined by a number of factors such as the length of bone required, the

number and location of epithelial surfaces that need to be repaired, the volume and location of the soft-tissue defect, and patient factors (availability of adjacent recipient vessels, peripheral vascular disease, need to avoid certain donor sites because of occupation, hobbies, or other reasons).
- The subscapular system offers a wide variety of options for osseous and soft-tissue reconstruction.

CASE 62

Rizwan Aslam and Yash Patil

History of Present Illness

A 70-year-old male with a one-pack-per-day smoking history and a history of significant alcohol consumption presents to the clinic for evaluation of an upper lip lesion. His past medical history is otherwise noncontributory. On physical examination there is an ulcerative process that appears fixed to the anterior maxilla. CT scan is performed

and demonstrates cortical erosion involving the premaxilla and hard palate. The patient's maxillary sinuses, periorbital area, and nasal vault are uninvolved. The planned resection of the anterior hard palate including the upper lip is shown in Figure 62.1.

Question: What is the optimal option for reconstruction (assuming a composite resection is completed)?

- Local rotational lip repair: yes/**no**

CASE 62   (continued)

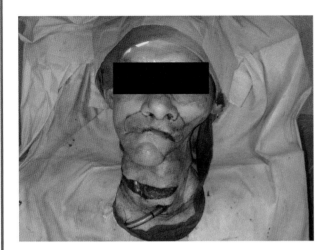

FIGURE 62.1 This intraoperative photo shows the proposed outline of the soft-tissue resection. The patient's premaxilla was involved as well and required resection.

Given involvement of the premaxilla, reconstruction will require both bone and soft tissue. A local rotation lip flap would therefore be inadequate.

- Soft-tissue free flap: yes/**no**

As above.

- Obturator: yes/**no**

Obturation works well for dentate patients with posterior and lateral defects of the maxilla and hard palate.

- Composite free flap: **yes**/no

For defects involving the maxilla with significant bone and soft-tissue loss, composite free flaps are the optimal choice for reconstruction. While local lip repairs can be used for less extensive lip defects, in this instance, when combining a subtotal upper lip repair with reconstruction of the anterior hard palate, use of a bone-containing free flap is the best option.

Question: Which of these are appropriate free-flap reconstructive options for this defect?

- Osteocutaneous radial forearm: **yes**/no
- Iliac crest: **yes**/no
- Fibula free flap: **yes**/no
- Scapula: **yes**/no

The flaps listed are all composite free flaps. While the osteocutaneous radial forearm free flap (OCRFFF) provides the best option with regards to soft-tissue pliability for lip repair, dental restoration is limited due to the reduced bone stock provided.

Following tumor ablation, it appears you will need a segment of bone with two osteotomies and adequate soft tissue to replace the entire upper lip. You select an OCRFFF as depicted in the images below (Figure 62.2a and b).

Question: You see the patient back in the office for his first postoperative visit and he is doing well. In counseling him about potential long-term complications of midface reconstruction, what would be important recipient site complications to mention?

- Oronasal fistula: **yes**/no

Oronasal fistula is a common complication in patients who undergo midface reconstruction with OCRFFFs. In a

(a)

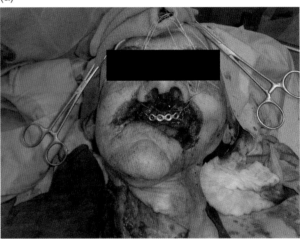

(b)

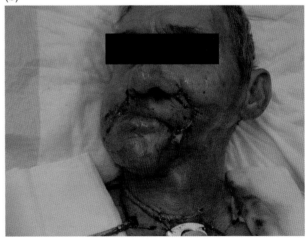

FIGURE 62.2 This intraoperative photo (a) demonstrates the use of a load-bearing plate to secure the radial bone. Following microvascular anastomosis, the skin paddle is used to reconstruct the inner and outer lining of the total upper lip defect (b).

(Continued)

CASE 62 (continued)

series of 24 patients who underwent midface reconstruction, 12% of developed this complication.

- Dystopia: yes/**no**
- Severe ectropion: yes/**no**

Severe ectropion and dystopia are also common complications occurring in 24% and 8% of patients; however, this patient would not be at risk for these complications as the defect did not involve the orbit.

Key Points

- For total or near-total lip defects, free-flap reconstruction often yields the best results.
- When performing midface reconstruction, factors to consider include the components of the defect (lining, soft-tissue deficit, and bone deficit), whether or not there is adequate remaining dentition to retain an obturator, whether or not the anterior or lateral projecting element needs to be repaired, and if the orbital floor support has been lost.
- Maintenance of the ipsilateral canine tooth is important to adequately retain a maxillary obturator postoperatively.
- Radial forearm osteocutaneous free flaps are ideal for premaxillary reconstruction.
- Larger-volume composite defects of the midface are effectively reconstructed with iliac crest free flaps or flaps from the subscapular system.
- In all cases of midface reconstruction using free flaps, it is critical to ensure adequate pedicle length is present to meet the desired recipient vessels in the face or neck.

CASE 63

Chase Heaton

History of Present Illness

A 57-year-old woman with an extensive smoking history is referred to head and neck surgery by her dentist for a painful right lateral tongue lesion. This has been present for 4 months. It was initially thought to be due to rubbing against her molar caps, but it has persisted after having the caps smoothed. An oral surgeon performed an incisional biopsy that showed invasive SCC.

Past Medical History

She has type II diabetes and coronary artery disease and is on a daily 81 mg aspirin.

Physical Examination

Two-centimeter right lateral tongue lesion, slightly exophytic, with leukoplakic changes on the periphery (see Figure 63.1).
There is no floor of mouth or mandible involvement.
Neck examination is normal.
The remainder of the head and neck examination is normal.

Management

A same-day CT scan is performed. Due to dental artifact, the tongue lesion is not visualized. There is no suspicious neck lymphadenopathy.
The case is reviewed at a multidisciplinary head and neck tumor board – recommendation is for partial glossectomy and ipsilateral selective neck dissection.

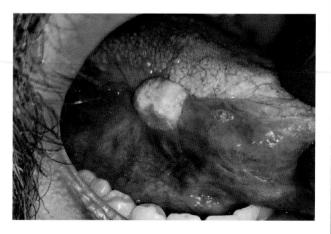

FIGURE 63.1 **This clinical photograph shows the patient's right lateral tongue cancer.**

Your colleague has scheduled the case, and has asked for your help with reconstruction of the tongue. Given the small size of the lesion (cT1), you believe primary closure is adequate.

Question: What are some important considerations when regarding primary closure following partial glossectomy?

- Defects involving up to ~1/3 of the tongue may be closed primarily without affecting speech and swallow function: **yes**/no
- Floor of mouth involvement is a relative contraindication to primary closure as tongue tethering may occur: **yes**.

CASE 63   (continued)

- Preservation of the tongue tip is key to retention of speech quality; loss of the tip in a partial glossectomy is as disruptive to speech as a hemi-glossectomy: **yes**/no
- Significant speech degradation is noted with primary closure as compared to free-flap repair following partial glossectomy: yes/**no**

An ideal tongue reconstruction is a single-stage, low-morbidity procedure that will restore tongue volume and prevent significant tethering to maintain adequate speech and swallowing function. With small cT1-2 tumors that involve less than 1/3 of the tongue volume and do not involve the floor of mouth, primary closure has been shown to have acceptable functional outcomes when compared to free-flap and local flap reconstruction.

The patient does well after surgery with primary closure, and has no functional complaints after healing. Final pathology shows a 1.2 cm primary tumor, margins negative, but extensive perineural invasion (PNI), and 3/23 lymph nodes positive. Radiation is recommended. There is an unfortunate delay in starting radiation due to issues with insurance authorization. Radiation is started 10 weeks after surgery and she completes the full course.

The patient does well until 1.5 years later, when she notes the presence and persistence of an ulcer on her lateral tongue at the site of the primary closure that she thought was from the tongue rubbing against her teeth. A biopsy is performed that shows invasive SCC. Imaging shows an extensive recurrence crossing the tongue midline and invading the floor of mouth musculature (see Figure 63.2). The ablative surgeon recommends a near-total glossectomy with preservation of the contralateral base of tongue.

Question: Which of the following options would be the most appropriate option for reconstruction in this patient?

- Radial forearm free flap: yes/**no**

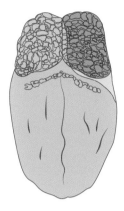

Subtotal Glossectomy

FIGURE 63.2   Depiction of tongue involvement with recurrent cancer.

A radial forearm free flap can provide good replacement of epithelial surface loss but had inadequate bulk for this defect.

- Supraclavicular rotational flap: yes/**no**
- A pectoralis major myocutaneous rotational flap: no. While the pectoralis major and supraclavicular flaps can be used in this repair, they result in significant tethering of the remnant tongue and immobile bulk and an unacceptable speech and swallowing result.
- Anterolateral thigh free flap: **yes**/no
  This patient will have a subtotal glossectomy defect and will need significant replacement of lost tongue bulk to optimize speech and swallowing recovery after surgery. Note that flap harvest should include a significant bulk of subcutaneous fat rather than muscle, as this will result in less flap atrophy over time.

Key Points

- When performing soft-tissue tongue reconstruction (not including a mandibulectomy defect), important considerations include the amount of epithelial surface and bulk loss that is expected, the associated loss of the adjacent floor of mouth mucosa, and the patient's body habitus.
- For glossectomy defects less than 1/3 of the tongue, with minimal associated loss of floor of mouth mucosa, primary closure can provide excellent long-term speech and swallowing results.
- For larger glossectomy defects such as a hemiglossectomy with or without loss of the adjacent floor of mouth, flap repair is often necessary to provide replacement of lost bulk and to avoid tethering of the remnant tongue. Excellent options include radial forearm, ulnar, lateral arm, and submental island flaps, with flap choice often being dictated by the specifics of the defect, the degree of nodal disease, and the patient's body habitus.
- For subtotal or total glossectomy reconstructions, flaps with increased bulk such as the anterolateral thigh or deep inferior epigastric family of flaps should be considered.

CASE 64

Rusha Patel

History of Present Illness

A 55-year-old patient is sent to you for evaluation. He has a history of a T2N0M0 glottic SCC and completed primary radiation therapy 6 months ago. He has recently been having left ear pain and hoarseness. He has been having more difficulty with swallowing and feels that he has lost weight. He also has a history of hypertension, currently controlled on medication. Flexible laryngoscopy was done in clinic and shows a left glottic ulcer with extension to the arytenoid.

Question: What is the next most appropriate step in workup?

- Due to the concern for radiation necrosis, plan for observation with close interval follow-up: yes/**no.**
  Though radiation necrosis of the larynx is possible, the patient history is highly concerning for recurrent cancer and this must be ruled out first.
- Operative endoscopy and biopsy: **yes**/no.
  The patient's symptoms and history warrant an operative endoscopy and biopsy. While radiation necrosis is a possibility, the possibility of recurrent cancer should be ruled out.
  - Videostroboscopy: yes/**no.** There is no role for videostroboscopy in this patient.
  - Referral to speech therapy: yes/**no.** Speech therapy may be appropriate but will not address the ulcer.

The patient undergoes endoscopy and biopsies in the operating room. Pathology returns as SCC. The patient undergoes imaging that does not show any distant disease.

Question: What finding from the patient's endoscopy would be the most important in deciding the extent of pharyngeal reconstruction?

- Involvement of the true and false vocal cords: yes/**no**
- Tumor extension to laryngeal surface of the epiglottis: no.
- Fixation of the left vocal cord: no.

The degree of endolaryngeal involvement has limited implications for the reconstruction following laryngectomy given the en bloc resection of the larynx.

- Tumor extension to the posterior pharynx: **yes**/no
  The degree of remaining pharyngeal mucosa is important in planning reconstruction. Extension of the tumor to the posterior pharynx may necessitate a total laryngopharyngectomy, requiring the use of a 360° tissue reconstruction. Involvement of the true and false cords and extension to the laryngeal surface of the epiglottis do not change the type of reconstruction. While fixation of the vocal cord and associated paraglottic space involvement

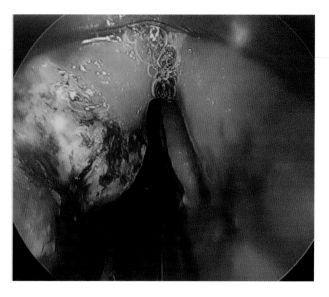

FIGURE 64.1 This intraoperative photo from the patient's microsuspension laryngoscopy shows a left glottic ulcer with extension to the left arytenoid. There was no evidence of significant hypopharyngeal extension.

can reduce the amount of available mucosa for reconstruction, this alone would not necessitate a tubed reconstruction.

On review of the patient's endoscopy (see Figure 64.1), the tumor is confined to the glottis on the left with mucosal extension to the left arytenoid. The pyriform sinuses are not involved and the remainder of the pharyngeal mucosa is intact.

After extensive counseling the patient is consented for a total laryngectomy. Question: Which of the following statements best reflects the benefit of using vascularized tissue for salvage laryngectomy?

- Vascularized tissue reconstruction is known to prevent locoregional recurrence: yes/**no**
- Vascularized tissue reconstruction is associated with decreased postsurgical pain: yes/**no**
- Vascularized tissue reconstruction has no proven benefit in salvage laryngectomy: yes/**no**
- Vascularized tissue reconstruction reduces the rate of pharyngocutaneous fistula: **yes**/no

The main benefit of vascularized tissue in salvage laryngectomy is decreasing the rate of fistula. Multiple studies have shown the benefit of vascularized tissue from the pectoralis major as well as free tissue transfer in preventing the rate of postoperative fistula and wound complication in salvage laryngectomy patients. Given the weight of evidence, all patients

CASE 64   (continued)

undergoing salvage laryngectomy should be offered vascularized tissue reconstruction.

Question: On further questioning the patient reveals that he is an avid bow hunter and wishes to continue this hobby after his surgery. He is active and intends to continue working as a construction manager after surgery. Which of the following is the most appropriate donor site for pharyngeal reconstruction in this patient?

- Radial forearm: yes/**no**

   Radial forearm free-flap harvest can be associated with measurable differences in wrist motion, pinch strength and sensation, all of which may impair this patient's ability to participate in his hobbies.

- Pectoralis major: yes/**no**

   Similarly, pectoralis major harvest is associated with decreased neck range of motion and loss of ipsilateral shoulder strength.

- Colonic interposition: yes/**no**

   Colonic interposition is reserved for circumferential defects and not appropriate in this situation

- Anterolateral thigh: **yes**/no

   Donor site morbidity should be taken into consideration when evaluating a patient for reconstruction. As such an anterolateral thigh reconstruction is preferable in patients who rely on their hands for their occupation or recreational interests.

The patient undergoes resection with the pharyngeal defect as shown in Figure 64.2a. You proceed with an ALT reconstruction with primary tracheoesophageal puncture (TEP) and incorporate the flap into your repair (Figure 64.2b and c).

Question: The patient has an uncomplicated postoperative course until postoperative day 5 (POD5), when his neck becomes more edematous. On POD6 there is a peristomal incisional dehiscence on exam, and probing reveals clear saliva from the wound. How would you manage the patient?

- Initiate a prolong course of IV antibiotics: yes/**no**
   Antibiotics are not necessary for uncomplicated fistula and do not significantly impact rates of resolution
- Initiate conservative management: patient NPO and performing BID or TID wound packing: **yes**/no
   Fistula rates in salvage laryngectomy after free tissue transfer remain between 20 and 30%. Initial management includes assessment of flap viability, NPO status, and wound packing. The majority of fistulae in this situation resolve with wound packing within several weeks.
- Vacuum-assisted closure has no role in fistula after laryngectomy: **yes**/no
   Vacuum-assisted closure has been described in the literature and can be a useful adjunct for specific cases of postlaryngectomy fistula.

(a) (b) (c)

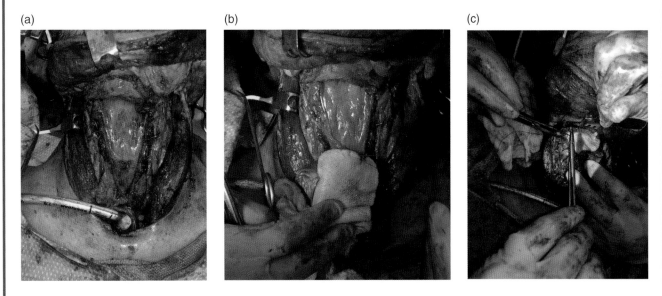

FIGURE 64.2   **(a) This intraoperative photo demonstrates the patient's salvage laryngectomy defect. (b) This intraoperative photo demonstrates the start of the skin paddle interposition inset to perform the pharyngeal repair. (c) This photo demonstrates the upper aspect of the ALT skin paddle inset for the pharyngeal repair.**

(Continued)

CASE 64 (continued)

• Immediate return to the operating room with pectoralis myocutaneous flap should be considered: yes/**no**
Additional reconstruction with a pectoralis myocutaneous flap can be considered after a trial of conservative management. In instances where there is significant carotid exposure and/or salivary contamination of the carotid space, especially in an irradiated wound, more proactive wound exploration and flap coverage may be needed to reduce the rate of carotid rupture.

Question: The patient is wondering about voicing after surgery and has explored options of speech rehabilitation. He specifically wants to discuss TEP. How would you counsel the patient regarding the benefits of primary versus secondary TEP placement?

• Primary TEP may be associated with a higher rate of wound complications in salvage laryngectomy patients than in treatment-naïve laryngectomy patients: **yes**/no
• Primary TEP in salvage laryngectomy patients is associated with a shorter time to speech than secondary TEP placement: **yes**/no

Primary TEP in salvage laryngectomy remains controversial. The overall complication rate of primary TEP in salvage laryngectomy patients has been reported as higher than in nonradiated patients, likely due to tissue vascularity and patient factors. However, large studies have shown that primary TEP can be performed safely in carefully selected patients in the salvage setting; therefore, it should be considered in the appropriate setting. The overall time to speech is significantly shorter for primary TEP patients, and it can be safely performed for patients undergoing pectoralis major reconstruction.

Key Points

• In patients being followed for surveillance after definitive head and neck cancer therapy, worsening throat/ear pain, difficulty swallowing, or new masses/ulcers or asymmetric swelling seen on physical exam should raise the suspicion for disease recurrence, and endoscopy with biopsy and/or imaging should be considered to rule it out.
• If cancer is identified, or if a laryngectomy is being considered for functional reasons or radiation necrosis, the patient should also be optimized for postoperative healing through control of any medical conditions such as diabetes mellitus, hypothyroidism, or malnutrition.
• In patients undergoing a salvage laryngectomy, reconstruction with nonradiated healthy tissue has been shown to significantly reduce the rate of pharyngocutaneous fistula formation.
• In patients who develop pharyngocutaneous fistula, the majority will close with local wound care and packing. More aggressive measures such as a regional muscle flap should be considered for refractory cases or in instances of carotid exposure.
• TEP is a standard method for voice rehabilitation following laryngectomy. While primary TEP has been shown to cause an increase in local wound complications in salvage laryngectomy patients, this approach can be safely used in carefully selected patients.

CASE 65

Jesse Ryan

History of Present Illness

A 62-year-old male presents for evaluation a facial lesion. Patient reports a 10-year history of a slowly enlarging right face mass. The lesion is not painful and has not been bleeding.

Past Medical History

Noncontributory.

Past Surgical History

Tonsillectomy as a child.

Social History

Patient is a current smoker (1.5 packs per day). He does not drink alcohol.
Review of systems is negative except for symptoms described above.

Physical Examination

Patient is a thin, healthy male in no apparent distress.
Ears: right TM normal. Left TM normal.
Face: right face with an approximately 6×6 cm ulcerative lesion covers most of right cheek (see Figure 65.1). Mass does not appear to involve nose, eye, or lips.

CASE 65   (continued)

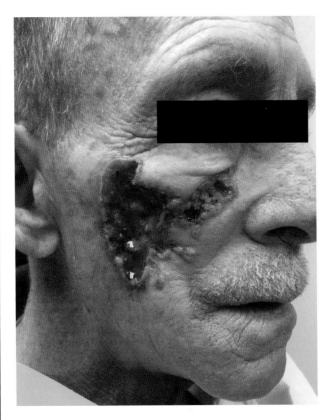

FIGURE 65.1   This photo taken in the clinic shows the ulcerative skin lesion of the patient's right cheek. It does not involve the lower lid and is slightly tethered but not fixed to the right zygoma.

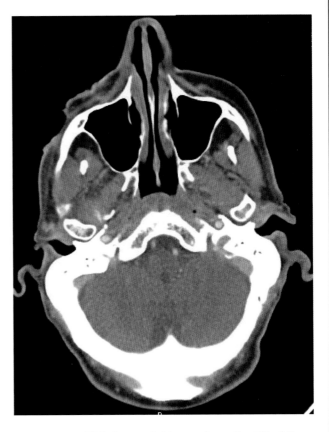

FIGURE 65.2   This is an axial image from the CT of the neck with IV contrast showing the primary lesion without obvious bone erosion. No lymphadenopathy is identified. The parotid gland does not appear to be involved.

Nasal cavity: septum straight, clear anteriorly, no masses visualized.

Oral cavity/oropharynx: no masses seen, absent tonsils, normal palate, normal tongue.

Neck: no palpable lymph nodes.

Cranial nerve exam: no deficits identified.

Question: Which of the following would be appropriate next steps in the evaluation and management of this patient? (Choose all that apply.)

- A punch biopsy of the skin lesion: **yes**/no. This is essential to confirm the pathologic diagnosis.
- CT of the neck with IV contrast: **yes**/no. This is an excellent way to assess for the depth of the primary lesion, to look for bone erosion, and also to assess for pathologic lymphadenopathy in the parotid gland and neck.

You obtain a CT scan of the neck, which shows the ulcerative mass of the right cheek abutting the maxilla (see Figure 65.2).

Question: Based on the history, physical examination, and imaging characteristics, what is the most likely diagnosis for this patient?

- SCC: yes/**no**
- Basal cell carcinoma: **yes**/no
  The extended time course (10 years) in addition to the ulcerative, endophytic nature of the tumor makes basal cell carcinoma the most likely of these options.
- Lymphoma: yes/**no**
- Merkel cell tumor: yes/**no**

Question: What would be an appropriate next step in the management of this patient?

- Wide local excision with immediate reconstruction with split thickness skin graft: yes/**no**
  Primary surgery (wide local excision) is recommended for treatment of basal cell carcinoma. The extension of the ulceration close to the maxilla on imaging is

(Continued)

CASE 65   (continued)

concerning, even though bone invasion is extremely rare with basal cell carcinoma. A split thickness skin graft would provide a sub-optimal reconstruction for this patient

- Vismodegib: yes/**no**
  Vismodegib is typically reserved for patients with unresectable or metastatic basal cell carcinoma or in cases where the morbidity of resection is unacceptable to the patient.
- Wide local excision, delayed reconstruction with radial forearm free tissue transfer (after margins cleared): **yes**/no
  Delayed reconstruction offers the opportunity to obtain clear circumferential margins and to assess the deep margin as well. Radial forearm donor site provides thin, pliable tissue for facial reconstruction.
- Radiation therapy: yes/**no**
  Basal cell carcinoma is typically sensitive to radiation therapy and this would offer a high chance of cure. However, given the extent of tissue loss from the tumor and proximity to bone, the patient may develop a chronic and difficult-to-manage facial wound.

The patient underwent wide local excision with defect seen in Figure 65.3a and b.

Question: Final margins are confirmed to be without cancer. The size of the defect is 8×7 cm in maximal dimension. Which of the following would be the best option for reconstruction?

- Cervicofacial advancement flap: yes/**no**
  In this instance, the defect is too large for primary closure and would be very challenging to repair with a cervicofacial advancement flap.
- Radial forearm free flap: **yes**/no
  Free-flap repair is likely going to yield the best result and a radial forearm free flap will provide a large amount of skin with minimal associated bulk.
- Anterolateral thigh free flap: yes/**no**
  An anterolateral thigh free flap may be a good option if there was as associated parotidectomy defect as there would be more of a need for volume replacement as well.

Question: If the resection included a radical parotidectomy with facial nerve sacrifice, which of the following flaps would offer the potential for a vascularized motor nerve graft to repair the facial nerve?

Answer: Anterolateral thigh free flap. The anterolateral thigh free flap can be harvested with the motor nerve to the vastus lateralis muscle. The branching pattern of this nerve is well suited to facial nerve construction particularly when the goal is to reconstruct multiple divisions of the nerve. This can be done with in continuity with the pedicle to maintain vascularity to the nerve and in discontinuity. The latissimus dorsi flap is typically harvested with the thoracodorsal nerve, which innervates the latissimus muscle; however, this flap is not well suited for a facial skin defect due to its bulk.

(a)

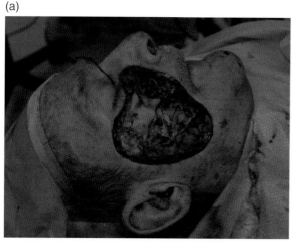

(b)

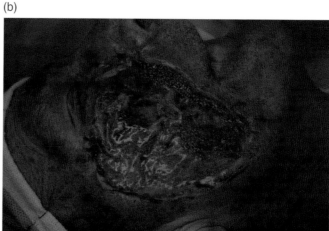

FIGURE 65.3   (a) This intraoperative photo shows the right cheek defect immediately after resection. (b) This intraoperative photo shows the right cheek wound after placement of an extracellular wound matrix to promote healing while margin assessment is being finalized.

CASE 65   (continued)

The defect in this patient was reconstructed with a templated radial forearm free flap in a delayed fashion after margins were cleared on permanent pathology (see Figure 65.4).

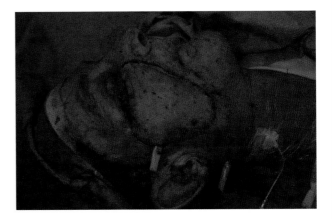

FIGURE 65.4   This photo demonstrates the result following reconstruction with a left-sided radial forearm fasciocutaneous free flap.

Key Points

- Basal cell carcinoma is the most common skin malignancy and should be considered for any slow-growing ulceration that has been present for more than a year.
- Following an office history and physical exam, a punch biopsy is usually recommended to obtain a tissue diagnosis. The periphery of the lesion is the ideal location for biopsy, as this best allows for confirmation of invasion.
- For extensive skin cancers of the face, free tissue transfer is a viable option and can achieve high-quality cosmetic results. Reconstruction can be done in either immediate or delayed fashion depending on the details of the individual case and level of concern regarding margins.
- Free-flap choice depends on the particular defect to be reconstructed, as well as patient factors. The radial forearm free flap offers thin pliable soft tissue that can help in repair of defects too large on not well positioned for local or regional repair.
- For larger volume soft tissue defects, options for reconstruction include regional options such as submental or supraclavicular rotational flaps, as well as bulkier free flaps such as anterolateral thigh, rectus abdominus, lateral arm, or subscapular system flaps.

Multiple Choice Questions

1. How much of the radius can be harvested as part of an OCRFFF?

   a. 10%.

   b. 25%.

   c. 50%.

   d. 75%.

   Answer: c. Up to 50% of the radius can be harvested up to a length of 12 cm. This bone segment is useful in defects that are non–load bearing and require minimal osteotomies. The remnant radius is then plated for reinforcement to minimize the risk of pathologic fracture after harvest.

2. How would you reconstruct a large midface defect involving soft tissue and the orbitomaxilla?

   a. Scapula free flap with latissimus dorsi.

   b. Iliac crest with internal oblique muscle.

   c. Rectus abdominus with calvarium.

   d. Either a or b.

   Answer: d. Large composite flaps are more reliable than soft-tissue and bone grafts, especially in instances where postoperative radiation therapy will be instituted. Of these options, the iliac crest flap is best able to accept dental implants; however, it comes with much more donor site morbidity.

3. In a patient where an iliac crest free flap was used to perform a hard palate reconstruction, the pedicle is not able to adequately

reach to the ipsilateral facial artery and vein. How could this have been avoided?

a. Use of a scapula tip free flap instead.

b. Use a saphenous vein graft.

c. Use the internal maxillary artery as a recipient artery for your anastomosis.

d. All of the above.

e. Both a and b.

Answer: e. One big challenge of midface reconstruction is having adequate pedicle length to reach the necessary recipient vessels. The iliac crest free flap, while it provides excellent bone stock and soft tissue, has a relatively short pedicle length. The scapula tip free flap provides a good bone source for hard palate reconstruction and has a long pedicle, as it is based on the angular branch off of the thoracodorsal vessels. An alternative option is to use the saphenous vein as an interposition graft. The internal maxillary artery, while a good caliber for reconstruction, lies deep to the mandibular ramus and is therefore not in an ideal location for a microvascular anastomosis. Moreover, in this location, there is no suitable recipient vein.

4. What are some of the benefits of using prosthetics in midface reconstruction?

a. Great aesthetic results.

b. Reduction of surgical times.

c. Lower morbidity.

d. Easier cancer surveillance.

e. All of the above.

Answer: e. In addition to the above findings, prosthetics are useful in medically infirm patients and helpful with earlier detection of cancer recurrences. However, prosthetics are expensive and not always available in financially restricted environments.

5. In explaining the anatomy of the ALT flap to your resident in clinic, you correctly state:

a. Type II perforators arising from the transverse branch of the lateral circumflex femoral artery (LCFA) occur in 80–90% of patients.

b. Sensory re-innervation of the skin paddle can be accomplished using the medial femoral cutaneous nerve.

c. Tissue types available for harvest with the ALT flap include skin, fat, fascia, muscle, and bone.

d. The maximum amount of skin accessible for harvest is 15×8 cm.

Answer: c. Given the long vascular pedicle, large available skin paddle, and diverse tissue types available, the ALT is increasingly becoming more popular and well suited for reconstruction of a variety of head and neck defects. Yu (2004) described a useful method for classification of the common variants of the ALT vascular anatomy. Cutaneous perforators to the ALT skin derive from three possible sites of origin: (i) type 1 perforators account for 90% and originate from the descending branch of the LCFA; (ii) type II perforators account for 4% and originate from the transverse branch of the LCFA;

and (iii) type III perforators account for 4% and arise directly from the profunda femoris.

Sensory innervation of the skin paddle can be accomplished using the lateral femoral cutaneous nerve.

Depending on skin perforator anatomy, an ALT of up to 20–30 cm in length may be harvested. The maximum flap width that allows for primary closure is estimated by pinching the skin of the thigh flap donor site between the thumb and fingers. In most patients this is 8–10 cm, but primary closure has been reported with defect widths up to 12 cm.

The osteocutaneous anterolateral thigh free flap (ALTO flap) has been described, where a partial thickness of the ipsilateral femur is harvested with the ALT flap based on the deep nutrient vessel to the mid femur off of the main flap pedicle. While a robust amount of bone can be obtained, there is a risk of fat embolus with the harvest, and prophylactic rod placement into the femur is recommended to avoid the risk of postoperative fracture.

6. Which of the following surgical maneuvers has been shown to negatively impact postoperative swallowing function?

a. Mandibular flap suspension sutures.

b. Transection of the suprahyoid musculature.

c. Tongue base preservation.

d. Overcorrection of volume loss with a large flap.

Answer: b. The tongue is crucial for propelling a food bolus to the pharynx. The oral phase of deglutition relies on contact of the tongue to the palate to drive the bolus. Following total glossectomy, the shape and bulk of the tongue are closely correlated with postoperative swallowing functional outcomes. Over-restoration of tongue volume, especially when postoperative radiation is indicated, may counteract the shrinkage of flaps that may occur. In addition, extensive resections involving the floor of mouth and suprahyoid musculature may lead to flap sagging, as well as disruption of the upward movement of the larynx and hyoid needed for a controlled swallow. Mandibular flap suspension sutures have been used with variable success for preventing sagging of the flap into the floor of mouth defect.

7. Which of the following is the most important lab test to obtain for preventing postoperative complications?

a. Testing for genetic coagulopathies.

b. Thyroid function testing.

c. Random blood glucose.

d. D-dimer.

Answer: b. The prevalence of hypothyroidism after primary radiation for laryngeal cancer can be as high as 45%. Hypothyroidism has been found to independently be associated with postoperative fistula after surgery; measuring a thyroid-stimulating hormone (TSH) and starting supplementation accordingly is a prudent part of preoperative management. Routine testing for genetic coagulopathies is not indicated in a patient who has no personal or family history of clotting. Diabetes is associated with wound complications, but in light of a normal HA1C, a random blood glucose has no benefit in this patient. Measurement of a D-dimer is not indicated in this case.

8. In considering reconstruction options for a lateral facial defect, which of the following would be an important consideration?

   a. The lateral arm provides a superior skin match to distal extremity free flaps.

   b. Though well suited to facial reconstruction, harvest of a submental island pedicle flap can compromise integrity of a level I nodal dissection.

   c. Supraclavicular island flaps offer excellent skin match; however, distal necrosis is the most commonly encountered postoperative complication.

   d. All of the above.

   Answer: d. All of the above are true statements and should be considered when performing complex soft-tissue reconstruction of a facial defect.

Suggested Reading

Andrades, P., Rosenthal, E.L., Carroll, W.R. et al. (2008). Zygomatic-maxillary buttress reconstruction of midface defects with the osteocutaneous radial forearm free flap. *Head Neck* 30 (10): 1295–1302.

Beckler, A.D., Ezzat, W.H., Seth, R. et al. (2015). Assessment of fibula flap skin perfusion in patients undergoing oromandibular reconstruction: comparison of clinical findings, fluorescein, and indocyanine green angiography. *JAMA Facial Plast. Surg.* 17 (6): 422–426.

Brown, J.S. and Shaw, R.J. (2010). Reconstruction of the maxilla and midface: introducing a new classification. *Lancet Oncol.* 11 (10): 1001–1008.

Ciolek, P.J., Prendes, B.L., and Fritz, M.A. (2018). Comprehensive approach to reestablishing form and function after radical parotidectomy. *Am. J. Otolaryngol.* 39 (5): 542–547.

Dowthwaite, S.A., Theurer, J., Belzile, M. et al. (2013). Comparison of fibular and scapular osseous free flaps for oromandibular reconstruction: a patient-centered approach to flap selection. *JAMA Otolaryngol. Head Neck Surg.* 139 (3): 285–292.

Hayashi, T., Furukawa, H., Oyama, A. et al. (2014). An analysis of cheek reconstruction after tumor excision in patients with melanoma. *J. Craniofac. Surg.* 25 (2): e98–e101.

Nicolletti, G., Soutar, D.S., Jackson, M.S. et al. (2004). Objective assessment of speech after surgical treatment for oral cancer; experience from 196 selected cases. *Plast. Reconstr. Surg.* 113: 114–125.

O'Connell, J.E., Bajwa, M.S., Schache, A.G., and Shaw, R.J. (2017). Head and neck reconstruction with free flaps based on the thoracodorsal system. *Oral Oncol.* 75: 46–53.

Patel, U.A., Moore, B.A., Wax, M. et al. (2013). Impact of pharyngeal closure technique on fistula after salvage laryngectomy. *JAMA Otolaryngol. Head Neck Surg.* 139 (11): 1156–1162.

Rapstine, E.D., Knaus, W.J. 2nd, and Thornton, J.F. (2012). Simplifying cheek reconstruction: a review of over 400 cases. *Plast. Reconstr. Surg.* 129 (6): 1291–1299.

Rosko, A.J., Birkeland, A.C., Bellile, E. et al. (2018). Hypothyroidism and wound healing after salvage laryngectomy. *Ann. Surg. Oncol.* 25 (5): 1288–1295.

Sayles, M. and Grant, D.G. (2014). Preventing pharyngocutaneous fistula in total laryngectomy: a systematic review and meta-analysis. *Laryngoscope* 124 (5): 1150–1163.

Sinclair, C.F., Rosenthal, E.L., McColloch, N.L. et al. (2011). Primary versus delayed tracheoesophageal puncture for laryngopharyngectomy with free flap reconstruction. *Laryngoscope* 121 (7): 1436–1440.

Sun, J., Weng, Y., Li, J. et al. (2007). Analysis of determinants on speech function after glossectomy. *J. Oral Maxillofac. Surg.* 65: 1944–1950.

Tang, A.L., Bearelly, S., and Mannion, K. (2017). The expanding role of scapular free-flaps. *Curr. Opin. Otolaryngol. Head Neck Surg.* 25 (5): 411–415.

Ung, F., Rocco, J.W., and Deschler, D.G. (2002). Temporary intraoperative fixation in mandibular reconstruction. *Laryngoscope* 112 (9): 1569–1573.

Urken, R. and Mark, L. (2012). *Multidisciplinary Head and Neck Reconstruction: A Defect-Oriented Approach*, 1e, vol. 1. LWW.

Wax, M.K., Burkey, B.B., Bascom, D., and Rosenthal, E.L. (2003). The role of free tissue transfer in the reconstruction of massive neglected skin cancers of the head and neck. *Arch. Facial Plast. Surg.* 5 (6): 479–482.

Yu, P. (2004). Characteristics of the anterolateral thigh flap in western population and its application in head and neck reconstruction. *Head Neck* 26: 1038–1044.

SECTION 15

Ethics

Andrew Shuman

CASE 66

Catherine T. Haring and Andrew G. Shuman

History of Present Illness

A 72-year-old man with T4bN2cM1 squamous cell carcinoma (SCC) of the oral cavity currently receiving palliative chemoradiation presents to the ER with worsening dyspnea. He is intubated in the ER for hypoxia. He is febrile, tachycardic to 120 seconds, and hypotensive to 70/40. Workup reveals a right-sided pneumonia and positive blood cultures. The patient is admitted to the ICU and started on IV antibiotics and intravenous fluids. His condition initially improves; however, over the next 2 weeks, he decompensates, developing renal failure that requires dialysis, and is ultimately unable to be weaned from the ventilator.

Past Medical History

He has a history of chronic obstructive pulmonary disease, hypertension, and hyperlipidemia.

Social History

He has a 50 pack-year smoking history but quit about 2 months ago at the time of his cancer diagnosis. He previously drank about a pint of whiskey per day but also quit at the time of his cancer diagnosis. He works in construction. The patient's wife died 1 year ago from breast cancer. He lives alone.

Question: What additional questions would you want to ask? (Choose all that apply.)

- Does the patient have an advance directive? **yes**/no. This is important to ask. The patient does not have an advance directive.

- Does the patient have a designated durable power of attorney (DPOA)? **yes**/no. This is necessary to determine. No, the patient does not have a DPOA.
- Does the patient have a surrogate decision-maker? **yes**/no. This is also critical to establish. The patient had not previously designated a surrogate decision-maker. His closest living relative is his adult daughter, who has been actively involved in his care since his cancer diagnosis. She has been at his bedside nearly every day since his admission.

Physical Examination

Vital signs: temp 37.1, HR 82, BP 100/50 (on vasopressors), RR 16, SpO2 95% on mechanical ventilation.

General: thin, cachectic appearing male, intubated and sedated.

Skin: no abnormal-appearing skin lesions.

Oral cavity: exophytic and ulcerative mass of the left oral tongue, extending to the left floor of mouth, causing tethering and trismus. Endotracheal tube in place.

Neck: 3 cm fixed mass in the left level Ib/II neck. Several additional enlarged lymph nodes bilaterally

Neuro: sedated. When sedation is weaned, he moves all extremities; however, he does not follow commands.

Management

Due to his poor prognosis, the multidisciplinary team recommends consideration of withdrawal of life-sustaining treatment in favor of focusing on comfort at the end of life.

(Continued)

Essential Cases in Head and Neck Oncology, First Edition. Edited by Michael G. Moore, Arnaud F. Bewley, and Babak Givi.
© 2022 American Head and Neck Society. Published 2022 by John Wiley & Sons Ltd.

CASE 66 (continued)

Question: What additional questions would you want to ask?

- Is there a chance for the patient to make a meaningful recovery? The Critical Care attending believes that the patient will be unable to be weaned from the ventilator. The Nephrology attending does not expect his kidney function to recover. His head and neck cancer is incurable, and barring other medical comorbidities, would have an anticipated prognosis measurable in months.
- What is his daughter's perspective? The patient's daughter has told the nurses that she is determined to continue aggressive treatment. She is adamantly opposed to transitioning to comfort care. She states that her father has "fought his cancer up to this point and would not want to give up now." She tells the nurses she would like to pursue all life-sustaining treatments including tracheostomy and gastrostomy tube placement.

Question: What is the definition of surrogate decision-maker?

Answer: A surrogate decision-maker, or proxy, is a person who has been named by the patient at the time when he/she has capacity or is a family member/close acquaintance who has been granted authority to make medical decisions for an incapacitated person who has not made a specific designation. In the United States, a hierarchy of health care surrogates may vary according to state laws.

Question: What would be the most appropriate next step in management of this patient?

Answer: The next best step is to schedule a family meeting with the patient's surrogate decision-maker to determine her understanding of the patient's current clinical situation.

Conflict in medical settings has been defined as "a dispute, disagreement, or difference of opinion related to the management of a patient involving more than one individual and requiring some decision or action." Conflict can occur between family and clinician, between clinician and clinician, between family and family, or between patient and clinician. In the ICU setting, conflict most commonly occurs between family and clinicians regarding life-sustaining measures at the end of life. Disagreement between providers and patients can create stress for everyone involved. Most disputes in the ICU arise from inadequate or ineffective communication, not from intractable value conflicts. Resolving conflict requires clinicians to move toward an understanding of why the family holds a particular viewpoint as opposed to trying to convince the family of a specific course of action.

A consensus statement by the American Thoracic Society, American Association for Critical Care Nurses, American College of Chest Physicians, European Society for Intensive Care Medicine, and Society of Critical Care states that clinicians should not provide potentially inappropriate or futile interventions. Interventions are defined as inappropriate when there is no reasonable expectation that the patient will improve sufficiently to survive outside the acute care setting. When responding to requests for futile interventions, clinicians should seek to understand the reason for such requests, provide emotional support, and explain why the requested intervention might not meet mutually agreed-upon goals. Saying "there is nothing more that can be done" can be perceived as a form of defiance or abandonment and is also likely to be inaccurate.

Question: During the family meeting, the patient's daughter shares that the patient's wife died about 1 year ago from metastatic breast cancer and he cared for her in her last days of life. He expressed to his family that he would never want to be maintained on a ventilator or live in a nursing facility. During the same conversation, the daughter becomes angry, stating she feels like the team is "giving up" and would like to continue maximum therapy. Given this new information, what is the most appropriate next step?

Answer: Surrogate decision-makers should base their decisions in accordance with a substituted judgment standard, which refers to a patient's wishes even if such wishes may not have been explicitly expressed.

Autonomy is a fundamental value in bioethics, and providers should strive to ground all decisions in autonomy even when the patient is no longer able to express an autonomous wish. When patients do not have advance directives or existing directives do not apply to the decisions at hand, providers should ask surrogate decision-makers what the patient would have wanted if he or she could express this opinion. Substituted judgment may also have psychological benefits. Surrogate decision-makers can feel a significant burden when authorizing decisions to forego life support for a loved one. Relying on a substituted judgment standard may instead remove some of the burden from the family by reframing the decision as the patient's own.

If disagreement persists despite conversation between the clinician and family, clinicians should obtain expert consultation to assist with conflict resolution and values clarification. It is important to incorporate multiple perspectives to minimize the risk that values of any one individual will carry undue weight. Empirical evidence indicates that ethics consultations can help deal with difficult conflicts and requests by surrogate decision-makers to provide potentially nonbeneficial interventions.

Question: After a long discussion with the multidisciplinary treatment team, the patient's surrogate decision-maker ultimately decides to focus on supportive management and symptom control at the end of life. What is the role for artificial nutrition in a moribund patient at the end of life?

CASE 66 (continued)

Answer: The literature demonstrates that artificial nutrition in the setting of a moribund patient with terminal cancer is unlikely to meaningfully prolong life and can potentially lead to medical complications and increased suffering. However, to date, there are no randomized controlled trials evaluating the effect of artificial nutrition at the end of life. No evidence has demonstrated an extension of life or improved quality of life with artificial nutrition, but considerable evidence indicates higher risk of complications, including aspiration, pneumonia, nausea, diarrhea, need for physical restraints, infection, and complications due to fluid overload.

Specific to the patient with head and neck cancer, progressive dysphagia is common at the time of diagnosis, during treatment, and at the end of life. Artificial nutrition may offer benefits in the acute setting, when there is reversible illness or as a component of chronic disease management, and otherwise when the benefits outweigh the complications. With terminal disease and prognosis of days to weeks, perceived benefits of artificial nutrition, including alleviation of thirst, can be achieved by less invasive measures including corticosteroids, oral care, and ice chips.

Key Points

- When a medical condition impairs a patient's decision-making capacity, it is necessary to identify an appropriate surrogate decision-maker to make decisions on the patient's behalf.
- Surrogate decision-makers should base their decisions in accordance with a substituted judgment standard, which refers to a patient's preference even if such wishes may not have been explicitly expressed.

- Recognizing and dealing with conflict to limit life-sustaining treatment can improve relationships and help guide family members and patients through difficult decisions.
- A physician should enlist help from an ethics consultant or committee when there remains discord regarding a decision that may not be in a patient's best interest.
- Clinicians are not obligated to provide potentially inappropriate or futile life-prolonging treatments.

CASE 67

Catherine T. Haring and Andrew G. Shuman

History of Present Illness

A 45-year-old man with newly diagnosed T3N1M0 (AJCC 8th ed.) p16+ SCC of the right tonsil presents to discuss his treatment options. His case was reviewed at tumor board and recommendations were made for chemoradiation versus enrollment in a clinical trial.

Past Medical History

He is otherwise healthy.

Social history

He is married and lives with his wife and two children, who are 9 and 13 years old. He works as an electrical engineer. He is a never-smoker. He drinks socially about two times per month.

Physical Examination

Vital signs: temp 37.2, HR 84, BP 140/50, RR 16, SpO$_2$ 98% on room air.

General: well-developed male, in no acute distress.

Skin: no abnormal-appearing skin lesions.

Oral cavity: no abnormal masses or lesions.

Oropharynx: 3 cm exophytic mass of the right tonsil, appears to extend to the retromolar trigone and base of tongue, not amenable to transoral resection.

Neck: 3 cm mobile mass in the right level II neck, several additional enlarged lymph nodes in right level III.

Neuro: cranial nerves are intact bilaterally.

Management

The treatment options including standard-of-care chemoradiation and a prospective treatment trial are discussed, including the relative risks and benefits of each.

Question: What additional questions would you want to ask? (Choose all that apply.)

- What is involved in the clinical trial? **yes**/no. The clinical trial involves radiation and treatment with an investigational chemotherapeutic agent versus standard of care.

(*Continued*)

CASE 67   (continued)

- What is the patient's preference for treatment? **yes**/no. He appreciates your guidance as his physician and would like to know your recommendations. He becomes tearful, stating that he has two young children and a wife who he loves very much, and he wants to pursue the option with best overall survival outcome. He is interested in hearing more about the "state-of-the-art" drug offered in the trial.

Question: What would be the most appropriate response to the patient in the case above?

Answer: The most appropriate response is to explain to the patient that the purpose of treatment trials is to produce generalizable knowledge and that the patient may or may not directly benefit from the intervention under study.

It is important for providers and patients to understand the inherent differences between clinical medicine and clinical research. Clinical medicine aims to provide individual patients with optimal care, whereas clinical research intends to contribute to the advancement of generalizable knowledge to serve future patients. In clinical research, therapeutic benefit to individuals who participate is secondary to the overriding goal of the study. Current research suggests that many research participants do not appreciate the important differences between treatment and research, a phenomenon called "therapeutic misconception." Therapeutic misconception exists when individuals do not understand that the defining purpose of clinical research is to produce generalizable knowledge regardless of whether the subjects enrolled in the trial may potentially benefit from the intervention under study or from other aspects of the clinical trial. Failure of participants to understand the goal of clinical research can compromise informed consent and trust in the research enterprise and create inaccurate expectations.

The objective of clinical research is to develop knowledge to improve health and/or increase understanding of human biology. There are seven requirements that provide a systematic and coherent framework for determining whether clinical research is ethical. To be ethical, clinical research must have (i) social or scientific value, (ii) scientific validity, (iii) fair subject selection, (iv) favorable risk–benefit ratio, (v) independent review, (vi) informed consent, and (vii) respect for potential and enrolled subjects. Value, validity, fair subject selection, favorable risk–benefit ratio, and respect for subjects are all necessary for clinical research. Clinical research that neglects or violates any of these requirements would be considered unethical. Informed consent is a procedural requirement intended to respect patient autonomy, minimize conflict of interest, and ensure concordance with patient interests. However, certain trial designs obviate the feasibility of informed consent. This may include retrospective analyses of existing or publicly available data or specific types of quality improvement research. In addition, research on emergency life-saving interventions for subjects who are unable to consent for interventions and for whom family is not immediately available may be conducted without consent. In some circumstances, consent can be waived.

With regard to fair subject selection, there are several components to consider. The scientific goals of the study should be the primary basis for fair subject selection as opposed to the vulnerability or privilege of the subject. In the past, vulnerable populations were sometimes enrolled in research, especially for research that entailed risks, because they were unable to advocate for themselves. Similarly, groups should not be excluded from the opportunity to participate in research without a good scientific reason or susceptibility to risk that justifies exclusion. It is important that results of research be generalizable, and thus diverse populations should be included in research. Subjects who are eligible to participate based on the scientific objectives of a study but who are at substantially higher risks of being harmed given medical comorbidities, functional status, or other reasons should be excluded. Selecting patients to maximize benefit of a study requires consideration of which subjects will most benefit from the intervention. If a potential drug or procedure is likely to be prescribed to a specific population, such as pregnant women or children, if proven safe and effective, then these groups should be included in the research study. In summary, fair subject selection should be guided by the scientific aims of the research and should ensure the equal distribution of potential risks and benefits.

Question: In the case above, suppose the tumor board recommended surgical extirpation of the oropharyngeal tumor and neck disease. You, as the surgeon, recently learned a new surgical technique that you believe will result in improved functional outcomes, and you would like to offer this technique to the patient. When does a surgical innovation require a formal institutional review board (IRB) approval?

Answer: The field of surgery has a unique culture and rich tradition of innovation. Surgeons constantly aim to perfect surgical techniques and improve surgical outcomes. Rapid advancements in technology inspire surgeons to innovate. Clinical research involving a new treatment, drug, or device clearly requires formal regulatory oversight. It is less clear when a minor modification of surgical technique is substantial enough to require disclosure to the patient or formal approval and oversight by a third party. The Society of University Surgeons Surgical Innovations Project team developed and published guidelines to define when surgical innovations require formal IRB approval. Formal review is required if an innovation is planned and the surgeon seeks to confirm a hunch or theory about innovation, the innovation differs significantly from the currently accepted local practice, outcomes of the innovation have not been previously described, the innovation entails potential risks for complications, or specific or additional patient consent appears appropriate.

Key Points

- Ethically appropriate clinical research must have scientific value, scientific validity, fair subject selection, favorable risk–benefit ratio, independent review, informed consent, and respect for potential and enrolled subjects.
- Fair subject selection in clinical research should be guided by the scientific aims of the research and should ensure the equal distribution of potential risks and benefits.
- Therapeutic misconception occurs when individuals do not understand that the defining purpose of clinical research is to produce generalizable knowledge, regardless of whether the subjects enrolled in the trial may potentially benefit from the intervention under study.
- Innovations involving a new treatment, drug, device or surgical innovation require regulatory oversight when there is an expectation to create and share generalizable knowledge.

CASE 68

Lulia A. Kana, Kevin J. Kovatch, and Andrew G. Shuman

History of Present Illness

A 50-year-old woman presents to clinic with a painful ulcer on her lateral tongue. She has a history of alcohol dependence and a 40 pack-year smoking history. She appears to be in poor health and endorses a 30-pound weight loss over the past 4 months along with odynophagia and dysphagia.

Past medical history

She has chronic obstructive pulmonary disease.

Surgical history

She has no significant surgical history.

Social history (living situation, support system, relationship with family members, religious and/or spiritual values): She lives alone and has a limited relationship with her two sons, both of whom live several hours away; she only sees them during the holidays. She works in a grocery store. She describes herself as an "independent woman" who likes to take care of matters on her own. She does not describe herself as religious, although she was raised in a Catholic household.

Physical Examination

Patient is sitting comfortably in no acute distress.

Ear exam: normal.

Anterior rhinoscopy is within normal limits.

Oral cavity shows a 3 × 3 cm ulcerative and deeply infiltrative lesion of the lateral tongue extending to the midline. Dentition is poor. Tonsils are symmetric without lesions, erythema, or exudate. Posterior pharyngeal wall without lesions or masses.

Cranial nerves II–XII are intact.

Neck exam shows no asymmetry, masses, or lymphadenopathy.

No abnormal skin lesions.

Flexible nasopharyngolaryngoscopy shows no base of tongue involvement. No other mucosal lesions.

Question: What other exam findings or test results are pertinent at this time? (Choose all that apply.)

- Tissue biopsy: **yes**/no. Biopsy of the lesion was positive for invasive SCC.
- Ross sectional imaging: **yes**/no. Cross-sectional imaging identifies the primary site as well as a 2 cm suspicious ipsilateral cervical lymph node; chest clear (cT2N1M0, stage III).
- Oral human papillomavirus (HPV) testing: yes/**no**. An oral HPV swab is not helpful here. It may give insight into if there is an oral HPV infection but will do little to guide in the diagnosis or management of this patient. Oral cancer is not frequently HPV-positive.

Management

Her head and neck surgeon strongly recommends subtotal glossectomy and bilateral neck dissection with free tissue transfer along with pathologic risk-adjusted adjuvant treatment.

She adamantly refuses surgery, stating that "life would not be worth living" if she could not speak or eat as she normally would.

(Continued)

CASE 68   (continued)

Question: What other information would be helpful to know? (Choose all that apply.)

- Advance directive: **yes**/no. Her advance directive, written years prior, limits the use of aggressive measures to be taken in the event of disease severity or poor prognosis.
- DPOA: **yes**/no. Her oldest son is her designated DPOA for medical decision-making.
- Patient understanding of her prognosis: **yes**/no. After a discussion, she relays back to you that she understands her best chance for cure would be surgery.
- Goals of care: **yes**/no. When asked about her goals of care, she states that she would rather maximize comfort and maintain dignity than undergo an invasive surgery with high morbidity. She states, "I lived long enough, and the cigarettes and booze caught up to me."
- Code status: **yes**/no. Code status was discussed. She would not like to have chest compressions performed or a breathing tube placed. She had seen a family friend undergo aggressive treatment for lung cancer, who had a prolonged treatment course with multiple hospitalizations and severe side effects from radiation and chemotherapy. This has weighed heavily on her decision.

Question: Which ethical principles are antagonistic in this scenario?

Answer: The four principles in medical ethics, as articulated by Beauchamp and Childress, include respect for autonomy, beneficence, nonmaleficence, and justice. The principle of autonomy is rooted in respecting a patient's values, wishes, and decisions with regard to medical care. Beneficence reflects the duty of a clinician to act in a patient's best interest. Nonmaleficence, put simply, is to "do no harm." Lastly, justice stipulates that patients should be treated fairly and equitably.

There are various frameworks that one can use when approaching ethical dilemmas. Principlism is a classic approach to problem-solving in medical ethics. It is based on the assumption that the four core ethical principles (autonomy, beneficence, nonmaleficence, and justice) are universal and can be used to describe and analyze moral and ethical problems. While there is no presumed hierarchy among the four principles, they are frequently in conflict.

In this case, there is a conflict between respecting a patient's right to autonomy (refusing surgery) and the surgeon's duty to "do good" (beneficence). This dilemma is a common conundrum. It is more challenging due to the contemporary negative connotation of acting paternalistically by prioritizing beneficence at the expense of autonomy.

From the surgeon's perspective, it may seem intuitive to strongly recommend proceeding with surgery. However, it can be helpful to solicit the patient's values to help understand the reasons for her refusal. What is she worried about? Is it fear of the unknown? Or is it her quality of life thereafter?

It is incumbent upon all clinicians to have a basic understanding of how to mitigate ethical dilemmas so that reasoned and appropriate decisions can be made.

Question: What is the most appropriate response to the patient's refusal of surgery?

Answer: Patients have the right to refuse any medical treatments that are not in agreement with their personal values and wishes, despite clinical recommendations. However, to make medical decisions individually, patients must also demonstrate having decision-making capacity. In the event that a patient loses capacity to make decisions, a surrogate decision-maker should be identified to help the medical team make decisions on behalf of the patient. To accomplish this, surrogate decision-makers should use the standard of substituted judgment, which requires decisions to take into account the wishes and values of the patient to ultimately facilitate a decision that the patient would have wanted for themselves had they still had decision-making capacity. In the event that a surrogate decision-maker is not designated through an advanced directive, a hierarchy of surrogates can exist in the following order but can vary state by state: guardian, spouse, adult son/daughter, parent, sibling, caregiver, other person with a close relationship.

In this situation, there is no reason to believe that the patient has lost capacity to make medical decisions. Therefore, the most appropriate response would be to discuss the patient's goals and values to further elucidate her primary reason for refusal.

Question: After listening more about the details of the surgery, the patient becomes distraught. She turns to you and asks, "what do you think I should do?" What is the most appropriate response in this instance?

Answer: Medical decisions should be made through shared decision-making and risk stratification with an emphasis on a patient's values and goals. Recently, there has been a concerted effort to move away from a paternalistic model of medical practice to a patient-centered model of decision-making. Discussions with patients about their treatment options should highlight the patient's preferences and interests even if it ultimately means proceeding with a plan of care that may not be consistent with clinical recommendations. It is critical for clinicians to have an understanding of a patient's personal values and thought process to help elucidate the reasoning behind the decisions that are ultimately being made.

To enable informed decision-making, it is imperative to provide enough information for patients to make reasonable decisions. During challenging life situations, patients often turn to their providers for guidance.

In an era in which patient autonomy is prized, it would behoove clinicians to be cognizant of the harm that can

CASE 68   (continued)

potentially be caused by burdening patients with the sole responsibility for making medical decisions. Instead, it is the duty of a physician to counsel and offer recommendations when appropriate. Ultimately, surgeons should use their expertise, training, and experience with other patients to confidently offer insight about what they think would be best for a patient.

Question: After further discussion, she says in tears, "I'm really scared, and I just don't want surgery!" What is the most appropriate next step?

Answer: Adult patients have the right to refuse medical treatments that are in accordance with their values and wishes; however, patients must have medical decision-making capacity to do so. Capacity is context-, situation-, and task-specific. Capacity requires the ability to communicate a decision, understand the information pertinent to the decision, appreciate the situation, understand the consequences of such decisions, and reason through various treatment options.

To allow patients to make fully informed decisions, clinicians should counsel patients thoroughly about an expected disease course when surgical treatment is refused. Patients must be educated on potential future symptoms, such as increasing pain, dysphagia, loss of communication, and airway compromise. Palliative therapy, including surgery, radiotherapy, chemotherapy, and sedation or pain management, should be discussed extensively with the patient, as well as available options for receiving care through inpatient, outpatient, and home care services. Ultimately, counseling patients with terminal head and neck cancers should involve a multidisciplinary team approach including professionals in the fields of palliative care, social work, psychology, and nursing, among others.

It would be reasonable to offer the patient some time to process the information and to come back to clinic, preferably with a trusted friend or family member, for a follow-up appointment to rediscuss her diagnosis as well as reflect upon her values and goals. Thereafter, the clinician can feel confident that if the patient ultimately refuses surgery, it was truly informed and in line with her values and wishes.

Key Points

- Head and neck cancers have distinct implications for patients because the disease process as well as treatment approaches involve compromising the senses, which leads to a loss of communication, threat to personal identity, and quality of life issues.
- Treatment refusals require careful consideration of trade-offs and expectations in the context of patient-centered values and preferences.

- Decision-making in the care of head and neck cancers can be very challenging due to the life-threatening and time-sensitive nature of the disease course.
- Clinicians should use their experience and expertise and feel empowered to offer patients clear recommendations with regard to treatment options.

CASE 69

Lulia A. Kana, Kevin J. Kovatch, and Andrew G. Shuman

History of Present Illness

A 70-year-old man presents with a 3-month history of dysphonia, odynophagia, and cough. The patient has been in a poor state of health, losing more than 30 pounds over the past 2 months and becoming cachectic.

Past medical history

He has a history of bladder cancer s/p chemoradiation, end-stage kidney disease on dialysis, and locoregionally advanced SCC of the larynx treated with chemoradiation 1 year ago.

Past surgical history

Noncontributory.

- Social history (living situation, support system, health behaviors, relationship with family members): He has a 30 pack-year smoking history with moderate alcohol use. The patient has good social support at home; he lives with his wife, who primarily takes care of his daily needs, and his three children visit him daily to help with his care. He spends most of the day in bed.

Physical Examination

Patient is frail and cachectic, sitting comfortably in no acute distress.

Oral cavity shows no ulcerative lesions or masses. Dentition is poor. Tonsils are symmetric without lesions, erythema, or exudate. Posterior pharyngeal wall without lesions or masses.

Cranial nerves II–XII are intact.

(Continued)

CASE 69   (continued)

Neck with bilateral bulky lymphadenopathy in levels III–IV. Voice is hoarse.

Flexible laryngoscopy demonstrates a large exophytic mass of the left vocal fold extending to the anterior commissure, with a fixed vocal fold.

Management

He was taken for direct laryngoscopy and biopsy, which revealed recurrent SCC of the larynx. Cross-sectional imaging demonstrates extralaryngeal tumor infiltration of the central compartment, bilateral pathologically enlarged lymph nodes encasing the left carotid artery and abutting the right carotid artery, and no distant metastases. The tumor was staged as T4aN3M0.

Question: What should be discussed at this time? What other information would be helpful to know? (Choose all that apply.)

- Discussion of prognosis and treatment options: **yes**/no. The patient is informed of his poor prognosis and the various treatment options available to him. The risks, morbidity, and anticipated toxicities of further cancer-directed treatment are discussed. A comfort-based treatment approach is also reviewed as an option.
- Patient understanding of prognosis and goals of care: **yes**/no. The patient insists on aggressive interventions and is most interested in salvage surgery. He has not had an end-of-life conversation to date. His code status is full code.
- Advance directive, DPOA: **yes**/no. This is important to assess up front. He has no advance directive and has not designated a DPOA.

Question: What is the most appropriate next step in the management of this patient?

Answer: The patient has a locoregionally advanced cancer with a high risk of recurrence and distant metastases. His current performance status is very poor as he is mostly bedbound. He will most likely not recover back to his original functional capabilities. The most appropriate next step would be to make sure that the patient understands the nature of his disease so as to mitigate the setting of unachievable goals or unrealistic expectations with regards to the curative potential of further cancer-directed treatment.

In the setting of terminal disease, clinicians should be prepared to share serious prognoses with patients and their loved ones with empathy and compassion. These discussions are often very difficult for patients and challenging for providers to conduct. Consideration should be given to which clinical teams will be present and which family members/supporting parties will be present for the discussion. Ideally, the discussion should take place in private and in quiet settings to help patients process prognostic information. While many models exist to help offer a framework to physicians for presenting difficult news, one of the models created by Walter Baile et al. uses the acronym SPIKES (setting, perception, invitation, knowledge, emotions, strategy, and summary). Recommendations from this model include asking open-ended questions, eliciting patient understanding and preferences regarding their diagnosis, relaying information in small components, and crafting a follow-up plan with the patient.

In treating patients with terminal disease, providers may consider alternative modes of therapy, such as palliative care and hospice. Palliative care, comfort care, and hospice are often confused or erroneously used interchangeably. In oncology, palliative care is indicated when patients present with symptoms due to the cancer, disease recurrence, hospitalization, or palliative radiation. Involvement of palliative care neither implies nor requires that the patient is on hospice care or imminently nearing death. In contrast, the goal of comfort care is to optimize a patient's quality of life through symptom control and relief of pain in the setting of discontinued curative treatments. A variety of support staff can be used, including physicians, nurses, chaplains, and social workers, during this process. Hospice is a service legislated by Medicare and can be offered to patients whose life expectancy is deemed to be 6 months or less by two physicians. Similar to comfort care, the goal of hospice is to enhance comfort and provide an optimal quality of life by controlling symptoms and pain and avoiding aggressive and futile care.

Proactive patient–provider discussions about end-of-life care are associated with fewer nonbeneficial interventions at the end of life that can improve quality of death and reduce healthcare costs. These discussions should include discussion about patient values, prognosis, treatment options, and elements of advance care planning. Balaban provides a four-step approach that clinicians should use when having these discussions: initiating discussion, clarifying prognosis, identifying end-of-life goals, and developing a treatment plan. Having this discussion can not only help clarify a patient's preferences but can also be helpful in understanding why patients seem to be requesting certain interventions that may be inconsistent with their clinical trajectory and own stated goals.

Question: After extensive discussion, the patient expresses a good understanding of his options and still insists on proceeding with further cancer-directed treatment. What is the most appropriate next best step?

Answer: Multidisciplinary tumor board is an integral component in the care of head and neck cancer patients. Clinical data are presented in a group to radiation oncology, head and neck surgery, medical oncology, radiology, pathology, and

CASE 69   (continued)

other supportive services, such as psychology, social work, and speech-language pathology. Studies have shown that using a multidisciplinary tumor board framework is cost-effective and can improve survival in patients with head and neck cancer.

Palliative care consultation is ideally involved early in the treatment of patients with terminal disease. A study by Temel et al. involving patients with lung cancer with metastatic disease who had received either standard oncology care or standard oncology care in addition to palliative care showed that patients who received palliative care had a longer survival time and care at the end of life that was less aggressive.

In this case, while the involvement of palliative care would be beneficial given his poor prognosis and progressive symptoms, it is first important to prognosticate his disease through a multidisciplinary tumor board discussion, as finalized treatment plans can help future palliative care teams craft a therapy regimen that is best suited for the patient. In addition, prior to consulting other services, it is also important to discuss palliative care involvement with the patient to optimize shared decision-making.

Question: The patient is treated with immunotherapy, and his disease progresses quickly with the development of lung metastases. His functional status rapidly deteriorates. He is admitted with pneumonia and is intubated, requiring medication to support his blood pressure. His code status remains full code. His wife continues to insist that "everything be done." What is the most appropriate next step?

Answer: At the end of life, patients may demand treatments that are nonbeneficial, inappropriate, or futile. However, physicians are under no obligation to offer or proceed with treatments that they believe would not benefit a patient. However, identifying what interventions are beneficial can be very difficult as interventions that a physician believes to be nonbeneficial may appear to be helpful from a patient/family perspective.

It is important to recognize the burden that is placed on patients and families when making decisions at the end of life. When interventions are known to be nonbeneficial, it is unfair to charge patients and families who may be dealing with anticipatory grief to have to choose between "doing everything" or "giving up." While not offering such interventions may seem paternalistic, physicians need to assume responsibility of making medical decisions that fall within their expertise and only have patients and families make decisions that are appropriate for them to decide upon.

A multisociety consensus statement by the American Thoracic Society, American Association for Critical Care Nurses, American College of Chest Physicians, European Society for Intensive Care Medicine, and Society of Critical Care provided recommendations in terms of how to best respond to requests for demanding inappropriate treatments in the ICU. Some of the committee recommendations included developing strategies to prevent treatment conflicts at an institutional level through the involvement of expert consultants, having clinicians advocate for the treatment plan they believe to be best for the patient, and managing disagreements through communication and conflict resolution.

Key Points

- End-of-life care is a common consideration when treating patients with advanced or recurrent head and neck cancer. This conversation should involve discussion of code status and goals of care as early as possible.
- Clinicians should be prepared to deliver difficult news to patients and families in an empathetic, compassionate, and honest manner.
- It is imperative for providers to understand the differences between various therapy approaches, including palliative

care, hospice, and comfort care, so as to tailor treatment plans accordingly.
- Using a multidisciplinary tumor board in the care of head and neck cancer patients has been shown to be effective in both reducing cost and improving survival.
- Providers are under no obligation to offer or perform any interventions that are deemed to be nonbeneficial or harmful to a patient despite requests from patients and families.

Multiple Choice Questions

1. Which statement by a surrogate decision-maker is most consistent with the substituted judgment standard?
   a. "I don't want Dad to have a tracheostomy."
   b. "I don't think Dad will be able to take care of a tracheostomy."
   c. "I don't think Dad would want to live with a tracheostomy."
   d. "Life is not worth living with a tracheostomy."

Answer: c. "I don't think Dad would want to live with a tracheostomy." Substituted judgment refers to the act of making a decision on behalf of a patient according to the patient's preference even if such wishes may not have been explicitly expressed.

2. A patient with terminal cancer insists that if he loses decision-making capacity due to illness, he wants his clinicians to "do everything." What is an appropriate response?
   a. "Of course. We will honor your wishes."
   b. "What does it mean to you to 'do everything,' and what is most important to you moving forward?"

c. "I'm sorry, but we cannot perform interventions that are futile."

d. "If you cannot make your own decisions, it will be up to your wife to decide what happens."

Answer: b. "What does it mean to you to 'do everything,' and what is most important to you moving forward?"

3. All of the following requirements are necessary to perform ethically sound clinical research EXCEPT?

a. Social or scientific value.

b. Informed consent.

c. Scientific validity.

d. IRB involvement.

Answer: b. Consent can be waived in certain select circumstances. Examples of when consent can be waived include minimal risk studies, research in emergency settings, public benefit or service program studies.

4. Protection of human subjects is critical for performing ethical clinical research. All of the following are requirements for fair subject selection EXCEPT?

a. The scientific goals of the study should be the primary basis for determining individuals who will be recruited and enrolled.

b. Individuals should not be excluded from participation without good scientific reason.

c. Subjects should be excluded from participation if they are at substantially higher risk.

d. Minorities and children should be excluded from participation in clinical research.

Answer: d. Minorities and children can and should be included in research, when appropriate.

5. Which of the following is a prerequisite for decision-making capacity?

a. Ability to communicate a decision.

b. Understanding information pertinent to the decision.

c. Reasoning through various treatment options.

d. All of the above.

Answer: d. All of the above.

6. A patient adamantly refuses a recommended cancer operation. What is an appropriate next step?

a. Seek a court order to mandate surgery.

b. Ask the patient's next of kin to weigh in.

c. Determine the patient's understanding of the consequences of refusing surgery.

d. Honor her wish and do not operate.

Answer: c. Determine the patient's understanding of the consequences of refusing surgery.

Patients have the right to refuse any medical treatments that not are in agreement with their personal values and wishes despite clinical recommendations. However, to make medical decisions individually, patients must also demonstrate having decision-making capacity.

7. Which of the following statements is *incorrect*?

a. Palliative care can be used in patients who are not terminally ill.

b. Palliative care is not used in patients with cancer when the main goal of ongoing therapy is cure.

c. The main goal of comfort care is optimizing quality of life through symptom control and relief of pain.

d. Hospice can be provided in a variety of settings, including nursing homes, hospitals, and a patient's home.

Answer: b. Palliative care is not used in patients with cancer when the main goal of ongoing therapy is cure. In oncology, palliative care is indicated when patients present with symptoms due to the cancer, disease recurrence, hospitalization, or palliative radiation. Involvement of palliative care neither implies nor requires that the patient is on hospice care or imminently nearing death.

8. An 87-year-old woman requests that her existing "Do Not Resuscitate" order remain in place during a scheduled cancer surgery. How would you proceed?

a. Refuse to operate unless the DNR order is temporarily suspended during surgery.

b. Honor her request and maintain the DNR order during surgery.

c. Discuss her request further with the patient, surgical team, and anesthesiologist.

d. Refer the patient to a palliative care provider.

Answer: c. Discuss her request further with the patient, surgical team, and anesthesiologist.

Suggested Reading

Appelbaum, P.S. (2007). Assessment of patients' competence to consent to treatment. *N. Engl. J. Med.* 357 (18): 1834–1840. https://doi.org/10.1056/NEJMcp074045.

Back, A.L. and Arnold, R.M. (2005). Dealing with conflict in caring for the seriously ill, "It was just out of the question.". *JAMA* 293 (11): 1374–1381.

Baile, W.F., Buckman, R., Lenzi, R. et al. (2000). SPIKES – A six-step protocol for delivering bad news: application to the patient with cancer. *Oncologist* 5 (4): 302–311. https://doi.org/10.1634/theoncologist.5-4-302.

Balaban, R.B. (2000). A physician's guide to talking about end-of-life care. *J. Gen. Intern. Med.* 15 (3): 195–200. https://doi.org/10.1046/j.1525-1497.2000.07228.x.

Biffl, W.L., Spain, D.A., Reitsma, A.M. et al. Society of University Surgeons Surgical Innovations Project Team (2008). Responsible development and application of surgical innovations: a position statement of the Society of University Surgeons. *J. Am. Coll. Surg.* 206 (6): 1204–1209.

Bosslet, G.T., Pope, T.M., Rubenfeld, G.D. et al. (2015). An official ATS/AACN/ACCP/ESICM/SCCM policy statement: responding to requests for potentially inappropriate treatments in intensive care units. *Am. J. Respir. Crit. Care Med.* 191 (11): 1318–1330. https://doi.org/10.1164/rccm.201505-0924ST.

Brett, A.S. and Jersild, P. (2003). Inappropriate treatment near the end of life: conflict between religious convictions and clinical judgment. *Arch. Intern. Med.* 163 (14): 1645–1649.

Chan, Y., Irish, J.C., Wood, S.J. et al. (2002). Patient education and informed consent in head and neck surgery. *Arch. Otolaryngol. Neck Surg.* 128 (11): 1269. https://doi.org/10.1001/archotol.128.11.1269.

Dalal, S. and Bruera, E. (2017). End-of-life care matters: palliative cancer care results in better care and lower costs. *Oncologist* 22 (4): 361–368. https://doi.org/10.1634/theoncologist.2016-0277.

Emanuel, E.J., Wendler, D., and Grady, C. (2000). What makes clinical research ethical? *JAMA* 283 (20): 2701–2711.

Eves, M.M. and Esplin, B.S. (2015). "She just doesn't know him like we do": illuminating complexities in surrogate decision-making. *J. Clin. Ethics* 26 (4): 350–354.

Henderson, G.E., Churchill, L.R., Davis, A.M. et al. (2007). Clinical trials and medical care: defining the therapeutic misconception. *PLoS Med.* 4 (11): 1735–1738.

Hogikyan, N.D. and Shuman, A.G. (2019). Can the doctor still know better? Reflections upon professionalism and duty. *Otolaryngol. Neck Surg.* 160 (4): 616–618. https://doi.org/10.1177/0194599819831254.

Joffe, S. and Miller, F. (2008). Bench to bedside: mapping the moral terrain of clinical research. *Hast. Cent. Rep.* 38 (2): 30–42. https://doi.org/10.1353/hcr.2008.0019.

Kon, A.A., Shepard, E.K., Sederstrom, N.O. et al. (2016). Defining futile and potentially inappropriate interventions: a policy statement from the Society of Critical Care Medicine Ethics Committee. *Crit. Care Med.* 44: 1769–1774.

Miller, F.G. and Rosenstein, D.L. (2003). The therapeutic orientation to clinical trials. *NEJM* 348 (14): 1383–1386.

Schenck, D.P. (2002). Ethical considerations in the treatment of head and neck cancer. *Cancer Control* 9 (5): 410–419. https://doi.org/10.1177/107327480200900506.

Shuman, A.G., Fins, J.J., and Prince, M.E. (2012). Improving end-of-life care for head and neck cancer patients. *Expert. Rev. Anticancer. Ther.* 12 (3): 335–343. https://doi.org/10.1586/era.12.6.

Spatz, E.S., Krumholz, H.M., and Moulton, B.W. (2017). Prime time for shared decision making. *JAMA* 317 (13): 1309. https://doi.org/10.1001/jama.2017.0616.

Temel, J.S., Greer, J.A., Muzikansky, A. et al. (2010). Early palliative care for patients with metastatic non–small-cell lung cancer. *N. Engl. J. Med.* 363 (8): 733–742. https://doi.org/10.1056/NEJMoa1000678.

Walker, T. (2009). What principlism misses. *J. Med. Ethics* 35 (4): 229–231. https://doi.org/10.1136/jme.2008.027227.

Index

Essential Cases in Head and Neck Oncology, First Edition. Edited by Michael G. Moore, Arnaud F. Bewley, and Babak Givi.
© 2022 American Head and Neck Society. Published 2022 by John Wiley & Sons Ltd.